Rheumatic Rarities

Editor

JONATHAN KAY

RHEUMATIC DISEASE CLINICS OF NORTH AMERICA

www.rheumatic.theclinics.com

Consulting Editor
MICHAEL H. WEISMAN

May 2013 • Volume 39 • Number 2

ELSEVIER

1600 John F. Kennedy Boulevard • Suite 1800 • Philadelphia, Pennsylvania, 19103-2899
http://www.theclinics.com

RHEUMATIC DISEASE CLINICS OF NORTH AMERICA Volume 39, Number 2
May 2013 ISSN 0889-857X, ISBN 13: 978-1-4557-7383-1

Editor: Pamela Hetherington

Rheumatic Disease Clinics of North America (ISSN 0889-857X) is published quarterly by Elsevier Inc., 360 Park Avenue South, New York, NY 10010-1710. Months of issue are February, May, August, and November. Business and editorial offices: 1600 John F. Kennedy Boulevard, Suite 1800, Philadelphia, PA 19103-2899. Periodicals postage paid at New York, NY and additional mailing offices. Subscription prices are USD 317.00 per year for US individuals, USD 555.00 per year for US institutions, USD 156.00 per year for US students and residents, USD 374.00 per year for Canadian individuals, USD 684.00 per year for Canadian institutions, USD 444.00 per year for international individuals, USD 684.00 per year for international institutions, and USD 218.00 per year for Canadian and foreign students/residents. To receive student/resident rate, orders must be accompanied by name of affiliated institution, date of term, and the *signature* of program/residency coordinator on institution letterhead. Orders will be billed at individual rate until proof of status received. Foreign air speed delivery is included in all *Clinics* subscription prices. All prices are subject to change without notice. **POSTMASTER:** Send address changes to *Rheumatic Disease Clinics of North America,* Elsevier Health Sciences Division, Subscription Customer Service, 3251 Riverport Lane, Maryland Heights, MO 63043. **Customer Service: 1-800-654-2452 (US and Canada). From outside of the US and Canada: 314-447-8871. Fax: 314-447-8029. For print support, e-mail: JournalsCustomerService-usa@elsevier.com. For online support, e-mail: JournalsOnline Support-usa@elsevier.com.**

Reprints. For copies of 100 or more of articles in this publication, please contact the Commercial Reprints Department, Elsevier Inc., 360 Park Avenue South, New York, New York, 10010-1710; Tel.: (+1) 212-633-3813, Fax: (+1) 212-462-1935, and E-mail: reprints@elsevier.com.

Rheumatic Disease Clinics of North America is covered in *MEDLINE/PubMed (Index Medicus), Current Contents/Clinical Medicine, Science Citation Index, ISI/BIOMED,* and *EMBASE/Excerpta Medica.*

Printed and bound by CPI Group (UK) Ltd, Croydon, CR0 4YY
Transferred to Digital Printing, 2013

Contributors

CONSULTING EDITOR

MICHAEL H. WEISMAN, MD
Director, Division of Rheumatology; Professor of Medicine, Cedars-Sinai Medical Center, Los Angeles, California

EDITOR

JONATHAN KAY, MD
Professor of Medicine and Director of Clinical Research, Division of Rheumatology, Department of Medicine, University of Massachusetts Medical School and UMass Memorial Medical Center, Worcester, Massachusetts

AUTHORS

ZAHIR AMOURA, MD
Department of Internal Medicine, French Reference Center for Rare Autoimmune and Systemic Diseases, Assistance Publique-Hôpitaux de Paris, Pitié-Salpêtrière Hospital; Université Pierre et Marie Curie, Paris, France

LAURENT ARNAUD, MD, PhD
Department of Internal Medicine, French Reference Center for Rare Autoimmune and Systemic Diseases, Assistance Publique-Hôpitaux de Paris, Pitié-Salpêtrière Hospital; Université Pierre et Marie Curie, Paris, France

QASIM AZIZ, PhD, FRCP
Professor, Wingate Institute of Neurogastroenterology, Centre for Gastroenterology, Blizard Institute, Barts and The London School of Medicine and Dentistry, Queen Mary University of London, London, United Kingdom

ALAN N. BAER, MD, FACP
Division of Rheumatology, Johns Hopkins University School of Medicine, Baltimore, Maryland

CINZIA MARIA BELLETTATO, PhD
Department of Pediatrics, Brains for Brain Foundation, University of Padua, Padua, Italy

SUELI CARNEIRO, MD, PhD
Associate Professor, School of Medical Sciences, State University of Rio de Janeiro; Assistant Dermatologist, University Hospital, Federal University of Rio de Janeiro, Rio de Janeiro, Brazil

FRÉDÉRIC CHARLOTTE, MD
Department of Anatomopathology, Assistance Publique-Hôpitaux de Paris, Pitié-Salpêtrière Hospital, Paris, France

NIDA CHAUDHARY, MD
Rhematology Fellow, Division of Rheumatology, Department of Medicine, University of Massachusetts Medical School and UMass Memorial Medical Center, Worcester, Massachusetts

RATNESH CHOPRA, MD
Rheumatology Fellow, Division of Rheumatology, Department of Medicine, University of Massachusetts Medical School and UMass Memorial Medical Center, Worcester, Massachusetts

LORINDA CHUNG, MD, MS
Assistant Professor, Division of Immunology and Rheumatology, Stanford University School of Medicine, Stanford, California

FLEUR COHEN-AUBART, MD, PhD
Department of Internal Medicine, French Reference Center for Rare Autoimmune and Systemic Diseases, Assistance Publique-Hôpitaux de Paris, Pitié-Salpêtrière Hospital; Université Pierre et Marie Curie, Paris, France

PAUL F. DELLARIPA, MD
Assistant Professor of Medicine, Division of Rheumatology, Brigham and Women's Hospital, Boston, Massachusetts

JEAN-FRANÇOIS EMILE, MD, PhD
Department of Pathology, Ambroise Paré Hospital, Assistance Publique Hôpitaux de Paris, Versailles University, Boulogne-Billancourt, France

NANCY FEELEY, CRNP
Division of Nephrology, The Johns Hopkins University School of Medicine, Baltimore, Maryland

ASMA FIKREE, BM BCh, MA, MRCP
Doctor, Wingate Institute of Neurogastroenterology, Centre for Gastroenterology, Blizard Institute, Barts and The London School of Medicine and Dentistry, Queen Mary University of London, London, United Kingdom

DAVID F. FIORENTINO, MD, PhD
Associate Professor, Department of Dermatology, Stanford University School of Medicine, Redwood City, California

GREGORY C. GARDNER, MD, FACP
Gilliland-Henderson Professor of Medicine, Division of Rheumatology, University of Washington, Seattle, Washington

RODNEY GRAHAME, CBE, MD, FRCP, FACP
Professor, Centre for Rheumatology, University College London Hospitals, London, United Kingdom

JULIEN HAROCHE, MD, PhD
Department of Internal Medicine, French Reference Center for Rare Autoimmune and Systemic Diseases, Assistance Publique-Hôpitaux de Paris, Pitié-Salpêtrière Hospital; Université Pierre et Marie Curie, Paris, France

GULEN HATEMI, MD
Associate Professor of Rheumatology, Division of Rheumatology, Department of Internal Medicine, Cerrahpasa Medical School, Istanbul University, Istanbul, Turkey

BOUKE P.C. HAZENBERG, MD, PhD
Assistant Professor, Department of Rheumatology and Clinical Immunology, University Medical Center Groningen, University of Groningen, Groningen, The Netherlands

BAPTISTE HERVIER, MD
Department of Internal Medicine, French Reference Center for Rare Autoimmune and Systemic Diseases, Assistance Publique-Hôpitaux de Paris, Pitié-Salpêtrière Hospital; Université Pierre et Marie Curie, Paris, France

NESRIN KARABUL, MD
Department of Pediatric and Adolescent Medicine, Villa Metabolica, University Medical Center of the Johannes Gutenberg-University of Mainz, Mainz, Germany

JONATHAN KAY, MD
Professor of Medicine and Director of Clinical Research, Division of Rheumatology, Department of Medicine, University of Massachusetts Medical School and UMass Memorial Medical Center, Worcester, Massachusetts

EYAL KEDAR, MD
Senior Fellow in Rheumatology, Division of Rheumatology, University of Washington, Seattle, Washington

CHRISTINA LAMPE, MD
Department of Pediatric and Adolescent Medicine, Villa Metabolica, University Medical Center of the Johannes Gutenberg-University of Mainz, Mainz, Germany

MANUEL MARTÍNEZ-LAVÍN, MD
Chief, Department of Rheumatology, Instituto Nacional de Cardiología Ignacio Chávez, Mexico City, Mexico

CARLOS PINEDA, MD
Director of Research, Instituto Nacional de Rehabilitación, Mexico City, Mexico

DEEPAK A. RAO, MD, PhD
Clinical Fellow, Division of Rheumatology, Brigham and Women's Hospital, Boston, Massachusetts

KERRI E. RIEGER, MD, PhD
Department of Pathology, Stanford University School of Medicine, Stanford Medical Center, Stanford, California

PERCIVAL D. SAMPAIO-BARROS, MD, PhD
Assistant Rheumatologist, Division of Rheumatology, Faculdade de Medicina, Universidade de São Paulo, São Paulo, Brazil

MAURIZIO SCARPA, MD, PhD
Department of Pediatrics, Brains for Brain Foundation, University of Padua, Padua, Italy

PAUL J. SCHEEL Jr, MD
Associate Professor of Medicine, Director, Division of Nephrology, The Johns Hopkins University School of Medicine, Baltimore, Maryland

MONICA SCHWARTZMAN, BA
Icahn School of Medicine, Mount Sinai Hospital, New York, New York

SERGIO SCHWARTZMAN, MD
Associate Attending Physician, Hospital for Special Surgery, Associate Professor, Weill Cornell Medical College, New York, New York

ROBERT L. WORTMANN, MD, FACP
Rheumatology Section, Geisel School of Medicine at Dartmouth, Lebanon, New Hampshire

AALIYA YAQUB, MD
Research Fellow, Division of Immunology and Rheumatology, Stanford University School of Medicine, Stanford, California

HASAN YAZICI, MD
Professor of Rheumatology (Retired), Division of Rheumatology, Department of Internal Medicine, Cerrahpasa Medical School, Istanbul University, Istanbul, Turkey

YUSUF YAZICI, MD
Assistant Professor of Medicine, Division of Rheumatology, Department of Internal Medicine, NYU Hospital for Joint Diseases, New York University School of Medicine, New York, New York

Contents

Behçet's syndrome (BS) shows a peculiar distribution, with a much higher prevalence in countries along the ancient Silk Road compared with rest of the world. BS also seems to follow a more severe course in ethnic groups with higher prevalence. Diagnosis depends on clinical findings. Criteria sets may not help in patients with less frequent types of involvement. Management strategies should be modified according to the age and sex of the patient and the organs involved. Being a serious health problem in endemic areas, BS also attracts global attention as a model to study inflammatory diseases of unknown cause.

Relapsing polychondritis (RP) is a rare systemic autoimmune disease characterized by episodic, progressive inflammatory destruction of cartilage. It can occur as an overlap syndrome in patients with other rheumatologic conditions. The disease usually follows an indolent relapsing-remitting course, but occasionally it can progress rapidly and even cause death. Although auricular or nasal chondritis or peripheral arthritis without other significant organ involvement are usually treated with low-dose corticosteroids, other more severe disease manifestations may require treatment with high-dose corticosteroids or other immunosuppressive agents. Biological targeted therapies might prove to be effective treatments of this condition.

Sarcoidosis is a systemic disease characterized by the development of epithelioid granulomas in various organs. Although the lungs are involved in most patients with sarcoidosis, virtually any organ can be affected. Recognition of extrapulmonary sarcoidosis requires awareness of the organs most commonly affected, such as the skin and the eyes, and vigilance for the most dangerous manifestations, such as cardiac and neurologic involvement. In this article, the common extrapulmonary manifestations of sarcoidosis are reviewed and organ-specific therapeutic considerations are discussed.

> Erdheim-Chester disease (ECD) is a rare form of non-Langerhans' cell his-
> tiocytosis. Diagnosis of ECD is based on the identification in tissue biopsy of
> histiocytes, which are typically foamy and immunostain for CD68+ CD1a−.
> Central nervous system involvement is a major prognostic factor in ECD.
> Interferon alpha may be the best first-line therapy and significantly improves
> survival of ECD. The BRAFV600E mutation is found in more than 50% of
> cases. Vemurafenib has been used for a small number of patients harbour-
> ing this mutation; inhibition of BRAF activation by vemurafenib was highly
> beneficial in these cases of severe multisystemic and refractory ECD.

> This article reviews the microbiology, pathophysiology, epidemiology, clin-
> ical manifestations, diagnostic testing, and treatment of Whipple's dis-
> ease, an illness caused by *Tropheryma whipplei* and characterized by
> multivariate clinical manifestations including an inflammatory arthropathy.
> Diagnosis is confirmed by tissue sampling with periodic acid-Schiff stain-
> ing and/or polymerase chain reaction. Clinical manifestations most fre-
> quently manifest in the gastrointestinal tract, musculoskeletal system,
> neurologic system, heart, and eyes, but can affect any site. Successful
> therapy with appropriate antibiotics is potentially curable, but recurrences
> may occur.

> Amyloidosis is the name for protein-folding diseases characterized by
> extracellular deposition of a specific soluble precursor protein that aggre-
> gates in the form of insoluble fibrils. The classification of amyloidosis is
> based on the chemical characterization of the precursor protein. Deposi-
> tion of amyloid is localized or systemic. The 4 main types of systemic
> amyloidosis are AL, AA, ATTR, and $A\beta_2M$ type. A schematic approach
> is proposed for the clinical management of systemic amyloidosis. The
> importance of typing amyloid with confidence, the usefulness of imaging
> techniques, the principles of treatment, and the need for well-planned
> treatment monitoring during follow-up are discussed.

> This article acquaints the reader with disorders of the skin that might mimic
> systemic sclerosis but whose pathology is localized to the skin and/or has
> extracutaneous manifestations that are different than systemic sclerosis.
> These disorders include localized scleroderma (morphea), eosinophilic
> fasciitis, scleredema, scleromyxedema, nephrogenic systemic fibrosis,
> and chronic graft-versus-host disease. Particular emphasis is placed on
> clinical and histopathologic features that help the clinician differentiate
> between these disorders. Treatment options are briefly reviewed.

Retroperitoneal fibrosis (RPF) is a condition characterized by the presence of inflammation and fibrosis in the retroperitoneal space, for which no standard diagnostic criteria exist. Historically, treatment has focused on relieving the obstruction with percutaneous or cystoscopic assisted placement of ureteral stents followed by more definitive resolution of ureteric obstruction with open or laparoscopic ureterolysis. However, over the past several years management has shifted from primarily a surgical approach to an immunosuppressive-based therapy aimed at modulation of the immune system. This review focuses on the recent advances in the classification, epidemiology, pathophysiology, pathology, imaging, and treatment of RPF.

This article presents an updated overview of hypertrophic osteoarthropathy and digital clubbing for the practicing rheumatologist. Discussion includes a brief historical perspective, its definition, incidence and prevalence, classification, pathology and pathophysiology, clinical manifestations, demographics, findings on physical examination, imaging techniques for its detection, differential diagnosis, and treatment modalities.

SAPHO syndrome is a disorder characterized by *S*ynovitis, *A*cne, *P*ustulosis, *H*yperostosis, and *O*steitis. As the osteoarticular and skin manifestations often do not occur simultaneously and there are no validated diagnostic criteria, the diagnosis can be difficult. Clinical and imaging investigation is necessary to establish the many differential diagnoses of SAPHO syndrome. The etiopathogenesis involves infectious (probably *Propionibacterium acnes*), immunologic, and genetic factors. Treatment is based on information gathered from case reports and small series, and is related to specific skin or articular symptoms.

Although perceived as a rare condition, joint hypermobility syndrome is common. Its prevalence in rheumatology clinics is extremely high. Early estimates suggest that it may be the most common of all rheumatologic conditions. The problem lies in the general lack of awareness of the syndrome, its means of recognition, and the resultant failure to diagnose it correctly when present. It is a worldwide problem. This article provides an overview of hypermobility and hypermobility syndrome, stressing its multisystemic nature and the negative impact that it may have on quality of life, with particular reference to gastrointestinal involvement.

RHEUMATIC DISEASE CLINICS OF NORTH AMERICA

Foreword

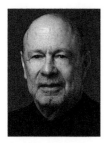

Michael H. Weisman, MD
Consulting Editor

When has a rheumatologist *not* been asked to see these patients described in this volume? The answer is pretty obvious as Jonathan Kay points out the bane of the existence of a rheumatologist; we are the go-to doctors when the rest are stumped or throw their hands up and say "this must be one of those autoimmune conditions."

That is probably why many of us chose this specialty—we like the challenge of grappling with a diagnosis or addressing the mechanisms of disease or figuring out why things happen rather than just dealing with physiologic explanations for organ failure.

Jonathan Kay has assembled a timely collection of articles that focus on a set of conditions whose manifestations (rashes, joint complaints, muscle and lung findings without explanation, etc) commonly fall within our purview. Each of these articles tries to address the conditions from epidemiology to treatment in a way to serve as a reference for the reader and a source of articles to look up the nuances of these conditions. He has done an excellent job in bringing this material to us in a fresh and stimulating way. That is why rheumatologists are most often the last word.

Michael H. Weisman, MD
Division of Rheumatology
Cedars-Sinai Medical Center
8700 Beverly Boulevard
Los Angeles, CA 90024, USA

E-mail address:
michael.weisman@cshs.org

Rheum Dis Clin N Am 39 (2013) xiii
http://dx.doi.org/10.1016/j.rdc.2013.03.009
0889-857X/13/$ – see front matter © 2013 Published by Elsevier Inc.

Preface

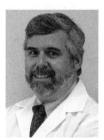

Jonathan Kay, MD
Editor

Many of the systemic diseases that are treated by rheumatologists present with protean manifestations involving multiple organ systems. In caring for patients with these conditions, the rheumatologist becomes highly skilled in the practice of internal medicine. Consequently, clinicians in other areas of medicine frequently identify the rheumatologist as the physician best suited to evaluate and treat patients who present with atypical features that repeatedly have eluded diagnosis. Although some such patients turn out to have conditions that traditionally are considered to be rheumatic diseases, others will have lesser known illnesses that do not fall directly into the province of any one subspecialty of internal medicine. This issue of the *Rheumatic Disease Clinics of North America* is devoted to reviewing those infrequently occurring conditions that the rheumatologist inevitably encounters during the course of clinical practice.

By virtue of their nature, no unifying pathophysiologic mechanism or clinical feature can be used to group these miscellaneous conditions. Some are diseases characterized by systemic inflammation, whereas the hallmark of others is localized fibrosis. Still others may be the consequence of metabolic abnormalities or result from mutations in genes for enzymes or components of extracellular matrix. The only commonality among patients experiencing this collection of illnesses is that the relative obscurity of their afflictions ultimately may prompt referral to a rheumatologist for diagnosis and treatment.

In this issue of the *Rheumatic Disease Clinics of North America,* we have assembled reviews written by expert clinicians about the epidemiology, pathophysiology, clinical presentation, diagnosis, and treatment of many of these less commonly recognized diseases. The authors have attempted to make each review comprehensive and of practical value to the clinician who encounters these patients. We have tried to group the articles by shared pathophysiologic mechanisms or clinical manifestations, as much as possible. However, if the organization of the articles seems somewhat disjointed, the culpability ultimately rests with me as guest editor.

I hope that this collection of reviews on the less common diseases that present intermittently to rheumatologists will aid in the evaluation and treatment of patients whose atypical constellation of clinical features might otherwise elude diagnosis. No longer should a patient with one of these conditions see a rheumatologist without

Rheum Dis Clin N Am 39 (2013) xv–xvi
http://dx.doi.org/10.1016/j.rdc.2013.03.008
0889-857X/13/$ – see front matter © 2013 Published by Elsevier Inc.

rheumatic.theclinics.com

the rheumatologist recognizing that she or he is seeing a patient with that disease. Most importantly, I hope that increased awareness and consideration of these disorders will result in advances in therapy and better outcomes for these patients in the future.

Jonathan Kay, MD
Rheumatology Center, Memorial Campus
UMass Memorial Medical Center
119 Belmont Street
Worcester, MA 01605, USA

E-mail address:
jonathan.kay@umassmemorial.org

Behçet's Syndrome

Gulen Hatemi, MD[a], Yusuf Yazici, MD[b], Hasan Yazici, MD[a],*

KEYWORDS

- Behçet's syndrome • Epidemiology • Eye involvement • Vascular involvement
- Genetics • Disease mechanisms • Diagnosis • Management

KEY POINTS

- Behçet's syndrome (BS) is a condition of unknown etiology, most prevalent in countries along the Old Silk Road.
- Epidemiologic data points to the role of both genetic and environmental factors in the etiology of BS.
- Pulmonary artery involvement in BS may consist of pulmonary artery aneurysms and/or pulmonary artery thrombosis, which may be accompanied by pulmonary hypertension during the acute stages.
- Pulmonary parenchymal lesions, which may accompany pulmonary vascular lesions, may be mistaken for pulmonary embolism or infections.
- There are distinct clusters in disease expression, such as the acne/arthritis/enthesopathy and the dural sinus thrombosis/pulmonary artery aneurysm/deep venous thrombosis/superficial venous thrombosis clusters, which possibly have distinct pathogenetic mechanisms.
- BS has a complex genetic background, and the most significant association is with HLA B51.
- Diagnosis of BS depends on clinical findings. There are no specific laboratory, radiologic, or histologic findings that help in diagnosing BS.
- Subsequent mucocutaneous and joint involvement may be bothersome and impair the quality of life, but do not cause organ-threatening damage. Their management depends on the type, frequency, and severity of the symptoms.
- Management of serious organ involvement such as ocular, vascular, gastrointestinal, and neurologic disease is with corticosteroids and immunosuppressives, which should be started early to prevent irreversible damage.
- More aggressive treatment of serious organ involvement with immunosuppressives and biologics has improved the outcome in BS patients.

Disclosures: Hasan Yazici and Gulen Hatemi do not have any conflict of interests related to the content of this article. Yusuf Yazici is a consultant for Celgene, BMS, and Genentech, and has received research support for Behçet's trials.

[a] Division of Rheumatology, Department of Internal Medicine, Cerrahpasa Medical School, Istanbul University, Cerrahpasa, Istanbul 34089, Turkey; [b] Division of Rheumatology, Department of Internal Medicine, NYU Hospital for Joint Diseases, New York University School of Medicine, 333 East 38th Street, New York, NY 10706, USA
* Corresponding author. Ic Hastaliklari Anabilim Dali, Cerrahpasa Tip Fakultesi, Aksaray, Istanbul, Turkey.
E-mail address: hyazici@attglobal.net

EPIDEMIOLOGY

The prevalence of Behçet's syndrome (BS) is highest in Turkey (1 in 250), where it was first described.[1,2] The comparative prevalences in other regions are shown in **Table 1**. Although the prevalence among Turkish immigrant workers and their offspring is lower than what has been reported from their native country, it is still higher than has been reported among ethnic Germans,[3] pointing to combined genetic and environmental factors in the pathogenesis. A comparative study of the frequency of BS among the ethnic Armenian population living in Istanbul, Turkey has shown that the frequency of familial Mediterranean fever (ΓΜΓ), a condition with a much better defined genetic component, was more common among Armenians than in the ethnic Turks, whereas the reverse was true for BS.[4]

In the United States, whereas an estimated rate of 0.33 in 10^5 was reported in Olmsted County, Rochester in 1978,[5] a higher rate (5.2 in 10^5) was calculated in the same region between 1996 and 2005.[6] The Behçet's Syndrome Evaluation, Treatment and Research Center at the NYU Hospital for Joint Diseases in New York has been

Table 1			
Prevalence of Behçet's syndrome in different countries			
Country	Authors, Year	Prevalence (per 100,000 Population)	HLA B51 Positivity (%)
Japan	Kurosawa et al,[86] 2004	11.9	
China	Zhang et al,[87] 2012	14	17
Iran	Davatchi et al,[88] 2008	80	NA
Iraq	Al-Rawi et al,[89] 2003	17	NA
Israel—Overall	Krause et al,[90] 2007	15.2	81
Druzes		146.4	NA
Arabs		26.2	NA
Jews		8.6	NA
Saudi Arabia	Al-dalaan et al,[91] 1997	20	NA
Egypt	Assaad Khalil et al,[92] 1997	7.6	58
Portugal	Crespo et al,[93] 1993	1.5	75
Spain	Gonzalez-Gay et al,[94] 2000	6.4	NA
Italy	Salvarani et al,[8] 2007	3.8	75
France—Overall	Mahr et al,[95] 2008	7.1	33
Europeans		2.4	NA
North African		34.6	NA
Asian		17.5	NA
Sub-Saharan African		5.1	NA
Noncontinental French		6.2	NA
Germany	Papoutsis et al,[3] 2006		
German		1.5	NA
Non-German		26.6	NA
Turks		77.4	NA
UK	Chamberlain, [96] 1977	0.64	18
Scotland	Jankowski et al,[97] 1992	0.3	13
Sweden	Ek et al,[98] 1993	3.5	80
USA	Calamia et al,[6] 2009	5.2	0

Abbreviation: NA, no data available.

collecting data on BS patients since 2005. Several interesting observations about disease manifestations have been noted. In this dedicated center, 197 consecutive patients were divided into 2 groups, Group 1 comprising patients with a northern European background and Group 2 consisting of patients ethnically from areas where Behçet's prevalence is high (Turkey, Greece, Israel, Middle East, and Far East). These groups were compared regarding their demography and disease manifestations.[7] There were significantly more females (78% vs 54%) in Group 1, made up of predominantly patients with skin and mucosal disease. About one-third of patients had eye disease in both groups; interestingly there were no patients who were blind in the whole cohort. Vascular involvement was seen in 3 patients in Group 2 and in none in Group 1. These data suggest that even though most manifestations of BS were similar in frequency between the 2 groups, some manifestations might be more severe in patients with backgrounds from endemic areas, such as the Middle East. Similarly, milder disease has also been reported among Italian patients from northern Italy.[8]

CLINICAL PRESENTATION

BS is seen with roughly equal frequency in males and females. Males have a distinctly more severe course, which particularly manifests itself in the morbidity associated with the disease as well as pulmonary vascular disease.[9] BS is relatively rare in childhood.

Comprehensive accounts of the clinical symptoms and signs of BS[10,11] are available. This article emphasizes the more recent developments in the understanding of the phenotype of BS, and discusses why BS might be a syndrome that is true to type, with perhaps more than one pathogenetic pathway responsible for its clinical expression.

Vascular Involvement

The most mortal manifestation of BS is the pulmonary artery aneurysm, which carries a mortality of around 25% to 30%.[12] It is now better appreciated that the pulmonary arterial aneurysm (PAA) is a manifestation of a more general pulmonary vascular disease. Some BS patients present mainly with the well-recognized PAA; in some the pulmonary artery thrombi (PAT) can accompany the PAA, and there is a third group who present with PAT only.[13] The main clinical feature of the third group is that they present with a less copious hemoptysis in comparison with the patients with PAA.

About 80% of patients with pulmonary vascular disease also have peripheral vascular disease, mainly in the form of thrombophlebitis. It has long been debated whether some of the lung lesions seen in BS patients are indeed pulmonary emboli. The authors' group has opposed this view mainly because: (1) in a condition with at least 30% to 40% venous thrombosis, pulmonary embolism at post mortem has not been observed[14]; (2) the venous thrombosis in BS, unlike common-variety venous thrombosis, involves long segments in the veins causing sticky thrombi; (3) although formal prospective studies testing the utility of anticoagulation are lacking, in 2 retrospective surveys it was found not to be useful.[15,16] The authors were able to observe the long-term (2–6 years) outcome of ventilation/perfusion mismatch in 6 patients whose initial lung scans had been interpreted as having pulmonary emboli.[13] This outcome is distinct from what one sees in pulmonary thromboembolism, where the defects seen on lung scans in true pulmonary embolism resolve mostly in a few months.

Many patients with pulmonary vascular disease in BS have parenchymal lesions in the lungs, which can easily arise as secondary infections in a patient using glucocorticoids and/or immunosuppressives, and some patients with pulmonary vascular disease also have mild to moderate pulmonary hypertension, as the authors have shown in a controlled study.[17] It may also be possible that among patients in the acute stage with PAA and/or PAT, the degree of this pulmonary hypertension will increase.

Symptom Clusters: Acne, Arthritis, and Enthesopathy

Some of the clinical features of BS tend to go together.[18] The most studied of these clusters has been the acne-arthritis cluster, which is interesting in the context of the well-known association of arthritis with acne (**Fig. 1**). However, it was noted that acne lesions were not sterile, as had been thought, and, rather unexpectedly, *Staphylococcus aureus* grew in the associated pustules, an uncommon occurrence in acne vulgaris.[19] This recurring theme of acne and arthritis led the authors to reconsider their initial stand on excluding BS from the seronegative spondarthritides, which some had thought was within the spectrum of BS. At this point the hypothesis that enthesitis, a common denominator in seronegative spondarthritides, was more frequent in BS was tested. Only those patients with arthritis and associated acne were found to have enthesitis more often.[20] However, on formally checking whether this same group also had an increased frequency of sacroiliitis or were more frequent HLA B27, it was discovered that this was not the case.[21]

More recently the authors have also shown that there was significant familial clustering of the acne/arthritis cluster,[22] suggesting that a common genetic pathway is involved in its clinical expression.

Symptom Clusters: Deep Venous Thrombosis, Superficial Venous Thrombosis, and Dural Sinus Thrombosis

In BS, superficial venous thrombosis (SVT) and deep venous thrombosis (DVT) also go together,[18] as well as dural sinus thrombosis (DST) and peripheral DVT.[23] The clustering of DST, DVT, and SVT is conceptually easy to understand. What is perhaps more intriguing is the association between PAA and DVT. It has repeatedly been shown that about 80% of patients with PAA also have peripheral DVT, an association that has for many years led many to incorrectly consider pulmonary emboli as an integral part of pulmonary vascular disease in BS. On the other hand, this association is perhaps not so difficult to surmise if one remembers that the pulmonary arteries, in their structure and

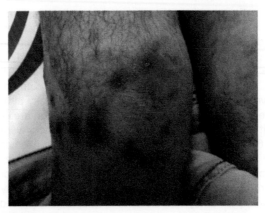

Fig. 1. Acne and arthritis.

content, are very similar to veins. As an extension of this PAA and DVT association, it is also worth noting that one-third of patients with DST have PAA,[23] whereas the frequency of PAA in the general population of BS patients is no more than 2% to 3%.[9]

The authors consider that within the phenotype of BS, acne and arthritis is surely one clinical cluster and, most probably, DST/PAA/DVT/SVT is another. The presence of such clusters obviously suggests that there might be more than one pathogenetic pathway in what today is known as BS.

What is identified as BS is probably the result of several different pathogenetic mechanisms, also finding support from the fact that, the same drug curiously can have different effects on different manifestations of this syndrome. As also discussed in the section on management, etanercept is effective for skin-mucosal manifestations but curiously has no effect on the pathergy reaction or the dermal response to sodium monourate crystals.[24] Gevokizumab, an interleukin (IL)-1β blocker, was reported as effective for eye disease in a small series of patients, whereas it seemed not very effective for oral ulcers.[25] In controlled studies colchicine, widely considered to be beneficial in BS, turned out to be mainly effective for arthritis, erythema nodosum, and genital ulceration, only among females.[26,27] On the other hand, if one looks at the effect of a single agent, such as glucocorticoids (GCS), in other inflammatory diseases such as rheumatoid arthritis (RA) or systemic lupus erythematosus (SLE), one finds that they are effective in managing active disease in any organ in either condition. In this context it is also important that in the only controlled study of GCS for BS, the authors' group showed that low-dose methylprednisolone was ineffective in controlling skin and mucosal manifestations.[28] In brief, there is good reason to suspect that pathways of inflammation are most probably not uniform and somewhat different to what is seen in other, more common inflammatory diseases such as like RA and SLE.

GENETICS AND DISEASE MECHANISMS

BS is genetically a complex disorder. A phenotype is associated with more than one gene locus. As the authors previously pointed out for BS,[29] it is, however, possible that at least a portion of this complexity might stem from attempts to ascribe multiple genetic associations to a single phenotype, whereas the phenotype at hand might not be homogeneous to begin with. Returning to the discussion about BS, it is well accepted that a simple Mandelian inheritance does not exist among adult patients with BS.[30] On the other hand, an autosomal recessive mode of inheritance has been suggested in childhood BS.[31] Although similar clinical features have been described in the pediatric and the adult forms, the frequency of genital ulceration and eye disease are less frequent among the pediatric cases.[32]

The most significant association of BS is with HLA B51.[33] However, this association explains around 20% to 30% of the heritability in a condition whereby only 1 in 10 patients identify a diseased relative. In a small (but the only) twin study, the concordance frequency among 4 monozygotic twins was 2 patients, and this did not change over the course of 8 years.[34] Recently IL-10 gene mutations have also been described in BS.[35] The contention that the mutation that causes a defect in the production of IL-10, an anti-inflammatory cytokine, is a risk factor in an inflammatory disease surely makes good sense. There is evidence that IL-10 levels do decrease with age,[36] whereas in BS disease activity distinctly lessens with age.[9]

DIAGNOSIS

There are no specific laboratory, radiologic, or histologic findings that help in diagnosing BS. The diagnosis, for all purposes, is entirely clinical. There have been various and heatedly debated sets of diagnostic and classification criteria, the most widely used of which are still the International Society for Behçet's Disease (ISBD) criteria of 1990.[37] While not aiming to describe the individual clinical manifestations, this article does discuss several points concerning the ISBD criteria that are worth reiterating for the purposes of diagnosis.

1. The ISBD criteria do not include gut disease, central nervous system disease, and pulmonary vascular disease, merely because these organ involvements had not been either specific or sensitive enough to have discriminatory value in separating BS from other diseases in the control groups.
2. In the ISBD criteria oral ulceration is assumed to be always present, so in a patient with no oral ulceration (<1%–2% of BS patients) these criteria are, strictly speaking, inapplicable.
3. Oral ulceration is the most sensitive lesion and genital ulceration is the most specific (**Fig. 2**). The latter therefore, like in all relatively rare conditions, is the most clinically useful lesion in diagnosing BS, according to the ISBD scheme.
4. If a patient presents with mainly intestinal inflammation, along with skin and mucosal manifestations, with perhaps the single exception of genital ulceration, it is singularly difficult to distinguish BS from Crohn disease. This difficulty does not diminish with endoscopy or histology.[38]
5. It is the authors' opinion that the notion of separation of diagnostic criteria from the classification is unfounded.[39] There is no difference in the cerebral process in either activity. In brief, diagnosis is nothing more or less than a classification for the individual patient.

MANAGEMENT

The European League Against Rheumatism (EULAR) recommendations for the management of BS and an accompanying systematic literature review were published some years ago.[40,41] There has been growing evidence since then regarding the use of biologics in BS (**Table 2**). In this review we tried to present an overview of the more robust management data.

The natural course of BS differs among patients depending on the age and sex of the patient, age at disease onset, and the organs involved. Therefore the management strategy should be customized accordingly. It was previously shown that young men

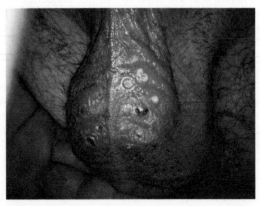

Fig. 2. Genital ulcers.

Table 2
EULAR recommendations for the management of BS

Recommendation	Category of Evidence	Strength of Recommendation
Eye Involvement Any patient with BS and inflammatory eye disease affecting the posterior segment should be on a treatment regime, which includes azathioprine and systemic corticosteroids	Ib	A/D
Refractory Eye Involvement If the patient has severe eye disease defined as >2 lines of drop in visual acuity on a 10/10 scale and/or retinal disease (retinal vasculitis or macular involvement), it is recommended that either cyclosporine A or infliximab be used in combination with azathioprine and corticosteroids; alternatively interferon-α with or without corticosteroids could be used instead	II	C/D
Vascular Involvement There is no firm evidence to guide the management of major vessel disease in BS. For the management of acute deep vein thrombosis in BS immunosuppressive agents such as corticosteroids, azathioprine, cyclophosphamide, or cyclosporine are recommended. For the management of both pulmonary and peripheral arterial aneurysms, cyclophosphamide and corticosteroids are recommended	III	C
Anticoagulation Similarly there are no controlled data on, or evidence of benefit from uncontrolled experience with, anticoagulant, antiplatelet, or antifibrinolytic agents in the management of deep vein thrombosis or for the use of anticoagulation for the arterial lesions of BS	IV	D
Gastrointestinal Involvement There is no evidence-based treatment that can be recommended for the management of gastrointestinal involvement of BS. Agents such as sulfasalazine, corticosteroids, azathioprine, TNF antagonists, and thalidomide should be tried first before surgery, except in emergencies	III	C
Joint Involvement In most patients with BS, arthritis can be managed with colchicine	Ib	A
Neurologic Involvement There are no controlled data to guide the management of CNS involvement in BS. For parenchymal involvement agents to be tried may include corticosteroids, interferon-α, azathioprine, cyclophosphamide, methotrexate, and TNF-α antagonists. For dural sinus thrombosis, corticosteroids are recommended	III	C/D
Cyclosporine A Neurotoxicity Cyclosporine should not be used in BS patients with CNS involvement unless necessary for intraocular inflammation	III	C

(continued on next page)

Table 2 (continued)		
Recommendation	**Category of Evidence**	**Strength of Recommendation**
Mucocutaneous Involvement	Ib	A/C
The decision to treat skin and mucosa involvement will depend on the perceived severity by the physician and the patient. Mucocutaneous involvement should be treated according to the dominant or codominant lesions present.		
Topical measures (ie, local steroids) should be the first line of treatment for isolated oral and genital ulcers		
Acne-like lesions are usually of cosmetic concern only. Thus, topical measures as used in acne vulgaris are sufficient		
Colchicine should be preferred when the dominant lesion is genital ulcer or erythema nodosum		
Leg ulcers in BS might have different causes. Treatment should be planned accordingly		
Azathioprine, interferon-α, and TNF antagonists may be considered in resistant cases		

Abbreviations: CNS, central nervous system; TNF, tumor necrosis factor.

Data from Hatemi G, Silman A, Bang D, et al, EULAR Expert Committee. EULAR recommendations for the management of Behçet's disease. Ann Rheum Dis 2008;67(12):1656–62.

have a more severe disease course, especially if their disease had started at an early age.[9] Mucocutaneous and joint involvement follows a relapsing and remitting course, can be disabling, and causes severe impairment of quality of life, but does not cause permanent damage. On the other hand, serious organ involvement, such as eye, nervous system, and gastrointestinal involvement, can cause severe irreversible harm. Eye involvement can lead to blindness in almost half of the patients, if left untreated. Similarly, nervous system involvement can result in neurologic deficits, and gastrointestinal perforations can necessitate the removal of large segments of small intestine and bowel. Moreover, vascular involvement can be life threatening, especially when arterial aneurysms are present. All of these factors should be taken into consideration when planning treatment. Rapid and effective suppression of inflammation should be aimed at when dealing with major organ involvement. Preventing recurrent attacks of mucocutaneous lesions and arthritis is important for preserving the daily functions and quality of life in BS patients, but how aggressive these lesions should be treated depends on how bothersome they are for the patient. A multidisciplinary approach is required for optimal management.

Mucocutaneous Disease

The management of mucocutaneous lesions of BS depends on the type, frequency, and severity of the symptoms. Some patients experience painful and frequent oral ulcers, genital ulcers, and erythema nodosum, which require systemic treatment, whereas others have occasional lesions that may be managed by topical measures.

The topical measures most frequently used are steroid preparations, sucralfate suspension, lidocaine gel, and antiseptics such as chlorhexidine. Among these, sucralfate was shown to be effective in oral and genital ulcers.[42] An open study showed that *Lactobacillus* lozenges may be effective for oral ulcers,[43] and good periodontal health and oral hygiene are important in disease management.[44]

Colchicine, 1 to 2 mg/d is probably the most frequently prescribed medication for mucocutaneous lesions in BS. Its effectiveness for genital ulcers and erythema nodosum, especially among women, has been shown in randomized controlled trials (RCTs).[26,27] However, there is no consensus on its effect on oral ulcers. Because of the relative lack of power of the 2 quoted studies, a subgroup of BS might indeed be responsive to colchicine, and a withdrawal study among the responders is required to show whether colchicine is beneficial for the treatment of oral ulcers in this subset.

Azathioprine[45] and interferon (IFN)-α[46] in a lower dose than that used for eye involvement, such as 3 MU, 3 times a week, may be preferred for mucocutaneous involvement. Thalidomide is effective for the treatment of oral and genital ulcers and papulopustular lesions, and a dose of 100 mg/d is usually sufficient. However, an increase in the number of nodular lesions was observed in the RCT with thalidomide.[47] Peripheral neuropathy and teratogenicity require caution. Mycophenolate may also be tried in patients with severe mucocutaneous lesions. Etanercept is the only tumor necrosis factor (TNF)-α inhibitor to be used in an RCT on BS.[24] Oral ulcers, genital ulcers, nodular lesions, and papulopustular lesions improved with etanercept. There are several case reports with infliximab and adalimumab, showing good results for mucocutaneous lesions.[48] GCS at moderate doses can be used for short periods during the active phases of genital ulcers and nodular lesions, and immunosuppressives are starting to show beneficial effects.[49]

In patients who have serious organ involvement, immunosuppressives prescribed for this indication such as azathioprine, IFN-α, and TNF-α inhibitors are usually effective for mucocutaneous lesions as well. However, this is not always true. Experience in few patients indicated a good response in serious organ involvement, such as eye and neurologic involvement, with gevokizumab and tocilizumab, respectively, but these drugs were probably not beneficial for mucocutaneous involvement.[25,50]

Other than immunosuppressives, antibiotics such as penicillin and minocycline, and other agents such as dapsone and rebamipide, have been studied and have shown some benefit for mucocutaneous lesions.

Joint Involvement

Arthritis in BS is usually in the form of a nondeforming, nonerosive oligoarthritis, which follows a recurrent course with exacerbations lasting a few weeks. Although sacroiliitis is not a feature of BS, enthesopathy may accompany arthritis in some patients. Colchicine is usually sufficient for preventing exacerbations of arthritis. Azathioprine may be added to colchicine in patients who continue to have arthritis attacks or whose attacks are prolonged. IFN-α, in lower doses similar to those for mucocutaneous involvement, and TNF-α inhibitors are usually effective in severe cases resistant to colchicine and azathioprine.

Low to moderate doses of GCS can be prescribed for short durations during acute and severe episodes of arthritis. Low-dose glucocorticoids were shown to be not beneficial for arthritis in an RCT; however, this is probably due to the small number of arthritis episodes in that study.[28] Nonsteroidal anti-inflammatory drugs (NSAIDs) may also be used during exacerbations; however, in the only RCT with an NSAID for BS (azapropazone), no benefit was apparent.[51]

Eye Involvement

Azathioprine and GCS are recommended as the initial therapy for all BS patients with posterior segment inflammation.[40] The usual dose of azathioprine is 2.5 mg/kg/d.

Azathioprine decreases the frequency of uveitis attacks and prevents visual loss. Moreover, in patients without eye involvement, development of new eye disease was less among those who used azathioprine, both during azathioprine treatment and afterward. These improvements were observed in an RCT and at long-term follow-up.[45,52,53] GCS are usually part of the initial treatment and are also used whenever attacks recur. However, they should be tapered as quickly as possible, because cataracts and glaucoma can complicate the ocular involvement in patients exposed to long-term GCS.

If the patient is refractory to azathioprine or has severe eye disease including retinal vasculitis and macular involvement at presentation, a more aggressive approach is mandated. Although there is no consensus on the best treatment strategy in such patients, frequently used alternatives cyclosporine A or infliximab together with azathioprine or the sole use of IFN-α.[40]

With cyclosporine A there is rapid improvement in visual acuity, and a decrease in the frequency and severity of ocular attacks.[40,54] The optimal dose is 2 to 5 mg/kg/d. Higher doses are toxic, and patients should be monitored for hypertension and renal function.

With IFN-α there is a substantial increase in visual acuity and a decrease in the frequency of uveitis attacks in BS patients with severe uveitis resistant to multiple immunosuppressives and corticosteroids.[55,56] This effect was observed to continue even after discontinuation of IFN-α. Although IFN-α is an effective treatment modality, compliance with this drug may be compromised by the difficulty in tolerating this agent, experienced by many patients. Influenza-like symptoms are frequent. Patients should be monitored for cytopenia, and concomitant use of azathioprine should be avoided because of serious myelosuppression. Depression is another adverse event that may be severe in some patients. The usual dose of IFN-α is 5 MU/d. A recent open study suggested that an initial dose of 3 MU/d for 2 weeks followed by 3 MU 3 times a week and increasing the dose to 4.5 MU, 6 MU, and 9 MU when relapses occur provided beneficial results with fewer adverse events.[57]

Although there are no controlled trials in eye disease, TNF-α inhibitors are beneficial in BS patients with eye involvement refractory to other immunosuppressives.[40] The usual dose of infliximab for this indication is 5 mg/kg every 6 to 8 weeks.[58] It is usually given together with azathioprine and/or cyclosporine A. Adalimumab was also used with good results in patients refractory or intolerant to infliximab.[59] One of the advantages of infliximab is its rapid suppression of inflammation.[60] A single intravitreal infliximab injection may also be beneficial,[61] and may be an advantage in preventing the potential adverse events of systemic infliximab. An important risk in these patients is tuberculosis, which may be more frequent with use of TNF-α inhibitors in BS than it is in other conditions, probably because of the similar geographic distribution of either condition.

A small study with gevokizumab, a recombinant humanized anti–IL-1β antibody, and a few case reports with canakinumab showed improvement in patients with uveitis and retinal vasculitis refractory to other immunosuppressives.[25,62,63]

Vascular Involvement

PAAs are treated aggressively with GCS and immunosuppressives. Cyclophosphamide, 1 g is given intravenously monthly up to 2 years, followed by maintenance treatment with azathioprine. GCS treatment is usually started with 3 pulses of 1 g intravenous methylprednisolone followed by oral prednisolone, 1 mg/kg/d. The beneficial results of this approach were demonstrated in 2 case series published 10 years apart, showing a significant decrease in mortality.[12,64] An alternative approach may be use of infliximab, which was reported to show good results in the management of PAAs in a few case reports.[65,66] Surgery is usually not preferred in PAA of BS, because of the high rate of mortality. Endovascular embolization may be tried during emergencies. However, this procedure may be complicated by venous thrombi, which have an increased frequency in patients with arterial aneurysms.

Peripheral artery aneurysms are usually treated with surgery. Immunosuppressives are also given concomitantly, with the aim of preventing relapses and improving surgical outcomes. A retrospective survey of BS patients with peripheral artery aneurysms showed that the preferred surgical procedure was aorto-biliac bypass when the aneurysm was located in the infrarenal aorta, and synthetic graft insertion when the aneurysm was located in an extremity.[67]

As pointed out earlier, the management of venous thrombosis is controversial. The authors' group maintains that anti-inflammatory immunosuppression is the mainstay of management, and a recent case series from France backs up this contention.[15] Systemic immunosuppressives, usually azathioprine 2.5 mg/kg, is used for preventing relapses.[40] Moreover, a decrease in the frequency of post-thrombophlebitic complications has been reported with immunosuppressives. Superior vena cava thrombosis and Budd-Chiari syndrome are usually treated more aggressively. Cyclophosphamide or TNF-α antagonists may be used in such cases. GCS may also be used for short periods during acute exacerbation of venous thrombosis.

An interesting survey among rheumatologists treating BS showed that most rheumatologists from the United States and Israel, countries with low and intermediate BS prevalence, stated that they would anticoagulate BS patients with major venous thrombosis, whereas in Turkey, where BS prevalence is much higher, more than half of rheumatologists indicated that they would not anticoagulate these patients.[68]

Gastrointestinal Involvement

There are no controlled trials in BS patients with gastrointestinal involvement. The clinical and endoscopic features of gastrointestinal involvement of BS closely resemble those of Crohn disease, and the same measures are effective in its treatment. GCS are used in moderate to high doses during acute exacerbations and tapered in 2 to 3 months. In mild cases 5-aminosalicylic acid (5-ASA) derivatives are usually preferred as first-line therapy. A recent retrospective survey of 143 patients from Korea showed that 32% of patients relapsed while being treated with 5-ASA derivatives.[69] A younger age at diagnosis, higher levels of C-reactive protein, and a higher disease activity index at baseline were the factors predicting relapse. Similarly, 9 of 13 (68%) Turkish patients with gastrointestinal involvement remained relapse free with 5-ASA derivatives during a mean follow-up of 44.3 ± 46.9 months.[70]

In more severe cases, or in patients nonresponsive to 5-ASA derivatives, the treatment of choice is azathioprine. In the authors' recent series, 22 of 33 (67%) patients who were prescribed azathioprine as first-line therapy and three-fourths of patients who used azathioprine after nonresponse to 5-ASA derivatives remained relapse free.[70]

Several case reports and case series reported that clinical and endoscopic remission could be obtained with thalidomide or TNF-α antagonists in resistant cases.[71–73] Most of the experience with TNF-α antagonists is with infliximab, 5 mg/kg/d. Rapid improvement in clinical findings such as abdominal pain and rectal bleeding, and endoscopic findings such as ulcers and fistulae have been observed. Both thalidomide and infliximab are usually given together with azathioprine.

Surgery may be required when deep penetrating ulcers perforate or cause severe bleeding. The use of immunosuppressives such as azathioprine in patients who require surgery decreases the frequency of relapses and postoperative complications, and improves the outcome.

Neurologic Involvement

The parenchymal neurologic involvement of BS is also treated with GCS and immunosuppressives. During the acute phase of neurologic involvement, GCS pulses are given as 1-g intravenous methylprednisolone infusions, 3 to 7 times on consecutive or alternate days, followed by 1 mg/kg/d prednisolone tapered slowly. Azathioprine, 2.5 mg/kg/d is the immunosuppressive of choice in most cases. It was shown to improve the long-term outcome of neurologic involvement in a large series.[74] Mycophenolate mofetil was tried and showed good results in few patients.[75] Cyclophosphamide used to be preferred for severe cases; however, IFN α and TNF α inhibitors are also good alternatives for such patients. A systematic review of infliximab in BS patients with neurologic involvement showed a good short and mid-term response.[76] The dose was 5 mg/kg in most of the patients in this review. Data are lacking regarding the long-term results in such patients. Tocilizumab is a promising agent, owing to the proposed role of IL-6 in the pathogenesis of neurologic involvement of BS. Few case reports with tocilizumab showing good results have been published.[77,78]

The other type of neurologic involvement in BS is caused by cerebral venous sinus thrombosis. Similar to the situation with DVT, there is also no consensus about the optimal treatment of this type of involvement. A systematic review identified 290 reported BS patients with cerebral venous thrombosis.[79] Around 90% of these patients were prescribed GCS with or without immunosuppressives and 74% were prescribed anticoagulants. In one of the largest series that favor anticoagulation, 62 of 64 BS patients with cerebral venous thrombosis were anticoagulated.[80] A relapse of thrombosis was observed in 31% of the patients in this series. Moreover, there were serious bleeding complications such as psoas hematoma, leg hematoma, and subdural hematoma in 6.5% of the patients who were anticoagulated.

In BS patients with neurologic involvement, the use of cyclosporine A is problematic because neurotoxicity caused by cyclosporine A itself is well described in BS patients. Case-control studies have suggested an increased frequency of neurologic involvement among those who use cyclosporine A.[81–83] These findings may be confounded by indication, because there is an association between neurologic involvement and eye involvement, which is the main indication for the use of cyclosporine A in BS. However, in a larger series in which only patients with eye involvement who used and did not use cyclosporine A, and who were matched for severity of eye involvement were compared, neurologic involvement was also more common in the cyclosporine A group.[84] It is thus possible that there is a true association.

SUMMARY

There has been an improvement in the management of BS, with more insight into the better use of older agents and the development of newer remedies including biologics. This trend is especially important for serious organ disorders with eye, neurologic, vascular, and gastrointestinal involvement. It is nowadays uncommon for a BS patient to become blind unless there has been a delay in the diagnosis or the onset of effective treatment. In part, this may be attributed to a possible decrease in the severity of BS over decades. However, the main reason is most probably the rapid and aggressive treatment of these patients.[85]

REFERENCES

1. Yurdakul S, Günaydin I, Tüzün Y, et al. The prevalence of Behçet's syndrome in a rural area in northern Turkey. J Rheumatol 1988;15(5):820–2.

2. Azizlerli G, Köse AA, Sarica R, et al. Prevalence of Behçet's disease in Istanbul, Turkey. Int J Dermatol 2003;42(10):803–6.
3. Papoutsis NG, Abdel-Naser MB, Altenburg A, et al. Prevalence of Adamantiades-Behçet's disease in Germany and the municipality of Berlin: results of a nation-wide survey. Clin Exp Rheumatol 2006;24(5 Suppl 42):S125.
4. Seyahi E, Tahir Turanli E, Mangan MS, et al. The prevalence of Behçet's syndrome, familial Mediterranean fever, HLA-B51 and MEFV gene mutations among ethnic Armenians living in Istanbul, Turkey. Clin Exp Rheumatol 2010; 28(4 Suppl 60):S67–75.
5. O'Duffy JD. Summary of international symposium on Behçet's disease. Istanbul, September 29-30, 1977. J Rheumatol 1978;5:229–33.
6. Calamia KT, Wilson FC, Icen M, et al. Epidemiology and clinical characteristics of Behçet's disease in the US: a population-based study. Arthritis Rheum 2009;61: 600–4.
7. Yazici Y, Moses N. Clinical manifestations and ethnic background of patients with Behçet's syndrome in a US Cohort. Arthritis Rheum 2007;56:S502.
8. Salvarani C, Pipitone N, Catanoso MG, et al. Epidemiology and clinical course of Behçet's disease in the Reggio Emilia area of Northern Italy: a seventeen-year population-based study. Arthritis Rheum 2007;57(1):171–8.
9. Kural-Seyahi E, Fresko I, Seyahi N, et al. The long-term mortality and morbidity of Behçet syndrome: a 2-decade outcome survey of 387 patients followed at a dedicated center. Medicine (Baltimore) 2003;82:60–76.
10. Ambrose NL, Haskard DO. Differential diagnosis and management of Behçet syndrome. Nat Rev Rheumatol 2013;9(2):79–89.
11. Yazici Y, Yurdakul S, Yazici H. Behçet's syndrome. Curr Rheumatol Rep 2010; 12(6):429–35.
12. Hamuryudan V, Er T, Seyahi E, et al. Pulmonary artery aneurysms in Behçet syndrome. Am J Med 2004;117(11):867–70.
13. Seyahi E, Melikoglu M, Akman C, et al. Pulmonary artery involvement and associated lung disease in Behçet disease: a series of 47 patients. Medicine (Baltimore) 2012;91(1):35–48.
14. Lakhanpal S, Tani K, Lie JT, et al. Pathologic features of Behçet's syndrome: a review of Japanese autopsy registry data. Hum Pathol 1985;16(8):790–5.
15. Desbois AC, Wechsler B, Resche-Rigon M, et al. Immunosuppressants reduce venous thrombosis relapse in Behçet's disease. Arthritis Rheum 2012;64(8):2753–60.
16. Ahn JK, Lee YS, Jeon CH, et al. Treatment of venous thrombosis associated with Behçet's disease: immunosuppressive therapy alone versus immunosuppressive therapy plus anticoagulation. Clin Rheumatol 2008;27(2):201–5.
17. Seyahi E, Baskurt M, Melikoglu M, et al. The estimated pulmonary artery pressure can be elevated in Behçet's syndrome. Respir Med 2011;105(11):1739–47.
18. Tunc R, Keyman E, Melikoglu M, et al. Target organ associations in Turkish patients with Behçet's disease: a cross sectional study by exploratory factor analysis. J Rheumatol 2002;29(11):2393–6.
19. Hatemi G, Bahar H, Uysal S, et al. The pustular skin lesions in Behçet's syndrome are not sterile. Ann Rheum Dis 2004;63:1450–2.
20. Hatemi G, Fresko I, Tascilar K, et al. Increased enthesopathy among Behçet's syndrome patients with acne and arthritis: an ultrasonography study. Arthritis Rheum 2008;58:1539–45.
21. Hatemi G, Fresko I, Yurdakul S, et al. Reply to letter by Priori et al commenting on whether Behçet's syndrome patients with acne and arthritis comprise a true subset. Arthritis Rheum 2010;62:305–6.

22. Karaca M, Hatemi G, Sut N, et al. The papulopustular lesion/arthritis cluster of Behçet's syndrome also clusters in families. Rheumatology (Oxford) 2012;51(6): 1053–60.
23. Melikoglu M, Ugurlu S, Tascilar K, et al. Large vessel involvement in Behçet's syndrome: a retrospective survey. Ann Rheum Dis 2008;67(Suppl II):67.
24. Melikoglu M, Fresko I, Mat C, et al. Short-term trial of etanercept in Behçet's disease: a double blind, placebo controlled study. J Rheumatol 2005;32(1): 98–105.
25. Gül A, Tugal-Tutkun I, Dinarello CA, et al. Interleukin-1β-regulating antibody XOMA 052 (gevokizumab) in the treatment of acute exacerbations of resistant uveitis of Behçet's disease: an open-label pilot study. Ann Rheum Dis 2012; 71(4):563–6.
26. Aktulga E, Altaç M, Müftüoglu A, et al. A double blind study of colchicine in Behçet's disease. Haematologica 1980;65(3):399–402.
27. Yurdakul S, Mat C, Tüzün Y, et al. A double-blind trial of colchicine in Behçet's syndrome. Arthritis Rheum 2001;44(11):2686–92.
28. Mat C, Yurdakul S, Uysal S, et al. A double-blind trial of depot corticosteroids in Behçet's syndrome. Rheumatology (Oxford) 2006;45(3):348–52.
29. Yazici H, Ugurlu S, Seyahi E. Behçet syndrome: is it one condition? Clin Rev Allergy Immunol 2012;43(3):275–80.
30. Bird Stewart JA. Genetic analysis of families of patients with Behçet's syndrome: data incompatible with autosomal recessive inheritance. Ann Rheum Dis 1986; 45(1):265 8.
31. Molinari N, Koné Paut I, Manna R, et al. Identification of an autosomal recessive mode of inheritance in paediatric Behçet's families by segregation analysis. Am J Med Genet A 2003;122A(2):115–8.
32. Seyahi E, Ozdogan H. Juvenile Behçet's syndrome. In: Yazici Y, Yazici H, editors. Behçet's syndrome. New York: Springer; 2010. p. 205–14.
33. Gul A, Ohno S. Genetics of Behçet's disease. In: Yazici Y, Yazici H, editors. Behçet's syndrome. New York: Springer; 2010. p. 265–76.
34. Masatlioglu S, Seyahi E, Tahir Turanli E, et al. A twin study in Behçet's syndrome. Clin Exp Rheumatol 2010;28(4 Suppl 60):S62–6.
35. Remmers EF, Cosan F, Kirino Y, et al. Genome-wide association study identifies variants in the MHC class I, IL10, and IL23R-IL12RB2 regions associated with Behçet's disease. Nat Genet 2010;42(8):698–702.
36. de Craen AJ, Posthuma D, Remarque EJ, et al. Heritability estimates of innate immunity: an extended twin study. Genes Immun 2005;6:167–70.
37. Criteria for diagnosis of Behçet's disease. International Study Group for Behçet's Disease. Lancet 1990;335(8697):1078–80.
38. Cheon JH, Çelik AF, Kim WH. Behçet's disease: gastrointestinal involvement. In: Yazici Y, Yazici H, editors. Behçet's syndrome. New York: Springer; 2010. p. 165–89.
39. Yazici H. A critical look at diagnostic criteria: time for a change? Bull NYU Hosp Jt Dis 2011;69(2):101–3.
40. Hatemi G, Silman A, Bang D, et al, EULAR Expert Committee. EULAR recommendations for the management of Behçet disease. Ann Rheum Dis 2008;67(12): 1656–62.
41. Hatemi G, Silman A, Bang D, et al. Management of Behçet disease: a systematic literature review for the European League Against Rheumatism evidence-based recommendations for the management of Behçet disease. Ann Rheum Dis 2009;68(10):1528–34.

42. Alpsoy E, Er H, Durusoy C, et al. The use of sucralfate suspension in the treatment of oral and genital ulceration of Behçet disease: a randomized, placebo-controlled, double-blind study. Arch Dermatol 1999;135:529–32.
43. Tasli L, Mat C, De Simone C, et al. Lactobacilli lozenges in the management of oral ulcers of Behçet's syndrome. Clin Exp Rheumatol 2006;24(5 Suppl 42): S83–6.
44. Karacayli U, Mumcu G, Simsek I, et al. The close association between dental and periodontal treatments and oral ulcer course in Behçet's disease: a prospective clinical study. J Oral Pathol Med 2009;38(5):410–5.
45. Yazici H, Pazarli H, Barnes CG, et al. A controlled trial of azathioprine in Behçet's syndrome. N Engl J Med 1990;322:281–5.
46. Alpsoy E, Durusoy C, Yilmaz E, et al. Interferon alfa-2a in the treatment of Behçet disease: a randomized placebo-controlled and double-blind study. Arch Dermatol 2002;138:467–71.
47. Hamuryudan V, Mat C, Saip S, et al. Thalidomide in the treatment of the mucocutaneous lesions of the Behçet syndrome. A randomized, double-blind, placebo-controlled trial. Ann Intern Med 1998;128:443–50.
48. Arida A, Fragiadaki K, Giavri E, et al. Anti-TNF agents for Behçet's disease: analysis of published data on 369 patients. Semin Arthritis Rheum 2011;41(1):61–70.
49. Mat CM, Bang D, Melikoglu M. The mucocutaneous manifestations and pathergy reaction in Behçet's Disease. In: Yazici Y, Yazici H, editors. Behçet's syndrome. New York: Springer; 2010. p. 53–72.
50. Diamantopoulos AP, Hatemi G. Lack of efficacy of tocilizumab in mucocutaneous Behçet's syndrome: report of 2 cases. Rheumatology (Oxford), in press.
51. Moral F, Hamuryudan V, Yurdakul S, et al. Inefficacy of azapropazone in the acute arthritis of Behçet's syndrome: a randomized, double blind, placebo controlled study. Clin Exp Rheumatol 1995;13:493–5.
52. Hamuryudan V, Ozyazgan Y, Hizli N, et al. Azathioprine in Behçet's syndrome: effects on long-term prognosis. Arthritis Rheum 1997;40:769–74.
53. Saadoun D, Wechsler B, Terrada C, et al. Azathioprine in severe uveitis of Behçet's disease. Arthritis Care Res (Hoboken) 2010;62(12):1733–8.
54. Masuda K, Nakajima A, Urayama A, et al. Double-masked trial of cyclosporin versus colchicine and long-term open study of cyclosporin in Behçet's disease. Lancet 1989;1:1093–6.
55. Kotter I, Vonthein R, Zierhut M, et al. Differential efficacy of human recombinant interferon-alpha2a on ocular and extraocular manifestations of Behçet disease: results of an open 4-center trial. Semin Arthritis Rheum 2004;33:311–9.
56. Kötter I, Hamuryudan V, Oztürk ZE, et al. Interferon therapy in rheumatic diseases: state-of-the-art 2010. Curr Opin Rheumatol 2010;22(3):278–83.
57. Onal S, Kazokoglu H, Koc A, et al. Long-term efficacy and safety of low-dose and dose escalating interferon alfa-2a therapy in refractory Behçet uveitis. Arch Ophthalmol 2011;129:288–94.
58. Keino H, Okada AA, Watanabe T, et al. Decreased ocular inflammatory attacks and background retinal and disc vascular leakage in patients with Behçet disease on infliximab therapy. Br J Ophthalmol 2011;95:1245–50.
59. Olivieri I, Leccese P, D'Angelo S, et al. Efficacy of adalimumab in patients with Behçet's disease unsuccessfully treated with infliximab. Clin Exp Rheumatol 2011;29(Suppl 67):S54–7.
60. Markomichelakis N, Delicha E, Masselos S, et al. A single infliximab infusion vs corticosteroids for acute panuveitis attacks in Behçet's disease: a comparative 4-week study. Rheumatology (Oxford) 2011;50:593–7.

61. Markomichelakis N, Delicha E, Masselos S, et al. Intravitreal infliximab for sight threatening relapsing uveitis in Behçet disease: a pilot study in 15 patients. Am J Ophthalmol 2012;154:534–541.e1.

62. Ugurlu S, Ucar D, Seyahi E, et al. Canakinumab in a patient with juvenile Behçet's syndrome with refractory eye disease. Ann Rheum Dis 2012;71(9):1589–91.

63. Cantarini L, Vitale A, Borri M, et al. Successful use of canakinumab in a patient with resistant Behçet's disease. Clin Exp Rheumatol 2012;30(3 Suppl 72): S115.

64. Hamuryudan V, Yurdakul S, Moral F, et al. Pulmonary arterial aneurysms in Behçet's syndrome: a report of 24 cases. Br J Rheumatol 1994;33(1):48–51.

65. Adler S, Baumgartner I, Villiger PM. Behçet's disease: successful treatment with infliximab in 7 patients with severe vascular manifestations. A retrospective analysis. Arthritis Care Res 2012;64:607–11.

66. Schreiber BE, Noor N, Juli CF, et al. Resolution of Behçet's syndrome associated pulmonary arterial aneurysms with infliximab. Semin Arthritis Rheum 2011;41: 482–7.

67. Tuzun H, Seyahi E, Arslan C, et al. Management and prognosis of nonpulmonary large arterial disease in patients with Behçet disease. J Vasc Surg 2012;55(1): 157–63.

68. Tayer-Shifman OE, Seyahi E, Nowatzky J, et al. Major vessel thrombosis in Behçet's disease: the dilemma of anticoagulant therapy—the approach of rheumatologists from different countries. Clin Exp Rheumatol 2012;30(5):735–40.

69. Jung YS, Hong SP, Kim TI, et al. Long-term clinical outcomes and factors predictive of relapse after 5-aminosalicylate or sulfasalazine therapy in patients with intestinal Behçet disease. J Clin Gastroenterol 2012;46:e38–45.

70. Hatemi I, Hatemi G, Erzin Y, et al. Characteristics, treatment and outcome of gastrointestinal involvement of Behçet's syndrome: experience in a dedicated center. Ann Rheum Dis 2012;71(Suppl 3):391.

71. Sayarlioglu M, Kotan MC, Topcu N, et al. Treatment of recurrent perforating intestinal ulcers with thalidomide in Behçet's disease. Ann Pharmacother 2004;38(5): 808–11.

72. Maruyama Y, Hisamatsu T, Matsuoka K, et al. A case of intestinal Behçet's disease treated with infliximab monotherapy who successfully maintained clinical remission and complete mucosal healing for six years. Intern Med 2012;51(16): 2125–9.

73. Shimizu Y, Takeda T, Matsumoto R, et al. Clinical efficacy of adalimumab for a postoperative marginal ulcer in gastrointestinal Behçet disease. Nihon Shokakibyo Gakkai Zasshi 2012;109(5):774–80 [in Japanese].

74. Kurtuncu M, Tuzun E, Mutlu M, et al. Clinical patterns and course of neuro-Behçet's disease: analysis of 354 patients comparing cases presented before and after 1990. Clin Exp Rheumatol 2008;26(4 Suppl 50):S17.

75. Shugaiv E, Tüzün E, Mutlu M, et al. Mycophenolate mofetil as a novel immunosuppressant in the treatment of neuro-Behçet's disease with parenchymal involvement: presentation of four cases. Clin Exp Rheumatol 2011;29(4 Suppl 67):S64–7.

76. Fasano A, D'Agostino M, Caldarola G, et al. Infliximab monotherapy in neuro-Behçet's disease: four year follow-up in a long-standing case resistant to conventional therapies. J Neuroimmunol 2011;239(1–2):105–7.

77. Urbaniak P, Hasler P, Kretzschmar S. Refractory neuro-Behçet treated by tocilizumab: a case report. Clin Exp Rheumatol 2012;30(3 Suppl 72):S73–5.

78. Shapiro LS, Farrell J, Haghighi AB. Tocilizumab treatment for neuro-Behçet's disease, the first report. Clin Neurol Neurosurg 2012;114(3):297–8.

79. Aguiar de Sousa D, Mestre T, Ferro JM. Cerebral venous thrombosis in Behçet's disease: a systematic review. J Neurol 2011;258(5):719–27.
80. Saadoun D, Wechsler B, Resche-Rigon M, et al. Cerebral venous thrombosis in Behçet's disease. Arthritis Rheum 2009;61(4):518–26.
81. Kotake S, Higashi K, Yoshikawa K, et al. Central nervous system symptoms in patients with Behçet disease receiving cyclosporine therapy. Ophthalmology 1999;106:586–9.
82. Kotter I, Gunaydin I, Batra M, et al. CNS involvement occurs more frequently in patients with Behçet's disease under cyclosporin A (CSA) than under other medications—results of a retrospective analysis of 117 cases. Clin Rheumatol 2006;25:482–6.
83. Kato Y, Numaga J, Kato S, et al. Central nervous system symptoms in a population of Behçet's disease patients with refractory uveitis treated with cyclosporine A. Clin Experiment Ophthalmol 2001;29:335–6.
84. Akman-Demir G, Ayranci O, Kurtuncu M, et al. Cyclosporine for Behçet's uveitis: is it associated with an increased risk of neurological involvement? Clin Exp Rheumatol 2008;26(4 Suppl 50):S84–90.
85. Turkstra F, van Vugt RM, Dijkmans BA, et al. Results of a questionnaire on the treatment of patients with Behçet's syndrome: a trend for more intensive treatment. Clin Exp Rheumatol 2012;30(3 Suppl 72):S10–3.
86. Kurosawa M, Inaba Y, Nishibu A, et al. Nationwide epidemiological survey of Behçet's disease in 2003 in Japanese. Clinical Experimental Rheumatology 2004;22(4 Suppl 34):S84.
87. Zhang Z, He F, Shi Y. Behcet's disease seen in China: analysis of 334 cases. Rheumatol Int 2012. [Epub ahead of print].
88. Davatchi F, Jamshidi AR, Banihashemi AT, et al. WHO-ILAR COPCORD Study (Stage 1, Urban Study) in Iran. J Rheumatol 2008;35(7):1384.
89. Al-Rawi ZS, Neda AH. Prevalence of Behçet's disease among Iraqis. Adv Exp Med Biol 2003;528:37–41.
90. Krause I, Yankevich A, Fraser A, et al. Prevalence and clinical aspects of Behcet's disease in the north of Israel. Clin Rheumatol 2007;26(4):555–60.
91. Al dalaan A, Al Ballaa S, Al Sukati M, et al. The prevalence of Behçet's disease in Al-Qassim region of Saudi Arabia. In: Hamza M, editor. Behçet's Disease. Tunis: Pub Adhoua; 1997. p. 170–2.
92. Assaad Khalil SH, Kamel FA, Ismail EA. Starting a regional registry for patients with Behçet's disease in North West Nile Delta region in Egypt. In: Hamza M, editor. Behçet's Disease. Tunis: Pub Adhoua; 1997. p. 173–6.
93. Crespo J, Ribeiro J, Jesus E, et al. Behçet's disease: particular features at the central zone of Portugal. In: Wechsler B, Godeau P, editors. Behçet's Disease: International Congress series 1037. Amsterdam: Excerpta Medica; 1993. p. 207–10.
94. González-Gay MA, García-Porrúa C, Brañas F, et al. Epidemiologic and clinical aspects of Behçet's disease in a defined area of Northwestern Spain, 1988-1997. J Rheumatol 2000;27(3):703–7.
95. Mahr A, Belarbi L, Wechsler B, et al. Population-based prevalence study of Behçet's disease: differences by ethnic origin and low variation by age at immigration. Arthritis Rheum 2008;58(12):3951–9.
96. Chamberlain MA. Behcet's syndrome in 32 patients in Yorkshire. Ann Rheum Dis 1977;36(6):491–9.
97. Jankowski J, Crombie I, Jankowski R. Behçet's syndrome in Scotland. Postgrad Med J 1992;68(801):566–70.
98. Ek L, Hedfors E. Behçet's disease: a review and a report of 12 cases from Sweden. Acta Derm Venereol 1993;73(4):251–4.

Relapsing Polychondritis

Ratnesh Chopra, MD, Nida Chaudhary, MD, Jonathan Kay, MD*

KEYWORDS

- Cartilage • Type II collagen • Auricular chondritis • Scleritis
- Tracheobronchomalacia • Myelodysplastic syndrome

KEY POINTS

- Relapsing polychondritis (RP) is a rare systemic autoimmune disease characterized by episodic, progressive inflammatory destruction of cartilage.
- RP can be primary or exist as an overlap syndrome with other rheumatologic conditions such as rheumatoid arthritis, spondyloarthropathies, and vasculitis, or as a paraneoplastic manifestation of myelodysplastic syndromes.
- No specific laboratory test is diagnostic for RP, but increased levels of acute phase reactants may indicate the presence of systemic inflammation. The diagnosis is confirmed by showing characteristic histologic features of RP on biopsy of affected tissues.
- Systemic immunosuppression is the mainstay of treatment of RP, but recent case reports suggest efficacy of tumor necrosis factor inhibitors and of the anti–interleukin-6 receptor monoclonal antibody tocilizumab.

INTRODUCTION

Relapsing polychondritis (RP) is an infrequently occurring systemic autoimmune disease that is characterized by episodic, progressive inflammatory destruction of cartilage. The cartilaginous structures most often involved include the elastic cartilage of the ears, the hyaline cartilage of the tracheobronchial tree and the joints, and the fibrocartilage of the axial skeleton. Immune-mediated damage can spread to involve noncartilaginous tissues that are rich in proteoglycans, such as that of the eyes, the inner ear, the heart, blood vessels, and the kidney. RP may occur alone (primary RP) or in association with other diseases. It follows a fluctuating, but progressive, course that may result in significant morbidity and sometimes death.

HISTORY

Rudolf Jaksch von Wartenhorst,[1] an Austrian internist, first described this disease in 1923. His patient was a 32-year-old male brewer who presented with fever,

Rheumatology Center, Memorial Campus, UMass Memorial Medical Center, 119 Belmont Street, Worcester, MA 01605, USA
* Corresponding author.
E-mail address: jonathan.kay@umassmemorial.org

Rheum Dis Clin N Am 39 (2013) 263–276
http://dx.doi.org/10.1016/j.rdc.2013.03.002
0889-857X/13/$ – see front matter © 2013 Elsevier Inc. All rights reserved.

asymmetric polyarthritis, and pain, swelling, and deformity of the ears and nose. Biopsy of nasal cartilage revealed loss of the cartilage matrix and a hyperplastic mucous membrane. Jaksch von Wartenhorst[1] characterized it as a degenerative disease of cartilage and named it polychondropathia. Taking his patient's occupation into consideration, he related the cause to excessive alcohol intake.

Since then, the disease has also been called diffuse perichondritis, chondromalacia, chronic atrophic polychondritis, diffuse chondrolysis, and dyschondroplasia. The current name, RP, was introduced by Pearson and colleagues[2] in 1960 to emphasize the episodic course of the disease.

EPIDEMIOLOGY

RP occurs predominantly in white people but has also been described in people of African, Asian, or Hispanic ancestry.[3,4] It occurs with equal frequency among men and women.[5] At the Mayo Clinic, the annual incidence has been estimated to be 3.5 cases per million.[6] Although RP may develop at any age, most reported cases have had onset between the ages of 20 and 60 years, with the highest incidence occurring between the ages of 40 and 50 years.[3] One case has been reported of a pregnant woman with RP whose baby was similarly affected at birth,[7] but no other cases suggest maternal-fetal transmission or a genetic predisposition to developing RP.

CAUSE AND PATHOGENESIS

The specific cause of RP is unknown, but the proposed pathogenesis involves both humoral and cellular immunity. Autoantibodies to collagen have been shown in the sera of patients with RP. Circulating antibodies to type II collagen were identified in 33% of patients with RP and acute cartilage inflammation.[8] Antibodies to type IX and type XI collagen also have been identified in patients with RP.[9] Antibodies to other cartilaginous proteins, including matrilin-I and cartilage oligomeric matrix proteins, have been identified in patients with RP.[10] Type II collagen neoepitope (TIINE), a 45-mer peptide fragment of type II collagen, has been detected in the urine of patients with RP and might be useful to follow as a biomarker of collagen destruction reflecting RP disease activity.[11]

It has been postulated that cell-mediated immunity may perpetuate cartilage inflammation.[2,4,5] CD4+ T lymphocytes, plasma cells,[12] immunoglobulin, and complement[13] have been isolated from RP lesions in cartilage. Incubation of lymphocytes obtained from patients with RP with cartilage mucopolysaccharides resulted in transformation of the lymphocytes into lymphoblasts.[14] Increased levels of chemokines, including monocyte chemotactic protein (MCP)-1, macrophage inflammatory protein (MIP)-1β, and interleukin (IL)-8, indicating activation of macrophages, have been observed in rodent models of RP.[15,16] In patients with RP, serum levels of macrophage inhibitory factor (MIF) were significantly increased compared with healthy controls.[17] This finding might account for the in vitro observation that migration of guinea pig macrophages to human laryngeal proteoglycan was inhibited when the macrophages were mixed with lymphocytes from patients with RP, compared with when they were mixed with lymphocytes obtained from healthy controls.[14] Tumor necrosis factor (TNF) α expression also is increased in patients with RP.[18]

The frequency of human leukocyte antigen (HLA) DR4 is significantly increased among patients with RP. However, oligonucleotide-based genotyping failed to show a predominance of any single HLA-DR4 subtype.[19] In contrast, the frequency of HLA-DR6 is decreased among patients with RP.[20,21]

CLASSIFICATION

It has been proposed that RP be considered as a syndrome, with the primary form occurring in isolation and the secondary form in association with one of the diseases listed in **Table 1**. Associated autoimmune diseases are present in 30% to 37% of patients with RP.[22,23] RP has occasionally developed following mechanical injury to cartilage, such as after piercing of the cartilaginous portion of the pinna of the ear.[24]

CLINICAL FEATURES

Auricular chondritis and arthritis are the most common presenting symptoms of RP, each of which is present in about 20% to 30% of patients at the time of diagnosis.[5,20] Another 10% to 15% of patients present with nasal chondritis, ocular inflammation, and/or respiratory tract involvement.[5,25,26] The diagnosis of RP may be delayed in patients who present only with nonspecific symptoms of fever, weight loss, fatigue, or lethargy and no signs of cartilage inflammation.

Auricular Manifestations

Auricular chondritis is the most characteristic presenting sign of RP. The pinna of the ear becomes painful, red, and swollen, but the earlobe is spared (**Fig. 1**). Attacks typically occur with subacute onset and follow a relapsing-remitting course. After recurrent attacks of inflammation, the pinna of the ear may become floppy and contorted,

Table 1 Diseases associated with RP	
Cutaneous	
Atopic dermatitis	Cutaneous leukocytoclastic vasculitis
Dermatitis herpetiformis	Lichen planus
Panniculitis	Psoriasis
Vitiligo	
Endocrine	
Diabetes mellitus	Graves' disease
Hashimoto's thyroiditis	Hypothyroidism
Gastrointestinal	
Inflammatory bowel disease	Primary biliary cirrhosis
Hematologic	
Acute lymphocytic leukemia	Cryoglobulinemia
Hodgkin's disease	MALT lymphoma
Myelodysplastic syndromes	Pernicious anemia
Genitourinary	
Glomerulonephritis	Retroperitoneal fibrosis
Rheumatologic	
Behçet's syndrome	Familial Mediterranean fever
Juvenile chronic arthritis	Rheumatoid arthritis
Spondyloarthropathies	Systemic vasculitis

Abbreviation: MALT, mucosa-associated lymphoid tissue.
   Data from Letko E, Zafirakis P, Baltatzis S, et al. Relapsing polychondritis: a clinical review. Semin Arthritis Rheum 2002;31(6):384–95; and Frances C, el Rassi R, Laporte JL, et al. Dermatologic manifestations of relapsing polychondritis. A study of 200 cases at a single center. Medicine 2001;80(3):173–9.

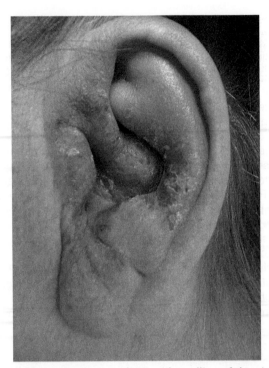

Fig. 1. Auricular chondritis in a patient with RP, with swelling of the pinna of the ear, but sparing of the earlobe. (*Courtesy of* Raymond Pertusi, DO, Worcester, MA.)

resembling the florets of a cauliflower.[3,5] Nearly all patients with RP eventually develop auricular chondritis; it involves both ears in all but a few patients. Stenosis of the external auditory canal, eustachian tube chondritis, and serous otitis media each can result in conductive hearing loss. Vasculitis of the internal auditory artery may cause acute sensorineural hearing loss, with or without vestibular dysfunction.[27]

Ocular Manifestations

The eye is involved in about 20% of patients with RP at the time of initial presentation; ocular involvement, most often episcleritis or scleritis, eventually develops in up to 65% of patients.[28] Inflammation with reactive lymphoid hyperplasia resulted in a mass similar to a salmon-patch on the conjunctiva of a patient with long-standing RP.[29] Recurrent or long-standing inflammation may cause thinning of the sclera, allowing the darker underlying choroid to appear as bluish discoloration through the thinned sclera. Keratoconjunctivitis sicca, keratitis, corneal perforation, iritis, retinopathy, and optic neuritis may occur in RP; each can result in blindness.[22,28] Inflammation external to the globe may present as orbital pseudotumor, lid edema, or extraocular muscle palsy.

Respiratory Tract Manifestations

Nasal chondritis is present in 10% to 15% of patients at the time of their initial presentation and eventually develops in 50% to 70% of patients with RP.[5,6] It presents with the acute onset of nasal swelling, warmth, and erythema, predominantly affecting the distal cartilaginous portion of the nasal septum. Patients experience a sensation of fullness of the nasal bridge and surrounding tissues. Recurrent episodes may result in a saddle nose deformity.[2,3,5]

Chondritis of the laryngotracheal cartilage causes respiratory tract symptoms in more than half of patients with RP. These symptoms include dyspnea, wheezing, cough, and, occasionally, a sensation of choking. Laryngeal inflammation can also cause vocal cord edema or paralysis, resulting in dysphonia or aphonia. The thyroid cartilage and anterior cervical trachea are tender to palpation. In later stages, ventilatory complications have been observed in half of patients with RP. These complications include fixed subglottic and bronchial stenosis with airway obstruction, thickening and calcification of the airways, obstructive bronchiectasis, and tracheal/bronchial collapse.[30–33]

Pulmonary function testing, including flow-volume curves, should be performed in all patients with RP to detect occult airway disease. If respiratory tract symptoms or abnormalities on pulmonary function testing are present, the patient should be imaged by computed tomography (CT) scanning of the chest.[34] Although bronchoscopy may help to distinguish active inflammation from changes caused by previous inflammation, this procedure may result in ventilatory decompensation and thus is not recommended.[32]

Musculoskeletal Manifestations

Patients with RP may experience arthralgias in the absence of objective evidence of joint inflammation. Inflammatory arthritis develops at some time during the disease course in 70% to 80% of patients with RP.[5] This seronegative arthritis typically presents with an asymmetric and migratory pattern of joint involvement, often involving the sternoclavicular, costochondral, and sternomanubrial joints, with intermittent flares. Aspiration of involved joints usually yields noninflammatory synovial fluid. Joint cartilage space narrowing and osteopenia may be observed on plain radiographs of appendicular joints, but bone erosion usually does not occur unless rheumatoid arthritis coexists. In severe cases, the clavicles and ribs may become dislocated and lysis of costochondral cartilage may result in a flail chest wall.[35,36]

Mucocutaneous Manifestations

Mucocutaneous signs and symptoms are present in half of patients with RP. Skin is involved in 20% to 30% of patients with primary RP[23] and in as many as 90% of patients with the combination of RP and a myelodysplastic syndrome (MDS).[7,34] Oral aphthous ulceration is the most common mucocutaneous manifestation associated with RP. The mouth and genital ulcers with inflamed cartilage (MAGIC) syndrome represents an overlap between Behçet's syndrome and RP.[37] Other cutaneous manifestations of RP include erythema nodosum, purpura, livedo reticularis, urticaria, angioedema, erythema multiforme, and panniculitis.[23] Histologic examination of skin biopsies from patients with RP most commonly reveals leukocytoclastic vasculitis, as well as thrombosis of cutaneous vessels, septal panniculitis, and neutrophilic dermatosis. The presence of mucocutaneous findings in a patient with RP should prompt a thorough evaluation for underlying myelodysplasia.[38]

Hematologic Manifestations

Despite its infrequent occurrence, RP presents in combination with MDS more frequently than would be expected by chance.[38] Thus, RP might be considered to be a paraneoplastic manifestation of MDS. Similar to those with a MDS alone, patients with the combination of RP and a MDS are typically men between the ages of

60 and 70 years. Older patients with newly diagnosed RP should therefore undergo a hematologic evaluation for a MDS.

The prognosis of RP occurring with a MDS is worse than that for primary RP. It depends primarily on the severity of the hematologic disease and whether the MDS undergoes leukemic transformation. In a patient with RP and a MDS that presented with a refractory anemia, the hematologic disease transformed to chronic myelomonocytic leukemia without the development of acute leukemia.[39] A case of pernicious anemia has been reported in association with RP.[5]

Cardiovascular Manifestations

Cardiovascular manifestations of RP typically occur in the setting of long-standing disease, even when patients have been receiving immunosuppressive therapy.[40] Aortic regurgitation is the most common cardiovascular complication of RP, occurring in 4% to 10% of patients.[41] Mitral regurgitation has been observed in 2% of patients with RP, more often in men.[42] Other cardiovascular manifestations of RP include aortitis, abdominal and thoracic aortic aneurysms with aneurysmal dilatation of the aortic root, cystic medial necrosis of the aorta, cardiac ischemia, cardiac conduction abnormalities, pericarditis, and thrombophlebitis.[43,44] Arterial thromboses have occurred in patients with secondary RP, typically in the setting of underlying antiphospholipid antibody syndrome.[45]

Biochemical analysis of diseased valves removed from patients with RP has revealed decreased amounts of hydroxyproline and glycine, which are amino acid constituents of collagen, suggesting that the valvular damage occurred as a result of chronic inflammation.[46,47] All patients with RP who present with a heart murmur or with otherwise unexplained dyspnea should have both an electrocardiogram and echocardiogram performed to investigate possible cardiovascular involvement.

Neurologic Manifestations

Neurologic involvement occurs in less than 3% of patients with RP and can present with either subacute or acute onset.[14] Cranial nerves are frequently involved, most commonly the second (manifesting as optic neuritis), the sixth (manifesting as lateral rectus palsy), the seventh (manifesting as facial weakness), and the eighth (manifesting as audiovestibular dysfunction).[48] Headaches, seizures, cerebellar dysfunction with ataxia, confusion, cerebral aneurysms, and aseptic meningitis have all been described in patients with RP.[49–51] As long as renal function is not impaired, gadolinium-containing contrast-enhanced magnetic resonance imaging (MRI) of the brain should be performed to evaluate a neurologic deficit that develops in a patient with RP. Multiple foci of gadolinium enhancement on brain MRI suggests the presence of active cerebral vasculitis.

Renal Manifestations

The kidney is infrequently involved in RP, with renal involvement occurring in 6% to 10% of patients with primary RP.[25,52] Renal abnormalities observed in patients with secondary RP are more often related to the associated disease, such as glomerulonephritis caused by systemic lupus erythematosus. Patients with RP with renal involvement typically have more severe systemic disease, including more severe arthritis and extrarenal vasculitis, which results in poorer survival.[52] Because an abnormal urinalysis was detected in about 25% of patients with RP and serum creatinine levels were increased in 10%,[6,52] the urine of patients with RP should be examined regularly to assess for the development of hematuria or worsening proteinuria that might herald the development of renal involvement (**Table 2**).

Table 2
Prevalence of clinical features in RP

Organ or Organ System	McAdam et al,[5] 1976 n = 159 (%)	Michet et al,[6] 1986 n = 112 (%)	Zeuner et al,[20] 1997 n = 62 (%)	Trentham and Le,[53] 1998 n = 66 (%)
Ear	89	85	94	95
Musculoskeletal	81	52	51	85
Nose	72	54	57	48
Eye	65	51	56	57
Laryngotracheal and pulmonary	56	48	30	67
Mucocutaneous	17	28	24	83
Cardiovascular	9	6	23	8
Neurologic	NR	NR	10	NR
Renal	NR	NR	6	NR

Abbreviation: NR, not reported.
Data from Refs.[5,6,20,53]

DIAGNOSIS

The diagnosis of RP is based on the presence of a characteristic combination of clinical findings. Laboratory and imaging studies provide support for the clinical diagnosis, and biopsy of involved cartilaginous tissue may confirm the diagnosis. Various diagnostic criteria have been proposed, but most are based on the criteria of McAdam (**Box 1**).[5] A recent modification of these diagnostic criteria requires 3 or more of the original McAdam criteria and also one of the following to make the diagnosis of RP[54,55]: (1) a clinical response to antiinflammatory drug therapy with either corticosteroids or dapsone, or (2) histologic confirmation of cartilage damage in a biopsy taken from auricular cartilage, the nasal cavity, or the tracheobronchial tree during a period when disease is inactive. Establishing the diagnosis of RP is often challenging and frequently protracted, with a mean delay from the time that medical attention was sought for symptoms until diagnosis of nearly 3 years.[53]

Box 1
The McAdam criteria for RP[a]

Bilateral auricular chondritis

Nonerosive, seronegative inflammatory polyarthritis

Nasal chondritis

Ocular inflammation (conjunctivitis, keratitis, scleritis and/or episcleritis, uveitis)

Respiratory tract chondritis (laryngeal and/or tracheal cartilages)

Cochlear and/or vestibular dysfunction (neurosensory hearing loss, tinnitus, and/or vertigo)

[a] RP is diagnosed when 3 of the 6 criteria are present.

Data from McAdam LP, O'Hanlan MA, Bluestone R, et al. Relapsing polychondritis: prospective study of 23 patients and a review of the literature. Medicine 1976;55(3):193–215; and Damiani JM, Levine HL. Relapsing polychondritis–report of ten cases. Laryngoscope 1979;89(6 Pt 1):929–46.

Laboratory Tests

No specific laboratory test establishes the diagnosis of RP. A complete blood count may reveal anemia, leukocytosis, thrombocytosis, or eosinophilia. Acute phase reactant levels are increased in almost all patients with RP, with the erythrocyte sedimentation rate being increased in about 80%.[2,4] When present, autoantibodies are usually caused by an associated disease rather than by RP. Circulating rheumatoid factor, antiphospholipid antibodies, and antineutrophil cytoplasmic antibodies (ANCA)[55] have been detected in fewer than half of patients with RP and circulating antinuclear antibodies have been identified in 20% to 60% of patients with RP. A urinalysis may reveal proteinuria or microhematuria if renal involvement is present.

Pathology

Showing inflammation on a biopsy of cartilage, usually from the pinna of the ear, confirms the diagnosis of RP. Characteristic histologic features observed on light microscopy include loss of basophilic staining, chondrocyte degeneration with accumulation of lysosomes and lipid-containing vacuoles, perivascular infiltrates of polymorphonuclear and mononuclear cells, perichondrial infiltrates of lymphocytes containing more plasma cells and CD4+ helper T cells than CD8+ cytotoxic T cells, and replacement of cartilage with fibrous tissue (**Fig. 2**).[56,57] By electron microscopy, an electron-lucent cytoplasm, swelling of cellular organelles, and loss of plasma membrane integrity may be observed.[58]

As the disease progresses, the normal architecture of cartilage-containing structures becomes disrupted. Granulation tissue, sometimes harboring sequestered islands of degenerated chondrocytes and extracellular matrix, invades the involved cartilage and lipid-containing cysts form. There may be focal areas of calcification and bone formation within the granulation tissue.[3,59,60]

Imaging

Plain chest radiographs and CT scanning of the chest, which may reveal evidence of occult large airway involvement, should be performed at baseline in all patients diagnosed with RP. Plain chest radiographs of patients with RP may show calcification of the tracheal or laryngeal cartilage, tracheal narrowing, and atelectasis caused by

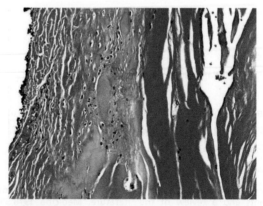

Fig. 2. Auricular cartilage showing degeneration with vacuolization of chondrocytes, fibrosis, and rare lymphocytes (200×, hematoxylin and eosin stain). (*Courtesy of* Kristine M. Cornejo, MD, Worcester, MA.)

bronchial obstruction. The most common changes observed in large airways on chest CT scanning include calcification and thickening of the airway walls, which may cause stenosis.[61] MRI may help to differentiate active airway inflammation from fibrosis.

Other imaging studies may aid in the assessment of patients with RP. Although limited in its availability, positron emission tomography (PET) scanning may reveal areas of occult tissue inflammation. In a patient who presented with fever of unknown origin, RP was diagnosed when increased radiotracer uptake was observed in costo-chondral and laryngotracheal cartilage on ^{18}F-fluorodeoxyglucose PET scanning.[62] When cardiac valvular inflammation is suspected, Doppler echocardiography should be performed.[40]

Ancillary Studies

Pulmonary function testing should include spirometry, a flow-volume loop, and resistance measurements. These studies may show evidence of upper airway obstruction, with decreases in forced expiratory volume in 1 second (FEV_1) and FEV_1/forced vital capacity even in asymptomatic patients. Bronchoscopy may be considered if there is a need to distinguish active inflammation from fibrotic changes caused by previous inflammation. However, because this procedure may result in ventilatory decompensation in patients with widespread laryngotracheal involvement, caution must be observed in patients with RP who have significant airway compromise.

DIFFERENTIAL DIAGNOSIS

Chondritis or inflammation of the external ear may also occur with trauma or infection. Unlike infectious chondritis, in which the ear lobe is usually also involved, the auricular chondritis of RP spares the soft lobule. If the auricular chondritis is bilateral, recurrent, resolves spontaneously, and is associated with other features of RP, the diagnosis of RP can be made with ease. However, in the patient who presents with a unilaterally inflamed ear, *Pseudomonas aeruginosa* infection with necrotizing external otitis should always be considered.[63] Nasal chondritis with subsequent collapse of the nasal septum and the resulting saddle nose deformity can also occur following trauma and in patients with granulomatosis with polyangiitis (GPA; previously known as Wegener granulomatosis), leprosy, or congenital syphilis.

Several systemic diseases, including reactive arthritis, rheumatoid arthritis (RA), GPA, and sarcoidosis share some clinical features with RP.[64,65] Patients with reactive arthritis may exhibit ocular, joint, and cardiovascular features similar to those seen in RP. However, the presence of psoriasiform skin changes and urethritis occurring in an individual with the HLA-B27 antigen suggests an appendicular spondyloarthropathy, such as reactive arthritis. RA is characterized histologically by chronic synovial inflammation and hypertrophy with pannus formation; subchondral bone loss occurs along with cartilage destruction. Patients with GPA may develop nasal septal collapse and involvement of the entire respiratory tract. However, on histologic evaluation of involved tissue, there is evidence of granulomatous vasculitis in patients with GPA, but not in those with RP. Patients with sarcoidosis may present with uveitis, middle ear involvement, and polyarthritis, but usually do not develop chondritis. Hilar adenopathy, interstitial pulmonary fibrosis, granuloma formation, and anergy, which are characteristic features of sarcoidosis, typically are not seen in patients with RP.

MANAGEMENT

Because of its infrequent occurrence, treatments for RP have not been evaluated in randomized, placebo-controlled clinical trials. Instead, the efficacy of various drugs has been reported in individual patients or in small case series. The response to treatment in RP is monitored by observing clinical improvement in disease activity and the reduction in acute phase reactant levels.

Oral nonsteroidal antiinflammatory drugs (NSAIDs) may be used to treat patients with RP with arthralgias or mild arthritis. Topical corticosteroids may be combined with oral NSAIDs to treat patients with mild ocular involvement, such as mild episcleritis, scleritis or iritis. Auricular chondritis has been treated with oral colchicine 0.6 mg twice daily.[66] However, mild to moderate disease that presents with, for example, auricular or nasal chondritis or peripheral arthritis without other significant organ involvement, is usually treated with low-dose corticosteroids, such as oral prednisone 10 to 20 mg daily. Oral dapsone 50 to 200 mg daily has been used to treat isolated nasal and auricular chondritis, but the common occurrence of side effects such as anemia, tachycardia, headache, and skin rash precludes its regular use to treat RP.[67]

Moderate to severe RP that presents with, for example, scleritis, audiovestibular nerve involvement, laryngotracheal chondritis, airway compromise, aortitis, or other significantly compromised organ function, should be treated with high-dose oral corticosteroids (such as prednisone 1 mg/kg/d), or pulse intravenous corticosteroids (1 gm/d for 3 days). The addition of nebulized racemic epinephrine to corticosteroid therapy may help to relieve acute airway obstruction.[68,69]

Methotrexate and azathioprine have each been used as a steroid-sparing agent with some success.[70] When organ-threatening pulmonary, renal, or cardiac disease is present, oral cyclophosphamide (1–2 mg/kg/d) or pulse intravenous cyclophosphamide (0.6 mg/m^2 monthly) may be given in addition to high-dose corticosteroids.[71,72] Oral cyclosporine A (5–15 mg/kg/d) has been used to treat patients with RP that had been refractory to treatment with corticosteroids, dapsone, aziathioprine, and cyclophosphamide.[73]

Several biological targeted therapies have been used with some success in patients with RP. Anti-CD4 monoclonal antibodies were the first biological agents used successfully to treat 2 patients with RP who had persistent disease activity despite conventional immunosuppressive therapy.[74,75] More recently, TNF inhibitors, such as adalimumab,[76] etanercept,[76,77] and infliximab,[78] and the anti–IL-6 receptor monoclonal antibody tocilizumab.[79] have shown efficacy in several patients with RP. However, the few published reports of patients with RP treated with biological agents are not sufficient to assess the efficacy and toxicity of these agents in RP.

Adjunctive therapy with biphasic positive airway pressure or continuous positive airway pressure, especially at night, may provide symptomatic relief to patients with tracheomalacia and bronchomalacia.[80] A tracheostomy may be required when there is subglottic involvement with respiratory distress. When there has been extensive tracheobrachial collapse, tracheal stenting or surgical tracheal reconstruction may be required.[81]

If valvular damage has resulted in heart failure that is refractory to medical management, valvuloplasty or valve replacement may be necessary. In patients with severe aortic insufficiency, the ascending aorta should be replaced with a graft that includes a prosthetic aortic valve to avoid aneurysm formation and periprosthetic valve leakage.[42] Pacemaker implantation is indicated when complete heart block is present.[82]

SUMMARY

RP is a rare systemic autoimmune disease characterized by episodic, progressive inflammatory destruction of cartilage. It can occur as an overlap syndrome in patients with other rheumatologic conditions such as rheumatoid arthritis, spondyloarthropathies, and vasculitis. Especially when it manifests with mucocutaneous involvement in elderly individuals, RP may present as a paraneoplastic manifestation of MDS. The disease usually follows an indolent relapsing-remitting course, but occasionally it can progress rapidly and even cause death, most often as a result of ventilatory compromise. Although auricular or nasal chondritis or peripheral arthritis without other significant organ involvement are usually treated with low-dose corticosteroids, other more severe disease manifestations may require treatment with high-dose corticosteroids or other immunosuppressive agents. Recent case reports of patients with RP who have responded well to TNF or IL-6 inhibitors suggest that biological targeted therapies might prove to be effective treatments for this condition.

REFERENCES

1. Jaksch-Wartenhorst R. Polychondropathia. Wien Arch Inn Med 1923;6:93–100.
2. Pearson CM, Kline HM, Newcomer VD. Relapsing polychondritis. N Engl J Med 1960;263(2):51–8.
3. Arkin CR, Masi AT. Relapsing polychondritis: review of current status and case report. Semin Arthritis Rheum 1975;5(1):41–62.
4. Hughes RA, Berry CL, Seifert M, et al. Relapsing polychondritis. Three cases with a clinico-pathological study and literature review. Q J Med 1972;41(163):363–80.
5. McAdam LP, O'Hanlan MA, Bluestone R, et al. Relapsing polychondritis: prospective study of 23 patients and a review of the literature. Medicine 1976; 55(3):193–215.
6. Michet CJ Jr, McKenna CH, Luthra HS, et al. Relapsing polychondritis. Survival and predictive role of early disease manifestations. Ann Intern Med 1986;104(1):74–8.
7. Arundell FD, Haserick JR. Familial chronic atrophic polychondritis. Arch Dermatol 1960;82(3):439–40.
8. Foidart JM, Abe S, Martin GR, et al. Antibodies to type II collagen in relapsing polychondritis. The New England journal of medicine 1978;299(22):1203–7.
9. Alsalameh S, Mollenhauer J, Scheuplein F, et al. Preferential cellular and humoral immune reactivities to native and denatured collagen types IX and XI in a patient with fatal relapsing polychondritis. J Rheumatol 1993;20(8):1419–24.
10. Klatt AR, Becker AK, Neacsu CD, et al. The matrilins: modulators of extracellular matrix assembly. Int J Biochem Cell Biol 2011;43(3):320–30.
11. Kraus VB, Stabler T, Le ET, et al. Urinary type II collagen neoepitope as an outcome measure for relapsing polychondritis. Arthritis Rheum 2003;48(10):2942–8.
12. Kindblom LG, Dalen P, Edmar G, et al. Relapsing polychondritis. A clinical, pathologic-anatomic and histochemical study of 2 cases. Acta Pathol Microbiol Scand A 1977;85(5):656–64.
13. Valenzuela R, Cooperrider PA, Gogate P, et al. Relapsing polychondritis. Immunomicroscopic findings in cartilage of ear biopsy specimens. Hum Pathol 1980;11(1):19–22.
14. Rajapakse DA, Bywaters EG. Cell-mediated immunity to cartilage proteoglycan in relapsing polychondritis. Clin Exp Immunol 1974;16(3):497–502.
15. Taneja V, Griffiths M, Behrens M, et al. Auricular chondritis in NOD.DQ8.Abetao (Ag7-/-) transgenic mice resembles human relapsing polychondritis. J Clin Invest 2003;112(12):1843–50.
16. Bradley DS, Das P, Griffiths MM, et al. HLA-DQ6/8 double transgenic mice develop auricular chondritis following type II collagen immunization: a model for human relapsing polychondritis. J Immunol 1998;161(9):5046–53.

17. Ohwatari R, Fukuda S, Iwabuchi K, et al. Serum level of macrophage migration inhibitory factor as a useful parameter of clinical course in patients with Wegener's granulomatosis and relapsing polychondritis. Ann Otol Rhinol Laryngol 2001; 110(11):1035–40.

18. Stabler T, Piette JC, Chevalier X, et al. Serum cytokine profiles in relapsing polychondritis suggest monocyte/macrophage activation. Arthritis Rheum 2004; 50(11):3663–7.

19. Luthra HS, McKenna CH, Terasaki PI, Lack of association of HLA-A and B locus antigens with relapsing polychondritis. Tissue Antigens 1981;17(4): 442–3.

20. Zeuner M, Straub R, Rauh G, et al. Relapsing polychondritis: clinical and immunogenetic analysis of 62 patients. J Rheumatol 1997;24(1):96–101.

21. Lang B, Rothenfusser A, Lanchbury JS, et al. Susceptibility to relapsing polychondritis is associated with HLA-DR4. Arthritis Rheum 1993;36(5):660–4.

22. Letko E, Zafirakis P, Baltatzis S, et al. Relapsing polychondritis: a clinical review. Semin Arthritis Rheum 2002;31(6):384–95.

23. Frances C, el Rassi R, Laporte JL, et al. Dermatologic manifestations of relapsing polychondritis. A study of 200 cases at a single center. Medicine 2001;80(3): 173–9.

24. Alissa H, Kadanoff R, Adams E. Does mechanical insult to cartilage trigger relapsing polychondritis? Scand J Rheumatol 2001;30(5):311.

25. Cohen PR, Rapini RP. Relapsing polychondritis. Int J Dermatol 1986;25(5):280–5.

26. O'Hanlan M, McAdam LP, Bluestone R, et al. The arthropathy of relapsing polychrondritis. Arthritis Rheum 1976;19(2):191–4.

27. Cody DT, Sones DA. Relapsing polychondritis: audiovestibular manifestations. Laryngoscope 1971;81(8):1208–22.

28. Isaak BL, Liesegang TJ, Michet CJ Jr. Ocular and systemic findings in relapsing polychondritis. Ophthalmology 1986;93(5):681–9.

29. Tucker SM, Linberg JV, Doshi HM. Relapsing polychondritis, another cause for a "salmon patch". Ann Ophthalmol 1993;25(10):389–91.

30. Krell WS, Staats BA, Hyatt RE. Pulmonary function in relapsing polychondritis. Am Rev Respir Dis 1986;133(6):1120–3.

31. Mohsenifar Z, Tashkin DP, Carson SA, et al. Pulmonary function in patients with relapsing polychondritis. Chest 1982;81(6):711–7.

32. Tillie-Leblond I, Wallaert B, Leblond D, et al. Respiratory involvement in relapsing polychondritis. Clinical, functional, endoscopic, and radiographic evaluations. Medicine 1998;77(3):168–76.

33. Davis SD, Berkmen YM, King T. Peripheral bronchial involvement in relapsing polychondritis: demonstration by thin-section CT. AJR Am J Roentgenol 1989; 153(5):953–4.

34. Kent PD, Michet CJ Jr, Luthra HS. Relapsing polychondritis. Curr Opin Rheumatol 2004;16(1):56–61.

35. Rosen T, Carr P. Relapsing polychondritis. Cutis 1981;28(3):274–6, 281–2.

36. Jawad AS, Burrel M, Lim KL, et al. Erosive arthritis in relapsing polychondritis. Postgrad Med J 1990;66(779):768–70.

37. Firestein GS, Gruber HE, Weisman MH, et al. Mouth and genital ulcers with inflamed cartilage: MAGIC syndrome. Five patients with features of relapsing polychondritis and Behcet's disease. Am J Med 1985;79(1):65–72.

38. Salahuddin N, Libman BS, Lunde JH, et al. The association of relapsing polychondritis and myelodysplastic syndrome: report of three cases. J Clin Rheumatol 2000;6(3):146–9.

39. Shirota T, Hayashi O, Uchida H, et al. Myelodysplastic syndrome associated with relapsing polychondritis: unusual transformation from refractory anemia to chronic myelomonocytic leukemia. Ann Hematol 1993;67(1):45–7.
40. Barretto SN, Oliveira GH, Michet CJ Jr, et al. Multiple cardiovascular complications in a patient with relapsing polychondritis. Mayo Clin Proc 2002;77(9):971–4.
41. Del Rosso A, Petix NR, Pratesi M, et al. Cardiovascular involvement in relapsing polychondritis. Semin Arthritis Rheum 1997;26(6):840–4.
42. Lang-Lazdunski L, Hvass U, Paillole C, et al. Cardiac valve replacement in relapsing polychondritis. A review. J Heart Valve Dis 1995;4(3):227–35.
43. Giordano M, Valentini G, Sodano A. Relapsing polychondritis with aortic arch aneurysm and aortic arch syndrome. Rheumatol Int 1984;4(4):191–3.
44. Bowness P, Hawley IC, Morris T, et al. Complete heart block and severe aortic incompetence in relapsing polychondritis: clinicopathologic findings. Arthritis Rheum 1991;34(1):97–100.
45. Balsa-Criado A, Garcia-Fernandez F, Roldan I. Cardiac involvement in relapsing polychondritis. Int J Cardiol 1987;14(3):381–3.
46. Esdaile J, Hawkins D, Gold P, et al. Vascular involvement in relapsing polychondritis. Can Med Assoc J 1977;116(9):1019–22.
47. Mestres CA, Igual A, Botey A, et al. Relapsing polychondritis with glomerulonephritis and severe aortic insufficiency surgically treated with success. Thorac Cardiovasc Surg 1983;31(5):307–9.
48. Sundaram MB, Rajput AH. Nervous system complications of relapsing polychondritis. Neurology 1983;33(4):513–5.
49. Willis J, Atack EA, Kraag G. Relapsing polychondritis with multifocal neurological abnormalities. Can J Neurol Sci 1984;11(3):402–4.
50. Strobel ES, Lang B, Schumacher M, et al. Cerebral aneurysm in relapsing polychondritis. J Rheumatol 1992;19(9):1482–3.
51. Wasserfallen JB, Schaller MD. Unusual rhombencephalitis in relapsing polychondritis. Ann Rheum Dis 1992;51(10):1184.
52. Chang-Miller A, Okamura M, Torres VE, et al. Renal involvement in relapsing polychondritis. Medicine 1987;66(3):202–17.
53. Trentham DE, Le CH. Relapsing polychondritis. Ann Intern Med 1993;129(2): 114–22.
54. Damiani JM, Levine HL. Relapsing polychondritis–report of ten cases. The Laryngoscope 1979;89(6 Pt 1):929–46.
55. Papo T, Piette JC, Le Thi Huong D, et al. Antineutrophil cytoplasmic antibodies in polychondritis. Ann Rheum Dis 1993;52(5):384–5.
56. Thompson LD. Relapsing polychondritis. Ear Nose Throat J 2002;81(10):705.
57. Buckner JH, Van Landeghen M, Kwok WW, et al. Identification of type II collagen peptide 261-273-specific T cell clones in a patient with relapsing polychondritis. Arthritis Rheum 2002;46(1):238–44.
58. Zong WX, Thompson CB. Necrotic death as a cell fate. Genes Dev 2006;20(1): 1–15.
59. Hashimoto K, Arkin CR, Kang AH. Relapsing polychondritis: an ultrastructural study. Arthritis Rheum 1977;20(1):91–9.
60. Herman JH, Dennis MV. Immunopathologic studies in relapsing polychondritis. J Clin Invest 1973;52(3):549–58.
61. Lin ZQ, Xu JR, Chen JJ, et al. Pulmonary CT findings in relapsing polychondritis. Acta radiologica 2010;51(5):522–6.
62. De Geeter F, Vandecasteele SJ. Fluorodeoxyglucose PET in relapsing polychondritis. N Engl J Med 2008;358(5):536–7.

63. Sander R. Otitis externa: a practical guide to treatment and prevention. Am Fam Physician 2001;63(5):927–36, 941–2.

64. Loehrl TA, Smith TL. Inflammatory and granulomatous lesions of the larynx and pharynx. Am J Med 2001;111(Suppl 8A):113S–7S.

65. Braman SS. Diffuse tracheal narrowing with recurrent bronchopulmonary infections. Relapsing polychondritis. Chest 2003;123(1):289, 290.

66. Askari AD. Colchicine for treatment of relapsing polychondritis. J Am Acad Dermatol 1984;10(3):507–10.

67. Barranco VP, Minor DB, Soloman H. Treatment of relapsing polychondritis with dapsone. Arch Dermatol 1976;112(9):1286–8.

68. Lipnick RN, Fink CW. Acute airway obstruction in relapsing polychondritis: treatment with pulse methylprednisolone. J Rheumatol 1991;18(1):98–9.

69. Gaffney RJ, Harrison M, Blayney AW. Nebulized racemic ephedrine in the treatment of acute exacerbations of laryngeal relapsing polychondritis. J Laryngol Otol 1992;106(1):63–4.

70. Park J, Gowin KM, Schumacher HR Jr. Steroid sparing effect of methotrexate in relapsing polychondritis. J Rheumatol 1996;23(5):937–8.

71. Stewart KA, Mazanec DJ. Pulse intravenous cyclophosphamide for kidney disease in relapsing polychondritis. J Rheumatol 1992;19(3):498–500.

72. Ruhlen JL, Huston KA, Wood WG. Relapsing polychondritis with glomerulonephritis. Improvement with prednisone and cyclophosphamide. JAMA 1981; 245(8):847–8.

73. Svenson KL, Holmdahl R, Klareskog L, et al. Cyclosporin A treatment in a case of relapsing polychondritis. Scand J Rheumatol 1984;13(4):329–33.

74. van der Lubbe PA, Miltenburg AM, Breedveld FC. Anti-CD4 monoclonal antibody for relapsing polychondritis. Lancet 1991;337(8753):1349.

75. Choy EH, Chikanza IC, Kingsley GH, et al. Chimaeric anti-CD4 monoclonal antibody for relapsing polychondritis. Lancet 1991;338(8764):450.

76. Lahmer T, Knopf A, Treiber M, et al. Treatment of relapsing polychondritis with the TNF-alpha antagonist adalimumab. Clin Rheumatol 2010;29(11):1331–4.

77. Carter JD. Treatment of relapsing polychondritis with a TNF antagonist. J Rheumatol 2005;32(7):1413.

78. Saadoun D, Deslandre CJ, Allanore Y, et al. Sustained response to infliximab in 2 patients with refractory relapsing polychondritis. J Rheumatol 2003;30(6):1394–5.

79. Kawai M, Hagihara K, Hirano T, et al. Sustained response to tocilizumab, anti-interleukin-6 receptor antibody, in two patients with refractory relapsing polychondritis. Rheumatology (Oxford) 2009;48(3):318–9.

80. Adliff M, Ngato D, Keshavjee S, et al. Treatment of diffuse tracheomalacia secondary to relapsing polychondritis with continuous positive airway pressure. Chest 1997;112(6):1701–4.

81. Karaman E, Duman C, Cansz H, et al. Laryngotracheal reconstruction at relapsing polychondritis. J Craniofac Surg 2010;21(1):211–2.

82. Hojaili B, Keiser HD. Relapsing polychondritis presenting with complete heart block. J Clin Rheumatol 2008;14(1):24–6.

Extrapulmonary Manifestations of Sarcoidosis

Deepak A. Rao, MD, PhD, Paul F. Dellaripa, MD*

KEYWORDS

- Sarcoidosis • Extrapulmonary • Granulomas • Granulomatous • Löfgren syndrome
- Neurosarcoidosis

KEY POINTS

- Sarcoidosis is a systemic granulomatous disease that most commonly affects the lungs, skin, and eyes.
- All patients with sarcoidosis should be evaluated for cardiac involvement, which may lead to life-threatening arrhythmias.
- Although many patients can be monitored without treatment, those with worsening pulmonary disease or cardiac, neurologic, or vision-threatening ocular disease require prompt therapy.
- Most manifestations of sarcoidosis can be treated with corticosteroids, with the highest doses used for cardiac and neurologic involvement.
- Disease-modifying antirheumatic drugs such as methotrexate and biological therapies such as antitumor necrosis factor agents are increasingly being used for refractory disease.

INTRODUCTION

Sarcoidosis is a systemic disorder characterized by the aberrant development of granulomas within various organs in the body. The lungs are involved in 90% of patients, and the skin, eyes, and heart are affected in a significant fraction of patients. The disease remits within 3 years in most patients, whereas 10% to 30% of patients develop chronic disease requiring ongoing treatment.[1] Significant variation in disease incidence and manifestations is well recognized. The incidence rate of sarcoidosis in Northern Europe is between 5 and 40 cases per 100,000 people, compared with a rate of 1 to 2 cases per 100,000 in Japan.[2] Cardiac and ocular disease are more common in Japanese patients, whereas joint symptoms and erythema nodosum are more common in northern Europeans.[3] In the United States, the age-adjusted annual

Disclosures: The authors have no relevant conflicts of interest to disclose.
Division of Rheumatology, Brigham and Women's Hospital, 45 Francis Street, PBB-3, Boston, MA 02115, USA
* Corresponding author.
E-mail address: pdellaripa@partners.org

incidence of sarcoidosis in black patients is 35.5 per 100,000, 3 times higher than that of white patients (10.9 per 100,000).[4] Black patients are more likely to develop ocular and granulomatous skin involvement and more frequently suffer chronic, debilitating disease.[4–6]

Although there are no universal criteria for the diagnosis of sarcoidosis, a diagnosis is likely when a patient presents with signs or symptoms consistent with sarcoidosis and has granulomas shown on tissue biopsy. Most patients with sarcoidosis develop pulmonary involvement, which may be asymptomatic or may cause dyspnea, dry cough, or chest discomfort. Chest radiographs show abnormalities classified into 5 stages (Table 1). Laboratory testing may reveal an increased angiotensin-converting enzyme (ACE) level; however, this test lacks sufficient specificity to make a diagnosis of sarcoidosis. Examination of bronchoalveolar lavage fluid may help in the diagnosis, because a markedly increased ratio of CD4+ T cells to CD8+ T cells in the bronchoalveolar lavage fluid is relatively specific for sarcoidosis; however, diagnosis is generally confirmed by showing epithelioid granulomas on transbronchial biopsy.[1,7] Diagnosis of sarcoidosis also requires the exclusion of other causes of granulomatous disease, including mycobacterial infections such as tuberculosis and leprosy, fungal infections such as coccidiomycosis and histoplasmosis, syphilis, exposures to particulates such as beryllium, and granulomatosis with polyangiitis.

Extrapulmonary disease may manifest before, concurrent with, or after development of pulmonary disease, thus patients with sarcoidosis come to the attention of a range of providers depending on the location of symptoms. Awareness of the common and protean manifestations of sarcoidosis is required to recognize the disease and monitor for additional disease complications. In this article, first, the immunopathology of sarcoidosis is reviewed. The common extrapulmonary manifestations of sarcoidosis are then reviewed, and organ-specific considerations in treatment are discussed.

IMMUNOPATHOLOGY

The hallmark of sarcoidosis is the development of epithelioid granulomas. Autopsy and imaging studies suggest that granulomatous involvement can be more widespread in patients with sarcoidosis than is apparent clinically.[8–10] Granulomas in different organs tend to conform to a similar histologic pattern, consisting of a dense collection of epithelioid macrophages and CD4+ T cells, with fewer CD8+ T cells restricted to the periphery. Part of the diagnostic challenge is that similar appearing granulomas may form in response to several different stimuli, some of which must be excluded to diagnose sarcoidosis. Exposure to beryllium causes a granulomatous disease similar in appearance to sarcoidosis; however, chronic beryllium disease is generally considered a distinct entity.[1]

Table 1 Chest radiographic staging	
Stage	Radiographic Findings
Stage 0	Normal radiograph
Stage I	Bilateral hilar lymphadenopathy
Stage II	Bilateral hilar adenopathy and parenchymal infiltrates
Stage III	Parenchymal infiltrates alone
Stage IV	Pulmonary fibrosis

Hints as to the cause of sarcoidosis have been derived from observations about the localization of lesions, spatial-temporal patterns of disease, immunophenotyping, and genetics; however, a cohesive understanding of the disease remains elusive. The pattern of tissue involvement, with a predominance of symptoms in the lungs, skin, and eyes, suggests that exposure to an external trigger plays a key role in initiating the disease. One potential set of triggers is environmental particulate matter. Just as particles of beryllium clearly cause a granulomatous reaction, other types of particulate matter have also been suspected in sarcoidosis. The most comprehensive evaluation for such a trigger was ACCESS (A Case Control Etiologic Study of Sarcoidosis),[11] which evaluated exposure histories of more than 700 patients with recently diagnosed sarcoidosis. The study found no association of sarcoidosis with occupational exposure to wood dust, metal, silica, or talc but did report that occupational exposure to insecticides was associated with a modestly increased risk of sarcoidosis. The increased frequency of sarcoidosis in people exposed to dust and debris from the World Trade Center collapse further supports the association between particulates and sarcoidosis.[12]

An infectious cause of sarcoidosis has also been long suspected, in particular because certain well-characterized infections, such as tuberculosis and leprosy, also induce granulomas. Presentations of Löfgren syndrome were noted to cluster in the spring and early summer, suggesting a possible infectious agent.[13] Person-to-person transmission was suggested by observations from the Isle of Man that patients diagnosed with sarcoidosis were more likely than healthy control patients to have been previously in contact with another person with sarcoidosis.[14,15] The ACCESS study also noted a positive association between sarcoidosis and occupational exposure to areas with musty odors, which perhaps carry higher loads of bioaerosols containing molds and mycobacteria.[11,12]

The case for a mycobacterial infection underlying at least some cases of sarcoidosis is particularly strong.[16] Several reports have described isolation of mycobacterial DNA from patients with sarcoidosis, and a meta-analysis of 31 studies[17] showed that detection of mycobacterial DNA by polymerase chain reaction (PCR) has been reported in about one-quarter of patients with sarcoidosis tested, although evidence of publication bias was noted. *Propionibacterium*, *Mycoplasma*, viruses, and *Borrelia* have been implicated in some patients. Given the variety of possible exposures associated with this disease, it seems unlikely that a single trigger explains all of sarcoidosis. Rather, it is more likely that several triggers may be able to initiate a granulomatous response in a susceptible host, causing a clinical presentation of sarcoidosis.

EXTRAPULMONARY MANIFESTATIONS
Cardiac

Cardiac sarcoidosis is a leading cause of death in sarcoidosis, responsible for 13% to 25% of deaths caused by sarcoidosis in US patients with sarcoidosis, and strikingly, 58% to 85% of deaths in Japanese patients with sarcoidosis.[4,9,18] Thus, evaluation for cardiac disease in all patients with sarcoidosis is particularly important. Cardiac involvement does not correlate with the severity of pulmonary involvement and can be difficult to diagnose in the context of active pulmonary disease.[19] In the United States, about 5% of patients with sarcoidosis have clinical manifestations of cardiac sarcoidosis; however, autopsy analyses show that myocardial granulomas can be found in 20% to 30% of patients.[1,9] More severe cardiac disease correlates with an increased risk of severe arrhythmias.[9] Symptoms suggestive of conduction disease include significant palpitations, presyncope, and syncope. The presence of such symptoms increases the likelihood of cardiac sarcoidosis by 8-fold, with significant palpitations being the most informative symptom.[19] Sarcoidosis has been found as a cause of previously unexplained atrioventricular block or early pacemaker dependence.[20] Sarcoidosis may also cause a dilated cardiomyopathy, associated with typical symptoms of heart failure such as dyspnea, weight gain, and edema, and can rarely cause valvular involvement.

All patients with sarcoidosis should have an electrocardiogram as part of the initial evaluation, although electrocardiograms are an insensitive method of evaluating for cardiac sarcoidosis.[19] Electrocardiographic abnormalities may include PR prolongation, atrioventricular nodal blockade, or atrial or ventricular premature beats. Patients suspected of having conduction disease from symptoms or an abnormal electrocardiogram should also undergo Holter monitoring. Rhythm abnormalities detected by Holter monitoring increase the likelihood of finding imaging abnormalities consistent with sarcoidosis by almost 20-fold.[19] The presence of ventricular dysfunction can be evaluated by a transthoracic echocardiogram.

Imaging by cardiac magnetic resonance imaging (MRI) and positron emission tomography (PET) have facilitated detection of cardiac sarcoidosis, and the combination of clinical assessment plus imaging has been reported to show cardiac involvement in almost 40% of patients with sarcoidosis.[19] Cardiac MRI may show a pattern of late gadolinium enhancement in the basolateral area of the left ventricle, with lesions most frequently seen in the midcardial to epicardial regions, distinct from the subendocardial regions commonly affected by ischemia.[21,22] The ability of cardiac MRI to differentiate active inflammation from previous injury is not fully defined; however, serial cardiac MRI evaluation has been suggested to have usefulness in following the response of cardiac sarcoidosis to corticosteroid treatment.[23]

Nuclear imaging by PET shows focally increased uptake of the radioactive tracer ^{18}F-fluorodeoxyglucose (FDG), most often in the basal and midanteroseptal-lateral areas of the left ventricle.[24,25] This method seems more sensitive than cardiac MRI in detecting cardiac sarcoidosis, with a reported sensitivity of 89% and specificity of 78%.[26] Because FDG PET theoretically depends on the presence of inflammatory cells to take up the radiolabeled tracer, this modality may be particularly useful in monitoring disease activity.[27] Recently, high-sensitivity cardiac troponin T has also been suggested as a means of assessing the presence and activity of cardiac sarcoidosis.[28]

The presence of granulomatous disease infiltrating the myocardium may be confirmed by endocardial biopsy. However, cardiac sarcoidosis is patchy and favors areas of the left ventricle, whereas endocardial biopsies are typically taken from the right side of the interventricular septum; thus, false-negative results are common because of limitations of sampling.[29]

Cutaneous

The skin is affected in 20% to 35% of patients with sarcoidosis, and skin lesions are often present at the time of diagnosis.[30,31] Cutaneous manifestations of sarcoidosis that are caused by granulomas are referred to as specific for sarcoidosis, whereas other lesions are considered nonspecific. The most common nonspecific cutaneous manifestation is erythema nodosum, which typically manifests as painful nodules on the lower legs, usually in the setting of an acute presentation of sarcoidosis. Erythema nodosum is more common in women and northern Europeans, and is associated with a favorable overall prognosis.[6,32] Histologically, the lesions show a septal panniculitis rather than granulomas.

Specific forms of cutaneous sarcoidosis occur in many patterns, with the most common being papular, maculopapular, and plaque lesions. Papular lesions occur commonly on the face, often around the eyes, whereas maculopapular lesions tend to favor the neck and trunk (**Fig. 1**).[30] Both are associated with milder pulmonary disease and a good prognosis, whereas plaque lesions are more often associated with chronic disease requiring steroid treatment.[33] Variants of papular and plaque sarcoidosis can take on many forms, including lesions that resemble psoriasis, lichen planus, verrucae, and lupus.[30]

A unique lesion of sarcoidosis, termed lupus pernio (unrelated to systemic lupus erythematosus) causes distinctive violaceous, indurated lesions on the face, often on the nasal alae. These lesions are often disfiguring and may damage underlying soft tissue and bony structures, causing nasal ulcerations, septal perforation, and deformity.[34] Bony cysts may develop under affected areas.[35] Lupus pernio occurs more frequently in female patients and is associated with more frequent pulmonary parenchymal involvement and more aggressive systemic disease.[34,36]

Cutaneous lesions in sarcoidosis may also be precipitated by skin trauma. So-called scar sarcoidosis can occur in response to abrasions, punctures, or tattoos. Reactions to tattoos may form in response to 1 or multiple colors within a tattoo, and may develop even years after placement of the tattoo.[37] Such reactions can be the initial presentation of sarcoidosis and should prompt the investigation of systemic manifestations of sarcoidosis. Granulomas may also occur in the subcutaneous tissue below otherwise normal-appearing skin, causing painless or only mildly tender nodules.[38,39] Such nodules, which may be the presenting sign of sarcoidosis, can be evaluated by ultrasonography or MRI, and biopsy reveals granulomas within the panniculus.[38,40] Most patients with subcutaneous sarcoidosis have hilar lymphadenopathy, and many are subsequently found to have granulomas in other organs.[39,41] Recognition of skin lesions is important in sarcoidosis, because identification of the disease by skin biopsy may obviate more invasive diagnostic procedures.

Ophthalmologic

The eye is the third most frequently involved organ, affected in between 10% and 60% of patients. Granulomatous disease may cause inflammation either within the eye or in adnexal structures. Ocular involvement occurs at higher rates in women and African Americans, and seems more common in Japanese cohorts.[6,42]

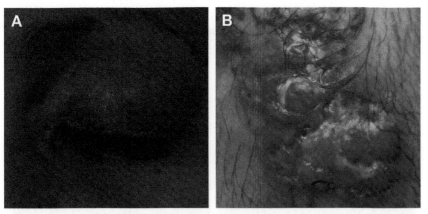

Fig. 1. Examples of cutaneous sarcoidosis. (*A*) Waxy papules over the eyelid of a patient with systemic sarcoidosis. (*B*) Granulomatous inflammation within the area of 1 color of a tattoo in a patient with systemic sarcoidosis. (*Courtesy of* Dr J. Merola, Brigham and Women's Hospital, Boston, MA.)

Uveitis is the most common ocular manifestation and can be vision-threatening; thus, all patients diagnosed with sarcoidosis should have an ophthalmologic evaluation (**Fig. 2**). Symptoms of uveitis may include tearing, photophobia, pain, and injection; however, about one-third of patients with uveitis caused by sarcoidosis have no ocular symptoms.[43] There are 2 peaks of incidence: the first in the third decade (more often associated with an acute course) and the latter in the sixth to seventh decade (more often associated with a chronic course).[43] Ocular inflammation is most often bilateral, and the anterior segment is involved in 70% to 85% of cases.[44] Involvement of the posterior segment occurs less frequently but is seen more often in whites, particularly elderly women, and is associated with a higher risk of central nervous system (CNS) involvement.[43,44] Symptoms of blurry vision, hyperopia, visual field deficits, or floaters may suggest the development of retinal vasculitis, which in sarcoidosis is usually a retinal periphlebitis, sparing the retinal arteries.[45] Uveitis occurring concomitant with fever, parotitis, and facial nerve paralysis has been termed uveoparotid fever or Heerfordt syndrome.

Ocular inflammation may be the presenting symptom of sarcoidosis; however, showing granulomatous disease in the eye is often not feasible, because biopsy is generally not pursued in patients presenting with uveitis. Biopsy of another involved site, if available, is useful. Given the frequent lack of ocular histologic evidence, an international consensus conference delineated criteria for the diagnosis of ocular sarcoidosis, which include a description of 7 clinical signs on ophthalmologic examination suggestive of ocular sarcoidosis.[42] The conference also outlined different levels of certainty regarding the diagnosis of ocular sarcoidosis based on ophthalmologic evaluation, laboratory investigation, and imaging (**Table 2**).[42]

Involvement of the orbit and adnexal structures is less common than uveitis, occurring in 8% to 27% of cases, and occurs independently of uveitis.[46] Adnexal involvement occurs in the form of lacrimal gland infiltration, formation of an orbital mass, or less commonly, involvement of the lacrimal sac. The lacrimal gland is the most commonly affected site, with an estimated incidence of 5% to 16% in sarcoidosis.[46] Patients may present with edema or erythema of the eyelid or symptoms of dry eye, which may mimic Sjögren syndrome. Progressive lacrimal gland disease may cause insufficient tear production; however, sicca symptoms do not necessarily correlate with lacrimal gland infiltration.[47,48] Occasionally, patients may present with a palpable

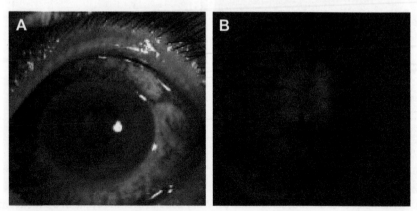

Fig. 2. Examples of ocular sarcoidosis. (*A*) Scleritis in a patient with sarcoidosis. (*B*) Optic nerve swelling on fundoscopic exam. (*Courtesy of* Dr G. Papaliodis, Massachusetts Eye and Ear Infirmary, Boston, MA.)

Table 2
Diagnosis of ocular sarcoidosis

Certainty of Ocular Sarcoidosis Diagnosis[42]	Findings
Definite	Uveitis compatible with sarcoidosis
	Biopsy of another organ supporting sarcoidosis
Presumed	Uveitis compatible with sarcoidosis
	Biopsy not performed
	Bilateral hilar adenopathy on chest imaging
Probable	3 signs of uveitis compatible with sarcoidosis
	Biopsy not performed
	2 other investigations supporting sarcoidosis:
	Chest computed tomography abnormalities
	Increased ACE or lysozyme level
	Abnormal liver enzyme tests
	Negative PPD in a BCG-vaccinated or
	previously PPD-positive patient
Possible	4 signs of uveitis compatible with sarcoidosis
	Lung biopsy negative
	2 other investigations supporting sarcoidosis:
	Chest computed tomography abnormalities
	Increased ACE or lysozyme level
	Abnormal liver enzyme tests
	Negative PPD in a BCG-vaccinated or
	previously PPD-positive patient

In all cases, alternative causes of uveitis, in particular tuberculosis, must be excluded.
Abbreviations: BCG, bacille Calmette-Guérin; PPD, purified protein derivative.

eyelid mass. A solid orbital mass may be caused by sarcoidosis; however, it is debated whether an isolated, solitary orbital granulomas should be considered sarcoidosis or a distinct entity.[47]

Neurologic

Neurologic symptoms affect an estimated 5% of patients with sarcoidosis and may also be the presenting manifestation of systemic sarcoidosis.[31,49,50] Granulomatous inflammation can affect the cranial nerves, peripheral nerves, or brain parenchyma, and autopsy studies suggest that granulomas are frequently present in these areas in the absence of symptoms.[8] Cranial nerve dysfunction is the most common neurologic manifestation. The facial nerve is the most frequently affected cranial nerve, followed by the optic and vestibulocochlear nerves, although any cranial nerve can be involved.[51]

Lesions occurring in the peripheral nervous system most often cause an axonal or sensory peripheral neuropathy, although sensory-motor and myopathic patterns are also seen.[51] Suspected peripheral nerve lesions can be confirmed by evaluation with nerve conduction studies and electromyography. Histologically, granulomas form within the epineurium or perineurinum, frequently accompanied by some component of granulomatous angiitis.[52] Involvement of the endoneurium may also occur, perhaps via inflammatory cell invasion along septae or via microvessels, which inflicts more severe injury to the nerve.[52] Peripheral nervous system involvement tends to respond to corticosteroid treatment and carries a better prognosis than does CNS involvement.[51]

Granulomatous involvement of the brain parenchyma is one of the most serious complications of sarcoidosis. However, attributing neurologic dysfunction to sarcoidosis is challenging, particularly in the absence of identifiable granulomatous disease in other organs. Symptoms of headache, nausea, and ataxia raise suspicion for cerebellar or brainstem involvement. Visual impairment, diplopia, and seizures may also occur. The base of the brain is frequently affected, often with granulomatous infiltration of the hypothalamus and pituitary, leading to dysfunction of the hypothalamic-pituitary axis.[53] Leptomeningeal involvement may yield an appearance of aseptic meningitis, and involvement of the spinal cord may result in myelopathy. Spinal cord involvement tends to occur in older patients with sarcoidosis and can be difficult to distinguish from cervical spondylosis.[54] Neuropsychiatric symptoms are uncommon.[53]

Evaluation for neurosarcoidosis typically includes a lumbar puncture and brain MRI (**Fig. 3**). Cerebral spinal fluid analysis may reveal an increased cell count with a lymphocytic pleiocytosis, increased protein levels, and oligoclonal bands. A variety of lesions can be seen on brain MRI, including enhancing parenchymal lesions, leptomeningeal thickening or enhancement, and dural involvement.[50] Periventricular white matter

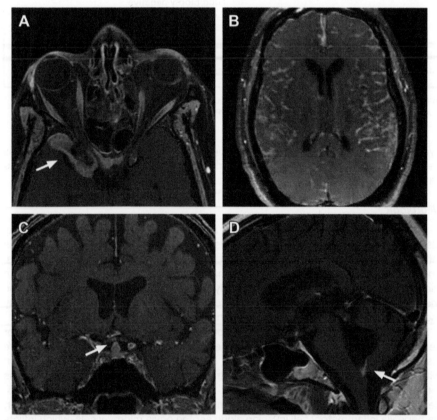

Fig. 3. Examples of neurosarcoidosis. (*A*) Orbital and dural involvement (*arrow*) on gadolinium-enhanced T1-weighted fat-saturated MRI. (*B*) Diffuse nodular meningeal lesions on gadolinium-enhanced T1-weighted fat-saturated MRI. (*C*) Involvement of the pituitary infundibulum (*arrow*) on gadolinium-enhanced T1-weighted fat-saturated MRI. (*D*) Involvement of the foramen of Magendie (*arrow*) causing hydrocephalus. (*Courtesy of* Dr K. Talekar, Thomas Jefferson University Hospital, Philadelphia, PA.)

lesions may be easily mistaken for lesions from multiple sclerosis.[55] A set of diagnostic criteria has been proposed to help classify patients as having definite, probable, or possible neurosarcoidosis (**Table 3**).[49,56]

Musculoskeletal

Sarcoidosis may involve joints, muscles, and bones, causing a variety of musculoskeletal complaints through different mechanisms. Arthritic syndromes in sarcoidosis can be categorized as acute or chronic. Acute sarcoid arthritis often occurs concomitant with bilateral hilar lymphadenopathy and erythema nodosum, a constellation termed Löfgren syndrome. In Löfgren syndrome, the ankles are most commonly affected, followed by the knees, wrists, elbows, wrists, and metacarpophalangeal joints.[57] Ultrasonographic evaluations have shown that swelling usually occurs in the soft tissue around joints, causing a periarthritis rather than a true arthritis.[58] Joint symptoms tend to precede or occur concomitantly with development of erythema nodosum, and even in the absence of erythema nodosum, the combination of hilar lymphadenopathy and ankle periarthritis can be considered a variant of Löfgren syndrome.[57,59] In a cohort of patients in the Netherlands, the presence of at least 3 of 4 criteria (symmetric ankle symptoms, age younger than 40 years, erythema nodosum, and symptoms of less than 2 months) had a 93% sensitivity and 99% specificity for the diagnosis of acute sarcoid arthritis.[60] Enthesitis also occurred in about one-third of patients with sarcoidosis in this cohort, mainly at the Achilles tendon and heels.[60] Soft tissue swelling at the ankles can be prominent, and biopsy of this soft tissue reveals a panniculitis similar to erythema nodosum, rather than granulomas.[61,62] Löfgren syndrome carries an excellent prognosis. Symptoms typically resolve without therapy, and joint destruction does not occur; however, a small subset of patients continue to experience arthralgias after the acute inflammatory state has resolved.[57]

In contrast to acute arthritis, chronic arthritis in sarcoidosis usually occurs in the setting of more diffuse organ involvement.[63] Ankles, knees, wrists, elbows, and hands

Table 3
Diagnosis of neurosarcoidosis

Certainty of Neurosarcoidosis Diagnosis[49]	Findings
Definite	Presentation suggestive of neurosarcoidosis Nervous system histology with granulomatous disease

Probable	Presentation suggestive of neurosarcoidosis
	One abnormality indicating CNS inflammation:
	  Increased CSF protein or cells
	  CSF oligoclonal bands
	  MRI findings consistent with sarcoidosis
	Either biopsy of another organ supporting sarcoidosis or 2 of the following[a]:
	  Increased ACE level
	  Abnormal chest imaging
	  Abnormal gallium scan

Possible	Presentation suggestive of neurosarcoidosis Criteria for probable neurosarcoidosis not met

In all cases, alternative diagnoses must be excluded.
Abbreviation: CSF, cerebrospinal fluid.
[a] Modifications have more recently been proposed to exclude the ACE level criterion and to include an increased CD4/CD8 T-cell ratio >3.5 in bronchoalveolar fluid or >5 in CSF.[56]

may all be affected, often in a polyarticular pattern.[63,64] Synovial fluid is usually noninflammatory or only mildly inflammatory, with a predominantly mononuclear infiltrate.[65] When obtained, synovial biopsies may show synovial granulomas or nonspecific mononuclear infiltrates and synovial hypertrophy.[65,66] Dactylitis similar to that seen in psoriatic arthritis, associated with pain, swelling, overlying skin erythema, and underlying bony changes may also occur.[67] Rarely, Jaccoud arthropathy, a nonerosive deformity, develops.[68,69]

Bony lesions of osseous sarcoidosis occur in 3% to 13% of patients with sarcoidosis.[31,70] The hands and feet are the most frequent sites of involvement, whereas the spine is less commonly affected (**Fig. 4**).[71,72] Only about half of patients with bony lesions have pain and stiffness, whereas the other half remain asymptomatic.[71] Radiographically, bone manifestations follow 3 distinct patterns, namely, lytic, permeative, and destructive. A lytic pattern results from focal areas of imbalanced bone destruction and bone formation, resulting in net bone resorption and cyst formation. Bone cysts are often associated with overlying skin disease, either on the hands and feet, for example associated with dactylitis, or on the face underlying skin lesions of lupus pernio.[34,67,73] The second pattern, termed permeative, results in a tunneled, reticular appearance of the cortex. The third pattern, termed destructive, is uncommon and causes severe bone damage and fractures. In some cases, MRI may be more sensitive in detecting bony lesions; however, sarcoidosis lesions on MRI can be difficult to distinguish from bony metastasis.[74]

Sarcoid myopathy occurs clinically in less than 5% of patients; however, granulomatous involvement of muscle can be found histologically in most patients with sarcoidosis.[75] Muscle involvement occurs in 3 general forms: acute myopathy, chronic myopathy, and nodular myopathy. Chronic myopathy, the most common form of sarcoid myopathy, typically causes symmetric proximal weakness. Creatine kinase levels are often normal but can be markedly increased.[76] Electromyography shows a myopathic pattern with abnormal spontaneous activity with fibrillation potentials.[76] MRI of affected muscles shows nonspecific muscle edema or fatty atrophy and is unlikely to indicate a specific diagnosis; however, such imaging may guide muscle biopsy site selection to avoid sampling atrophic areas.[77]

Additional imaging with radionucleotide scanning can be useful in sarcoidosis.[67] Gallium scanning has been reported to identify extensive areas of granulomatous muscle infiltration in the absence of significant musculoskeletal symptoms.[10] PET scanning has also been suggested to have usefulness in identifying muscle inflammation and in monitoring response to therapy.[78,79] Histologically, granulomas in sarcoid myopathies show a pattern similar to that seen in other organs, with collections of macrophages and activated CD4+ T cells throughout the granulomas.[80] In contrast to patterns seen in polymyositis, CD4+ cells outnumber CD8+ cells in sarcoid myopathy, and muscle fibers do not express increased levels of major histocompatibility complex class I.[80]

Nodular myopathy is an uncommon form of sarcoid myopathy characterized by the accumulation of large granulomas and dense connective tissue into nodules. These lesions, which can resemble tumors, may be painful but rarely cause weakness. On MRI, nodules are long and display a distinctive pattern on T2-weighted axial images of a dark, star-shaped lesion surrounded by a bright rim.[81]

Acute myopathy is the least common form of sarcoid myopathy. It presents with a rapid onset of proximal weakness and myalgias over several weeks, often associated with fever. The presentation may appear similar to polymyositis, with serum creatine kinase levels usually, although variably, increased.[82] Biopsy of acute sarcoid myopathy shows pronounced lymphocytic infiltration associated with granulomas.[82]

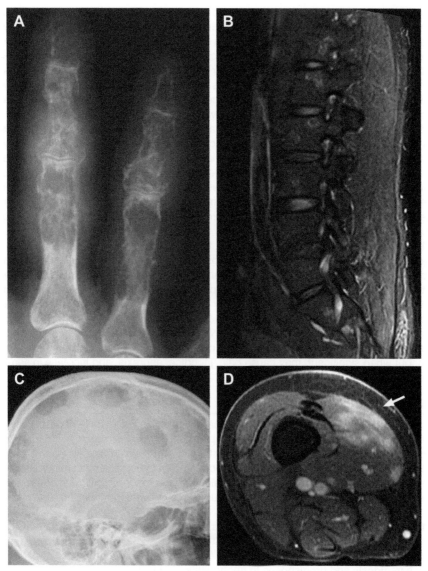

Fig. 4. Examples of musculoskeletal involvement in sarcoidosis. (*A*) Punched-out cortical lesions and coarsened trabeculae yield a characteristic lacelike pattern in the proximal, middle, and distal phalanges. (*B*) Focal targetlike lesions in the vertebral bodies seen on sagittal short-tau inversion recovery sequence MRI. (*C*) Multiple large, lytic lesions within the skull of a patient with sarcoidosis. (*D*) Lobular lesions (*arrow*) within the vastus medialis muscle on gadolinium-enhanced MRI. (*Courtesy of* [*A, C, D*] Dr S. Smith, Brigham and Women's Hospital, Boston, MA; and [*B*] Dr K. Talekar, Thomas Jefferson University Hospital, Philadelphia, PA.)

Gastrointestinal

Sarcoidosis frequently involves the liver; however, a variety of insults may induce liver granulomas; thus, it is important to distinguish granulomas caused by sarcoidosis from those with other causes. Generally, granulomatous disease in a second organ, plus exclusion of alternate causes, is needed to consider a patient with liver granulomas to have sarcoidosis.[83] Based on observations from autopsies and liver biopsies, granulomas within the liver can be found in 50% to 80% of patients with sarcoidosis, although the fraction of patients with clinically evident liver disease is smaller.[83] As with the eye, skin, and bone marrow, liver involvement is more common in African American patients than whites.[6] Symptoms from liver involvement include abdominal pain, pruritus, and less commonly, jaundice and ascites.[83] Increase in liver enzyme tests occur in about one-third of patients with sarcoidosis.[84]

Sarcoidosis may cause biliary disease and cholestasis via several mechanisms. Pathologic patterns resembling either sclerosing cholangitis or biliary cirrhosis have been described. Chronic damage may result in ductopenia, or loss of small biliary ducts, and once this stage is reached, treatment is unlikely to improve function. Granulomatous disease rarely progresses to cirrhosis; however, portal hypertension may still occur caused by granulomatous obstruction of blood flow through the portal circulation, or through development of portal vein thrombosis or Budd-Chiari syndrome.[83,85]

It is uncommon for sarcoidosis to affect the luminal gastrointestinal tract. When it occurs, the gastric antrum is the area most frequently affected.[83] Symptoms may include abdominal pain, nausea, early satiety, and progressive weight loss. Even without involvement of the gut wall, symptoms of obstruction may be caused by external compression of the gut lumen by enlarged lymph nodes or adjacent large granulomas.[83] Granulomas of sarcoidosis can be found within the pancreas in approximately 5% of patients with sarcoidosis.[86] Nodular lesions may infiltrate the pancreas diffusely or cause a mass in the head of the pancreas. The lesions are rarely symptomatic, but when significant, may cause pain, jaundice, anorexia, and increase in serum lipase levels.

Renal

Granulomatous involvement of the kidney can be found in 7% to 23% of patients with sarcoidosis; however, significant renal impairment is less common.[86,87] The most common lesion is a granulomatous interstitial nephritis, which usually occurs in the setting of more diffuse disease and is associated with hypercalcemia and hypergammaglobulinemia.[88,89] Sterile pyuria, proteinuria, and microscopic hematuria may occur.[87] Rarely, a granulomatous pseudotumor may develop, mimicking malignancy in 1 or both kidneys.[90]

Hypercalcemia is common in sarcoidosis, occurring in 10% to 20% of patients, as a result of excess conversion of 25(OH) vitamin D to 1,25(OH) vitamin D by macrophage 1-α-hydroxylase within granulomas.[91] Hypercalciuria occurs in half of patients with sarcoidosis and predisposes to nephrolithiasis, which develops in about 10% to 15% of patients.[87,89] Symptomatic nephrolithiasis may be the initial indication of systemic sarcoidosis in approximately 1% of sarcoidosis cases.[92]

TREATMENT
General Principles

It is important to recognize that not all patients with sarcoidosis require immunosuppressive treatment. Patients with acute presentations of Löfgren syndrome usually remit spontaneously and require only symptomatic therapy with nonsteroidal antiinflammatory drugs (NSAIDs). Patients with stable pulmonary function without symptoms and limited disease elsewhere, including an absence of cardiac, neurologic, and vision-threatening ocular involvement, may be monitored closely without therapy and often maintain a stable course.[93] On the other hand, patients with progressive pulmonary disease or cardiac, neurologic, or ocular involvement require prompt treatment. The mainstay of treatment of sarcoidosis is glucocorticoid therapy. Steroids can be used to treat virtually all manifestations of sarcoidosis; however, it is not clear that corticosteroid treatment has any beneficial effect on long-term disease outcomes.[94] Higher doses are used for neurologic and cardiac involvement, whereas lower doses usually suffice for other affected organs. Efforts should be made to minimize the potential complications of glucocorticoids by using the lowest effective dose, using local therapy when possible, and promptly initiating adjunctive therapies to prevent glucocorticoid-induced bone loss and opportunistic infections.

In cases in which the steroid dose cannot be tapered without disease recurrence, or when steroid therapy is not tolerated, steroid-sparing agents should be considered. Methotrexate has been frequently used in these situations and can be effective in both pulmonary and extrapulmonary disease.[95] Antimalarial agents such as chloroquine and hydroxychloroquine are also effective, particularly for cutaneous disease and hypercalcemia.[96] Use of immunosuppressive agents such as azathioprine, mycophenolate mofetil, and cyclophosphamide has also been described, although controlled trials are lacking. Given the importance of tumor necrosis factor (TNF) in granuloma formation, anti-TNF agents are increasingly being used to treat sarcoidosis.[97,98] The anti-TNF antibodies infliximab and adalimumab seem to be more effective than the soluble receptor etanercept.[99] However, reports of sarcoidosislike granulomatous reactions in patients treated with anti-TNF therapies for other indications have prompted heightened caution with this approach.[97,100] Recently, attention has also focused on the role of rituximab in treating sarcoidosis, with reports of efficacy in both ocular sarcoidosis and neurosarcoidosis.[101,102] In the following sections, some of the organ-specific considerations of sarcoidosis treatment are discussed.

Pulmonary

Patients with little or no change in respiratory symptoms and pulmonary function tests over the preceding 3 months can be monitored closely without corticosteroid treatment.[93] Patients with progressive disease based on symptoms, lung function tests, or radiography should be treated with systemic cortico steroids, usually in the range of 0.5 to 1 mg/kg of prednisone, tapered slowly over the course of a year. Inhaled corticosteroids have not been shown to reduce pulmonary disease but may help reduce cough and symptoms of airway hyperresponsiveness.[94,103]

Cardiac

Higher doses of corticosteroids, often in the range of 1 to 1.5 mg/kg of prednisone, are used to suppress cardiac inflammation and fibrosis, with the goal of limiting damage to the conduction system, reducing arrhythmias, and preventing the development of systolic dysfunction. Steroids are tapered slowly, and relapse once off steroids is not uncommon.[104] Optimal strategies for monitoring disease activity while tapering steroids have not been established, although serial evaluation by PET and monitoring of circulating cardiac troponin T have been proposed.[27,28] High-grade conduction system disease or complete heart block necessitates permanent pacemaker implantation. Placement of an implantable cardioverter-defibrillator (ICD) should be pursued in patients with sustained ventricular tachycardia or ventricular fibrillation and those who meet other standard criteria.[105] ICD implantation can also be considered in patients with cardiac sarcoidosis and evidence of active disease on cardiac imaging, although there is no consensus on this issue.[104] Symptoms of heart failure are managed with ACE inhibitors, β-blockers, and diuretics as with other causes of dilated cardiomyopathies. Cardiac transplantation is rarely necessary; however, when performed, transplants performed for cardiac sarcoidosis fare as well if not better than those performed for most other indications.[106]

Neurologic

Parenchymal brain disease also requires higher-dose corticosteroids, usually in the range of 1 to 1.5 mg/kg. Severe or rapidly progressive symptoms are treated initially with pulse-dose intravenous solumedrol in the range of 1 g per day for 3 days, followed by oral prednisone. Some have recommended continued weekly pulse-dose solumedrol for several weeks until symptoms are controlled.[49] Close monitoring of symptoms and serial evaluation of MRI abnormalities are monitored during steroid tapering. Multiple steroid-sparing agents have been used, with methotrexate and hydroxychloroquine being the most common.[49] Experiences with azathioprine, cyclophosphamide, cyclosporine, and mycophenolate mofetil have also been described, although controlled data are lacking. Anti-TNF therapy with infliximab has been reported to have efficacy in multiple case reports and small case series.[97] Patients with neurosarcoidosis should be monitored frequently for signs of hypothalamic-pituitary dysfunction and treated with hormone replacement as needed. Development of hydrocephalus may require placement of a ventriculoperitoneal shunt, although this carries an increased risk of CNS infection, in particular in immunosuppressed patients.[53] Cranial nerve disease and aseptic meningitis can be treated with less aggressive corticosteroid doses, often in the range of 0.5 to 1 mg/kg.[51]

Cutaneous

Treatment of cutaneous lesions is aimed at limiting disfigurement. Initial management is usually attempted with topical corticosteroids. Lesions on the trunk and extremities can be treated with high-potency topical corticosteroids with occlusion, whereas medium-potency corticosteroids are preferred on the face to reduce the risk of atrophy. However, facial lupus pernio lesions are particularly resistant to treatment and often require high-potency treatments. Lesions that do not respond to topical therapy can be treated with intralesional corticosteroids. For diffuse disease or lesions not responding to local therapies, systemic therapies are initiated. Recently, an algorithm has been described that suggests trying the steroid-sparing agents hydroxychloroquine, methotrexate, or tetracycline antibiotics first for mild to moderate disease, then moving to systemic corticosteroids, followed by combination therapy.[30] On the other hand, for severe disease, corticosteroids plus a steroid-sparing agent, such as methotrexate, hydroxychloroquine, or mycophenolate mofetil, are tried first, followed by an anti-TNF for treatment failures. For lupus pernio, retrospective analyses suggest that anti-TNF antibodies are more effective than corticosteroids; therefore, accelerated use of anti-TNF antibodies has been suggested if lupus pernio does not respond to corticosteroids.[30,107] Other agents that have been described include thalidomide, isotretinoin, allopurinol, and photodynamic therapy.

Ophthalmologic

Anterior uveitis is often treated first with topical corticosteroid eye drops. Cycloplegic agents are used in parallel to prevent formation of synechiae. Patients who do not respond to topical steroids may be treated with systemic steroids, usually at doses of 1 to 1.5 mg/kg of prednisone. Uveitis in the posterior compartment generally requires systemic therapy, given the increased risk of CNS involvement.[108] Optic neuritis also merits treatment with systemic corticosteroids. For chronic or refractory uveitis, several steroid-sparing agents can be considered, although there are few published data to support their efficacy.[99] Methotrexate has been reported to be an effective steroid-sparing agent in panuveitis.[109] Mycophenolate mofetil, azathioprine, cyclosporine, and anti-TNF therapies are also used.[99,110] Recently, rituximab was reported to improve granulomatous eye disease in 3 of 4 patients with ocular sarcoidosis.[102] Granulomatous disease in the lacrimal gland or orbit usually responds to systemic corticosteroids.

Musculoskeletal

Acute sarcoid arthritis can be treated symptomatically with high-dose NSAIDs alone and does not require corticosteroids. If control is inadequate, low-dose corticosteroids in the range of 10 to 20 mg per day of prednisone are often effective.[99] In a randomized clinical trial, methotrexate was shown to be effective in reducing musculoskeletal symptoms in acute sarcoidosis.[111] Although controlled data are lacking, methotrexate seems helpful in chronic arthritis as well.[112] Additional options include hydroxychloroquine, azathioprine, sulfasalazine, and biological therapies. Recently, an algorithmic approach to management of sarcoid arthritis incorporating these agents has been proposed.[112]

Gastrointestinal

Treatment of granulomatous liver disease in sarcoidosis is of uncertain usefulness, because corticosteroid treatment has not been clearly shown to improve abnormal liver enzyme tests.[85] Corticosteroids may be tried for symptomatic liver disease with intermediate doses in the range of 0.5 to 1 mg/kg, tapered slowly over the course of a year. Treatment with ursodeoxycholic acid, a naturally occurring bile acid, has been suggested to reduce symptoms and biochemical abnormalities of cholestasis in patients with hepatic sarcoidosis.[113–115]

Renal

All patients with sarcoidosis with hypercalcemia should be cautioned to limit dietary calcium, avoid vitamin D supplementation and sun exposure, and limit oxalate intake to reduce the risk of kidney stone formation.[87] Hypercalcemia usually requires corticosteroids, which can lower serum calcium within a few days.[99,116] Hydroxychloroquine can also be particularly effective in treating hypercalcemia.[117–119] Patients treated with hydroxychloroquine should undergo routine ophthalmologic evaluation monitoring for the accumulation of retinal deposits, although the risk is low with less than 5 years of therapy.[120,121] Persistent hypercalcemia can be treated with ketoconazole, which inhibits macrophage 1 α-hydroxylase, the enzyme that converts 25(OH) vitamin D to calcitriol in sarcoidosis granulomas.[87,122] Granulomatous interstitial nephritis tends to respond to corticosteroid therapy in the range of 1 mg/kg.[87,123]

SUMMARY

Granulomatous infiltration in systemic sarcoidosis may cause dysfunction in almost any organ; however, decades of observations have helped define the more common manifestations of sarcoidosis in various organs. An understanding of the typical patterns of involvement is critical for early detection and treatment of disease. Sarcoidosis is characteristically responsive to corticosteroids, which remain the mainstay of therapy. Disease-modifying antiinflammatory drugs, including anti-TNF agents, play an increasing role in managing refractory disease; however, further studies are required to clarify the roles of these agents in the treatment of systemic sarcoidosis.

ACKNOWLEDGMENTS

We thank Dr Joseph Merola and Dr Rebecca Hunter for helpful discussions and critical review of parts of the article. We are grateful to Dr Joseph Merola, Dr George Papaliodis, Dr Stacy Smith, and Dr Kiran Talekar for generous image contributions.

REFERENCES

1. Statement on sarcoidosis. Joint Statement of the American Thoracic Society (ATS), the European Respiratory Society (ERS) and the World Association of Sarcoidosis and Other Granulomatous Disorders (WASOG) adopted by the ATS Board of Directors and by the ERS Executive Committee, February 1999. Am J Respir Crit Care Med 1999;160:736–55.
2. Iannuzzi MC, Rybicki BA, Teirstein AS. Sarcoidosis. N Engl J Med 2007;357: 2153–65.
3. Pietinalho A, Hiraga Y, Hosoda Y, et al. The frequency of sarcoidosis in Finland and Hokkaido, Japan. A comparative epidemiological study. Sarcoidosis 1995; 12:61–7.
4. Rybicki BA, Major M, Popovich J Jr, et al. Racial differences in sarcoidosis incidence: a 5-year study in a health maintenance organization. Am J Epidemiol 1997;145:234–41.
5. Iannuzzi MC, Rybicki BA. Genetics of sarcoidosis: candidate genes and genome scans. Proc Am Thorac Soc 2007;4:108–16.
6. Baughman RP, Teirstein AS, Judson MA, et al. Clinical characteristics of patients in a case control study of sarcoidosis. Am J Respir Crit Care Med 2001;164:1885–9.
7. Costabel U. CD4/CD8 ratios in bronchoalveolar lavage fluid: of value for diagnosing sarcoidosis? Eur Respir J 1997;10:2699–700.
8. Manz HJ. Pathobiology of neurosarcoidosis and clinicopathologic correlation. Can J Neurol Sci 1983;10:50–5.
9. Silverman KJ, Hutchins GM, Bulkley BH. Cardiac sarcoid: a clinicopathologic study of 84 unselected patients with systemic sarcoidosis. Circulation 1978;58: 1204–11.
10. Suehiro S, Shiokawa S, Taniguchi S, et al. Gallium-67 scintigraphy in the diagnosis and management of chronic sarcoid myopathy. Clin Rheumatol 2003;22: 146–8.
11. Newman LS, Rose CS, Bresnitz EA, et al. A case control etiologic study of sarcoidosis: environmental and occupational risk factors. Am J Respir Crit Care Med 2004;170:1324–30.
12. Newman KL, Newman LS. Occupational causes of sarcoidosis. Curr Opin Allergy Clin Immunol 2012;12:145–50.
13. Badrinas F, Morera J, Fite E, et al. Seasonal clustering of sarcoidosis. Lancet 1989;2:455–6.
14. Hills SE, Parkes SA, Baker SB. Epidemiology of sarcoidosis in the Isle of Man–2: evidence for space-time clustering. Thorax 1987;42:427–30.
15. Parkes SA, Baker SB, Bourdillon RE, et al. Epidemiology of sarcoidosis in the Isle of Man–1: a case controlled study. Thorax 1987;42:420–6.
16. Brownell I, Ramirez-Valle F, Sanchez M, et al. Evidence for mycobacteria in sarcoidosis. Am J Respir Cell Mol Biol 2011;45:899–905.
17. Gupta D, Agarwal R, Aggarwal AN, et al. Molecular evidence for the role of mycobacteria in sarcoidosis: a meta-analysis. Eur Respir J 2007;30: 508–16.

18. Iwai K, Sekiguti M, Hosoda Y, et al. Racial difference in cardiac sarcoidosis incidence observed at autopsy. Sarcoidosis 1994;11:26–31.
19. Mehta D, Lubitz SA, Frankel Z, et al. Cardiac involvement in patients with sarcoidosis: diagnostic and prognostic value of outpatient testing. Chest 2008;133: 1426–35.
20. Kandolin R, Lehtonen J, Kupari M. Cardiac sarcoidosis and giant cell myocarditis as causes of atrioventricular block in young and middle-aged adults. Circ Arrhythm Electrophysiol 2011;4:303–9.
21. Smedema JP, Snoep G, van Kroonenburgh MP, et al. Evaluation of the accuracy of gadolinium-enhanced cardiovascular magnetic resonance in the diagnosis of cardiac sarcoidosis. J Am Coll Cardiol 2005;45:1683–90.
22. Matoh F, Satoh H, Shiraki K, et al. The usefulness of delayed enhancement magnetic resonance imaging for diagnosis and evaluation of cardiac function in patients with cardiac sarcoidosis. J Cardiol 2008;51:179–88.
23. Bussinguer M, Danielian A, Sharma OP. Cardiac sarcoidosis: diagnosis and management. Curr Treat Options Cardiovasc Med 2012;14:652–64.
24. Ishimaru S, Tsujino I, Takei T, et al. Focal uptake on 18F-fluoro-2-deoxyglucose positron emission tomography images indicates cardiac involvement of sarcoidosis. Eur Heart J 2005;26:1538–43.
25. Yamagishi H, Shirai N, Takagi M, et al. Identification of cardiac sarcoidosis with (13)N-NH(3)/(18)F-FDG PET. J Nucl Med 2003;44:1030–6.
26. Youssef G, Leung E, Mylonas I, et al. The use of 18F-FDG PET in the diagnosis of cardiac sarcoidosis: a systematic review and metaanalysis including the Ontario experience. J Nucl Med 2012;53:241–8.
27. Keijsers RG, Heuvel DA, Grutters JC. Imaging the inflammatory activity of sarcoidosis. Eur Respir J 2012. [Epub ahead of print].
28. Baba Y, Kubo T, Kitaoka H, et al. Usefulness of high-sensitive cardiac troponin T for evaluating the activity of cardiac sarcoidosis. Int Heart J 2012;53:287–92.
29. Uemura A, Morimoto S, Hiramitsu S, et al. Histologic diagnostic rate of cardiac sarcoidosis: evaluation of endomyocardial biopsies. Am Heart J 1999;138: 299–302.
30. Haimovic A, Sanchez M, Judson MA, et al. Sarcoidosis: a comprehensive review and update for the dermatologist: part I. Cutaneous disease. J Am Acad Dermatol 2012;66:699.e1–e18 [quiz: 717–8].
31. Siltzbach LE, James DG, Neville E, et al. Course and prognosis of sarcoidosis around the world. Am J Med 1974;57:847–52.
32. Honeybourne D. Ethnic differences in the clinical features of sarcoidosis in South-East London. Br J Dis Chest 1980;74:63–9.
33. Marcoval J, Mana J, Rubio M. Specific cutaneous lesions in patients with systemic sarcoidosis: relationship to severity and chronicity of disease. Clin Exp Dermatol 2011;36:739–44.
34. Spiteri MA, Matthey F, Gordon T, et al. Lupus pernio: a clinico-radiological study of thirty-five cases. Br J Dermatol 1985;112:315–22.
35. Marchell RM, Judson MA. Chronic cutaneous lesions of sarcoidosis. Clin Dermatol 2007;25:295–302.
36. Yanardag H, Pamuk ON, Pamuk GE. Lupus pernio in sarcoidosis: clinical features and treatment outcomes of 14 patients. J Clin Rheumatol 2003;9:72–6.
37. Antonovich DD, Callen JP. Development of sarcoidosis in cosmetic tattoos. Arch Dermatol 2005;141:869–72.
38. Vainsencher D, Winkelmann RK. Subcutaneous sarcoidosis. Arch Dermatol 1984;120:1028–31.

39. Ahmed I, Harshad SR. Subcutaneous sarcoidosis: is it a specific subset of cutaneous sarcoidosis frequently associated with systemic disease? J Am Acad Dermatol 2006;54:55–60.

40. Chen HH, Chen YM, Lan HH, et al. Sonographic appearance of subcutaneous sarcoidosis. J Ultrasound Med 2009;28:813–6.

41. Dalle Vedove C, Colato C, Girolomoni G. Subcutaneous sarcoidosis: report of two cases and review of the literature. Clin Rheumatol 2011;30:1123–8.

42. Herbort CP, Rao NA, Mochizuki M. International criteria for the diagnosis of ocular sarcoidosis: results of the first International Workshop on Ocular Sarcoidosis (IWOS). Ocul Immunol Inflamm 2009;17:160–9.

43. Rothova A. Ocular involvement in sarcoidosis. Br J Ophthalmol 2000;84:110–6.

44. Obenauf CD, Shaw HE, Sydnor CF, et al. Sarcoidosis and its ophthalmic manifestations. Am J Ophthalmol 1978;86:648–55.

45. Androudi S, Dastiridou A, Symeonidis C, et al. Retinal vasculitis in rheumatic diseases: an unseen burden. Clin Rheumatol 2013;32(1):7–13.

46. Demirci H, Christianson MD. Orbital and adnexal involvement in sarcoidosis: analysis of clinical features and systemic disease in 30 cases. Am J Ophthalmol 2011;151:1074–1080.e1.

47. Prabhakaran VC, Saeed P, Esmaeli B, et al. Orbital and adnexal sarcoidosis. Arch Ophthalmol 2007;125:1657–62.

48. Evans M, Sharma O, LaBree L, et al. Differences in clinical findings between Caucasians and African Americans with biopsy-proven sarcoidosis. Ophthalmology 2007;114:325–33.

49. Zajicek JP, Scolding NJ, Foster O, et al. Central nervous system sarcoidosis–diagnosis and management. QJM 1999;92:103–17.

50. Shah R, Roberson GH, Cure JK. Correlation of MR imaging findings and clinical manifestations in neurosarcoidosis. AJNR Am J Neuroradiol 2009;30:953–61.

51. Gascon-Bayarri J, Mana J, Martinez-Yelamos S, et al. Neurosarcoidosis: report of 30 cases and a literature survey. Eur J Intern Med 2011;22:e125–32.

52. Said G, Lacroix C, Plante-Bordeneuve V, et al. Nerve granulomas and vasculitis in sarcoid peripheral neuropathy: a clinicopathological study of 11 patients. Brain 2002;125:264–75.

53. Joseph FG, Scolding NJ. Neurosarcoidosis: a study of 30 new cases. J Neurol Neurosurg Psychiatry 2009;80:297–304.

54. Sakushima K, Yabe I, Nakano F, et al. Clinical features of spinal cord sarcoidosis: analysis of 17 neurosarcoidosis patients. J Neurol 2011;258:2163–7.

55. Scott TF, Yandora K, Kunschner LJ, et al. Neurosarcoidosis mimicry of multiple sclerosis: clinical, laboratory, and imaging characteristics. Neurologist 2010;16:386–9.

56. Marangoni S, Argentiero V, Tavolato B. Neurosarcoidosis. Clinical description of 7 cases with a proposal for a new diagnostic strategy. J Neurol 2006;253:488–95.

57. Gran JT, Bohmer E. Acute sarcoid arthritis: a favourable outcome? A retrospective survey of 49 patients with review of the literature. Scand J Rheumatol 1996;25:70–3.

58. Kellner H, Spathling S, Herzer P. Ultrasound findings in Lofgren's syndrome: is ankle swelling caused by arthritis, tenosynovitis or periarthritis? J Rheumatol 1992;19:38–41.

59. Mana J, Gomez-Vaquero C, Salazar A, et al. Periarticular ankle sarcoidosis: a variant of Lofgren's syndrome. J Rheumatol 1996;23:874–7.

60. Visser H, Vos K, Zanelli E, et al. Sarcoid arthritis: clinical characteristics, diagnostic aspects, and risk factors. Ann Rheum Dis 2002;61:499–504.
61. Grunewald J, Eklund A. Sex-specific manifestations of Lofgren's syndrome. Am J Respir Crit Care Med 2007;175:40–4.
62. Chatham W. Rheumatic manifestations of systemic disease: sarcoidosis. Curr Opin Rheumatol 2010;22:85–90.
63. Pettersson T. Rheumatic features of sarcoidosis. Curr Opin Rheumatol 1997;9: 62–7.
64. Abril A, Cohen MD. Rheumatologic manifestations of sarcoidosis. Curr Opin Rheumatol 2004;16:51–5.
65. Palmer DG, Schumacher HR. Synovitis with non-specific histological changes in synovium in chronic sarcoidosis. Ann Rheum Dis 1984;43:778–82.
66. Sokoloff L, Bunim JJ. Clinical and pathological studies of joint involvement in sarcoidosis. N Engl J Med 1959;260:841–7.
67. Pitt P, Hamilton EB, Innes EH, et al. Sarcoid dactylitis. Ann Rheum Dis 1983;42: 634–9.
68. Lima I, Ribeiro DS, Cesare A, et al. Typical Jaccoud's arthropathy in a patient with sarcoidosis. Rheumatol Int 2011. [Epub ahead of print].
69. Sukenik S, Hendler N, Yerushalmi B, et al. Jaccoud's-type arthropathy: an association with sarcoidosis. J Rheumatol 1991;18:915–7.
70. Wilcox A, Bharadwaj P, Sharma OP. Bone sarcoidosis. Curr Opin Rheumatol 2000;12:321–30.
71. Neville E, Carstairs LS, James DG. Sarcoidosis of bone. Q J Med 1977;46: 215–27.
72. Boyaci B, Hornicek F, Rosenthal D, et al. Sarcoidosis of the spine: a report of five cases and a review of the literature. J Bone Joint Surg Am 2012;94:e42.
73. Shorr AF, Murphy FT, Gilliland WR, et al. Osseous disease in patients with pulmonary sarcoidosis and musculoskeletal symptoms. Respir Med 2000;94:228–32.
74. Moore SL, Kransdorf MJ, Schweitzer ME, et al. Can sarcoidosis and metastatic bone lesions be reliably differentiated on routine MRI? AJR Am J Roentgenol 2012;198:1387–93.
75. Silverstein A, Siltzbach LE. Muscle involvement in sarcoidosis. Asymptomatic, myositis, and myopathy. Arch Neurol 1969;21:235–41.
76. Le Roux K, Streichenberger N, Vial C, et al. Granulomatous myositis: a clinical study of thirteen cases. Muscle Nerve 2007;35:171–7.
77. Moore SL, Teirstein A, Golimbu C. MRI of sarcoidosis patients with musculoskeletal symptoms. AJR Am J Roentgenol 2005;185:154–9.
78. Marie I, Lahaxe L, Vera P, et al. Follow-up of muscular sarcoidosis using fluorodeoxyglucose positron emission tomography. QJM 2010;103:1000–2.
79. Marie I, Levesque H, Manrique A, et al. Positron emission tomography in the diagnosis of muscular sarcoidosis. Am J Med 2007;120:e1–2.
80. Tews DS, Pongratz DE. Immunohistological analysis of sarcoid myopathy. J Neurol Neurosurg Psychiatry 1995;59:322–5.
81. Otake S. Sarcoidosis involving skeletal muscle: imaging findings and relative value of imaging procedures. AJR Am J Roentgenol 1994;162:369–75.
82. Fujita H, Ishimatsu Y, Motomura M, et al. A case of acute sarcoid myositis treated with weekly low-dose methotrexate. Muscle Nerve 2011;44:994–9.
83. Ebert EC, Kierson M, Hagspiel KD. Gastrointestinal and hepatic manifestations of sarcoidosis. Am J Gastroenterol 2008;103:3184–92 [quiz: 93].
84. Vatti R, Sharma OP. Course of asymptomatic liver involvement in sarcoidosis: role of therapy in selected cases. Sarcoidosis Vasc Diffuse Lung Dis 1997;14:73–6.

85. Valla D, Pessegueiro-Miranda H, Degott C, et al. Hepatic sarcoidosis with portal hypertension. A report of seven cases with a review of the literature. Q J Med 1987;63:531–44.
86. Longcope WT, Freiman DG. A study of sarcoidosis; based on a combined investigation of 160 cases including 30 autopsies from the Johns Hopkins Hospital and Massachusetts General Hospital. Medicine (Baltimore) 1952;31:1–132.
87. Berliner AR, Haas M, Choi MJ. Sarcoidosis: the nephrologist's perspective. Am J Kidney Dis 2006;48:856–70.
88. Bergner R, Hoffmann M, Waldherr R, et al. Frequency of kidney disease in chronic sarcoidosis. Sarcoidosis Vasc Diffuse Lung Dis 2003;20:126–32.
89. Lebacq E, Desmet V, Verhaegen H. Renal involvement in sarcoidosis. Postgrad Med J 1970;46:526–9.
90. La Rochelle JC, Coogan CL. Urological manifestations of sarcoidosis. J Urol 2012;187:18–24.
91. Sharma OP. Hypercalcemia in granulomatous disorders: a clinical review. Curr Opin Pulm Med 2000;6:442–7.
92. Rizzato G, Fraioli P, Montemurro L. Nephrolithiasis as a presenting feature of chronic sarcoidosis. Thorax 1995;50:555–9.
93. Hunninghake GW, Gilbert S, Pueringer R, et al. Outcome of the treatment for sarcoidosis. Am J Respir Crit Care Med 1994;149:893–8.
94. Paramothayan S, Jones PW. Corticosteroid therapy in pulmonary sarcoidosis: a systematic review. JAMA 2002;287:1301–7.
95. Baughman RP, Lower EE. A clinical approach to the use of methotrexate for sarcoidosis. Thorax 1999;54:742–6.
96. Baughman RP, Lower EE. Steroid-sparing alternative treatments for sarcoidosis. Clin Chest Med 1997;18:853–64.
97. Baughman RP, Lower EE, Drent M. Inhibitors of tumor necrosis factor (TNF) in sarcoidosis: who, what, and how to use them. Sarcoidosis Vasc Diffuse Lung Dis 2008;25:76–89.
98. Egen JG, Rothfuchs AG, Feng CG, et al. Macrophage and T cell dynamics during the development and disintegration of mycobacterial granulomas. Immunity 2008;28:271–84.
99. Murray PI, Bodaghi B, Sharma OP. Systemic treatment of sarcoidosis. Ocul Immunol Inflamm 2011;19:145–50.
100. Massara A, Cavazzini L, La Corte R, et al. Sarcoidosis appearing during anti-tumor necrosis factor alpha therapy: a new "class effect" paradoxical phenomenon. Two case reports and literature review. Semin Arthritis Rheum 2010;39: 313–9.
101. Bomprezzi R, Pati S, Chansakul C, et al. A case of neurosarcoidosis successfully treated with rituximab. Neurology 2010;75:568–70.
102. Lower EE, Baughman RP, Kaufman AH. Rituximab for refractory granulomatous eye disease. Clin Ophthalmol 2012;6:1613–8.
103. Baughman RP, Iannuzzi MC, Lower EE, et al. Use of fluticasone in acute symptomatic pulmonary sarcoidosis. Sarcoidosis Vasc Diffuse Lung Dis 2002;19: 198–204.
104. Dubrey SW, Falk RH. Diagnosis and management of cardiac sarcoidosis. Prog Cardiovasc Dis 2010;52:336–46.
105. Epstein AE, DiMarco JP, Ellenbogen KA, et al. ACC/AHA/HRS 2008 Guidelines for Device-Based Therapy of Cardiac Rhythm Abnormalities: a report of the American College of Cardiology/American Heart Association Task Force on Practice Guidelines (writing committee to revise the ACC/AHA/NASPE 2002

guideline update for implantation of cardiac pacemakers and antiarrhythmia devices) developed in collaboration with the American Association for Thoracic Surgery and Society of Thoracic Surgeons. J Am Coll Cardiol 2008;51:e1–62.

106. Zaidi AR, Zaidi A, Vaitkus PT. Outcome of heart transplantation in patients with sarcoid cardiomyopathy. J Heart Lung Transplant 2007;26:714–7.

107. Stagaki E, Mountford WK, Lackland DT, et al. The treatment of lupus pernio: results of 116 treatment courses in 54 patients. Chest 2009;135:468–76.

108. Rose AS, Tielker MA, Knox KS. Hepatic, ocular, and cutaneous sarcoidosis. Clin Chest Med 2008;29:509–24, ix.

109. Dev S, McCallum RM, Jaffe GJ. Methotrexate treatment for sarcoid-associated panuveitis. Ophthalmology 1999;106:111–8.

110. Wakefield D, Zierhut M. Controversy: ocular sarcoidosis. Ocul Immunol Inflamm 2010;18:5–9.

111. Baughman RP, Winget DB, Lower EE. Methotrexate is steroid sparing in acute sarcoidosis: results of a double blind, randomized trial. Sarcoidosis Vasc Diffuse Lung Dis 2000;17:60–6.

112. Sweiss NJ, Patterson K, Sawaqed R, et al. Rheumatologic manifestations of sarcoidosis. Semin Respir Crit Care Med 2010;31:463–73.

113. Becheur H, Dall'osto H, Chatellier G, et al. Effect of ursodeoxycholic acid on chronic intrahepatic cholestasis due to sarcoidosis. Dig Dis Sci 1997;42:789–91.

114. Baratta L, Cascino A, Delfino M, et al. Ursodeoxycholic acid treatment in abdominal sarcoidosis. Dig Dis Sci 2000;45:1559–62.

115. Alenezi B, Lamoureux E, Alpert L, et al. Effect of ursodeoxycholic acid on granulomatous liver disease due to sarcoidosis. Dig Dis Sci 2005;50:196–200.

116. Singer DR, Evans DJ. Renal impairment in sarcoidosis: granulomatous nephritis as an isolated cause (two case reports and review of the literature). Clin Nephrol 1986;26:250–6.

117. Adams JS, Diz MM, Sharma OP. Effective reduction in the serum 1,25-dihydroxyvitamin D and calcium concentration in sarcoidosis-associated hypercalcemia with short-course chloroquine therapy. Ann Intern Med 1989;111:437–8.

118. Barre PE, Gascon-Barre M, Meakins JL, et al. Hydroxychloroquine treatment of hypercalcemia in a patient with sarcoidosis undergoing hemodialysis. Am J Med 1987;82:1259–62.

119. O'Leary TJ, Jones G, Yip A, et al. The effects of chloroquine on serum 1,25-dihydroxyvitamin D and calcium metabolism in sarcoidosis. N Engl J Med 1986; 315:727–30.

120. Mavrikakis I, Sfikakis PP, Mavrikakis E, et al. The incidence of irreversible retinal toxicity in patients treated with hydroxychloroquine: a reappraisal. Ophthalmology 2003;110:1321–6.

121. Wolfe F, Marmor MF. Rates and predictors of hydroxychloroquine retinal toxicity in patients with rheumatoid arthritis and systemic lupus erythematosus. Arthritis Care Res (Hoboken) 2010;62:775–84.

122. Adams JS, Sharma OP, Diz MM, et al. Ketoconazole decreases the serum 1,25-dihydroxyvitamin D and calcium concentration in sarcoidosis-associated hypercalcemia. J Clin Endocrinol Metab 1990;70:1090–5.

123. Mahevas M, Lescure FX, Boffa JJ, et al. Renal sarcoidosis: clinical, laboratory, and histologic presentation and outcome in 47 patients. Medicine (Baltimore) 2009;88:98–106.

Erdheim-Chester Disease

Julien Haroche, MD, PhD[a,b,*], Laurent Arnaud, MD, PhD[a,b],
Fleur Cohen-Aubart, MD, PhD[a,b], Baptiste Hervier, MD[a,b],
Frédéric Charlotte, MD[c], Jean-François Emile, MD, PhD[d],
Zahir Amoura, MD[a,b]

KEYWORDS

- Erdheim-Chester disease • Histiocytosis • Langerhans cell histiocytosis
- Interferon α • BRAF

KEY POINTS

- Diagnosis of Erdheim-Chester disease (ECD) is based on the identification in tissue biopsy samples of histiocytes, which are typically foamy and immunostain for CD68+ CD1a–, whereas histiocytes in cases of Langerhans cell histiocytosis (LCH) are CD68+ CD1a+.
- Two signs highly suggestive of ECD are technetium Tc 99m bone scintigraphy showing nearly constant tracer uptake by the long bones and a hairy kidney appearance on abdominal computed tomography scan (observed in about half such cases).
- Central nervous system involvement is a key prognostic factor and an independent predictor of death in ECD.
- Interferon α (IFN-α) (or PEGylated IFN-α) may be the best first-line therapy for prolonged treatment of ECD and significantly improves survival. Tolerance of this treatment is poor in some cases.
- ECD is associated with intense systemic immune activation mainly involving IFN-α, interleukin 1 (IL-1)/IL-1 receptor antagonist, IL-6, IL-12, and monocyte chemotactic protein 1, consistent with the systemic immune Th-1-oriented disturbance associated with this disorder.
- The $BRAF^{V600E}$ mutation is an activating mutation of the proto-oncogene BRAF, and is found in more than 50% of cases of ECD. Vemurafenib has been used for a few patients harboring this mutation and with severe multisystemic and refractory ECD and LCH; inhibition of BRAF activation by vemurafenib was highly beneficial in these cases.

[a] Department of Internal Medicine, French Reference Center for Rare Autoimmune and Systemic Diseases, Assistance Publique-Hôpitaux de Paris, Pitié-Salpêtrière Hospital, 47-83 boulevard de l'Hôpital, 75651 Paris Cedex 13, France; [b] Université Pierre et Marie Curie, UPMC Univ Paris, Paris, France; [c] Department of Anatomopathology, Assistance Publique-Hôpitaux de Paris, Pitié-Salpêtrière Hospital, Paris, France; [d] Department of Pathology, Ambroise Paré Hospital, Assistance Publique Hôpitaux de Paris, Versailles University, 9 Avenue Charles de Gaulle, 92104 Boulogne-Billancourt, France
* Corresponding author. Department of Internal Medicine, French Reference Center for Rare Autoimmune and Systemic Diseases, Assistance Publique-Hôpitaux de Paris, Pitié-Salpêtrière Hospital, 47-83 boulevard de l'Hôpital, 75651 Paris Cedex 13, France.
E-mail address: julien.haroche@psl.aphp.fr

Rheum Dis Clin N Am 39 (2013) 299–311
http://dx.doi.org/10.1016/j.rdc.2013.02.011
0889-857X/13/$ – see front matter © 2013 Elsevier Inc. All rights reserved.

INTRODUCTION

Erdheim-Chester disease (ECD) is a rare, non-Langerhans form of histiocytosis of unknown origin. The disease was first described as the lipoid granulomatose by Jakob Erdheim's pupil William Chester in 1930.[1] Between then and January 2013, more than 500 cases were reported.[2–4] ECD is characterized by xanthomatous or xanthogranu-lomatous infiltration of tissues by foamy histiocytes, lipid-laden macrophages or histiocytes, surrounded by fibrosis.[5,6] The immunohistologic characteristics of histio-cytes can be used to distinguish ECD from Langerhans cell histiocytosis (LCH): in ECD, cells stain positive for CD68 and negative for CD1a; staining for the S-100 protein is also negative in most cases (80%).

ECD is a true multisystemic disease, with diverse manifestations, including skeletal involvement with bone pain, exophthalmos, diabetes insipidus, xanthelasma, intersti-tial lung disease, bilateral adrenal enlargement, retroperitoneal fibrosis with perirenal or ureteral obstruction, renal impairment, testis infiltration, and the involvement of the central nervous system (CNS) or cardiovascular system.[4,5]

The clinical course of ECD is largely dependent on the extent and distribution of the disease. It may involve only asymptomatic bone lesions or present as multisystemic, life-threatening forms with poor prognosis. This review focuses on the 53 patients published in 2011 (**Table 1**).[4] Our personal experience with ECD has increased rapidly since then. We have seen 95 patients with ECD at least once, and most of them were regularly assessed in our center, between 1991 and January 2013. Most of these patients live in France, although 21 come from abroad, mainly Europe, and some from Israel and South Africa. Twenty of these patients have died (21%).

Histiocytoses are heterogenous diseases and some patients present with associa-tions of various types of histiocytoses (most often ECD and LCH but also with Rosai-Dorfman disease (RDD), another non-Langerhans form of histiocytosis, with a generally more favorable outcome).[7–9] Such associations are found in about 15% of the 95 patients followed at our institution until January 2013: 11 patients had ECD

Table 1
Frequency of the main clinical and radiologic characteristics in ECD

	From the Literature (%)	Personal Experience (%)[a]
Bone pain	50	40[b]
Periaortic infiltration	60	66
Coated aorta (sheathing of the whole thoracoabdominal aorta)	30	23[b]
Pericardial involvement	45	42
Exophthalmos	27	25
Diabetes insipidus	27	25[b]
Xanthelasmas	19	28
Hairy kidney aspect	ND	68
CNS involvement	15–25	51
Pulmonary involvement	22	43
Death	60	26

Abbreviation: ND, no data available.
[a] In all cases, unless mention of comparison with another series, based on the 53 patients in the series published in 2011.[3]
[b] Compared with the 48 patients followed at Pitié-Salpêtrière Hospital (taken from the 53 patients from the series published in 2011[3]).

and LCH, 2 had ECD and RDD, and 1 had LCH, ECD, and RDD. The frequency of these overlap forms of LCH and ECD seems to be too high to be fortuitous, and suggests a pathogenic link between the various histiocytic disorders. Clinicians should be aware of this association and should consider the possibility of ECD in patients with LCH.

Diagnostic Criteria

The diagnosis of ECD is mainly based on the characteristic histology of the disease (**Fig. 1**): infiltration with foamy histiocytes nested among polymorphic granuloma and fibrosis or xanthogranulomatosis, with CD68-positive and CD1a-negative immunohistochemical staining.[5,6] Virtually any tissue can be infiltrated by histiocytes in ECD.

There are 2 signs that are highly suggestive of ECD: tracer uptake by the long bones is observed by technetium Tc 99m bone scintigraphy (**Fig. 2**) in almost all patients (96% of our 53 patients)[10,11]; and hairy kidney on abdominal computed tomography (CT) scan (**Fig. 3**) ($\approx$50% of cases).[12,13] Biopsy is required to diagnose ECD, so an elegant diagnostic approach is to use ultrasound-guided biopsy of the perirenal infiltration (when present, ie, 68% of our 53 patients).[14]

Our team has established possible diagnostic criteria for ECD:

1. Characteristic histologic findings (see **Fig. 1**): infiltration by foamy histiocytes into polymorphic granuloma and fibrosis or xanthogranulomatosis with CD68-positive and CD1a-negative immunohistochemistry, typical of ECD histiocytes;
2. Typical skeletal findings with (a) radiographs showing bilateral and symmetric cortical osteosclerosis of the diaphyseal and metaphyseal regions in the long bones or (b) technetium Tc 99m bone scintigraphy evidence of symmetric and abnormally strong labeling of the distal ends of the long bones of the lower limbs, and in some cases the upper limbs.

These ECD criteria were those used for our previous literature reviews in 1996, 2004, and 2011. All cases followed at our center fulfilled criterion 1 and all but 4 fulfilled criterion 2.

Thus, a few cases of true ECD lack the typical hallmark of the disease, defined by the long bone involvement; in these cases, bone scintigraphy, radiographs, magnetic resonance imaging (MRI) and positron emission tomography (PET)-CT investigations do not reveal abnormalities.

Epidemiology

The 95 patients currently followed at our center are mostly men (74% men and 26% women), consistent with our previous analysis in 2011.[4] The mean age at diagnosis in the 2 large series published by our team was relatively stable between 2004 and 2011: 55 years $\pm$ 14 (range, 16–80 years) in the 2011 series.[4,5] ECD is rarely described in children, and there have been only 8 pediatric cases reported, none of which had cardiac involvement.[15,16]

The mean delay before diagnosis for the patients included in our preliminary study in 2006 was between a few months and several years (up to 25 years). However, this delay has shortened substantially because of better awareness of the disease.[11]

Clinical Manifestations

Osseous involvement

Almost all patients with ECD present with skeletal involvement (96% of the 53 patients reported in the 2011 series), but only 50% of patients suffer bone pain, which is nevertheless the most common clinical feature of ECD (see **Table 1**).[11] The bone pain

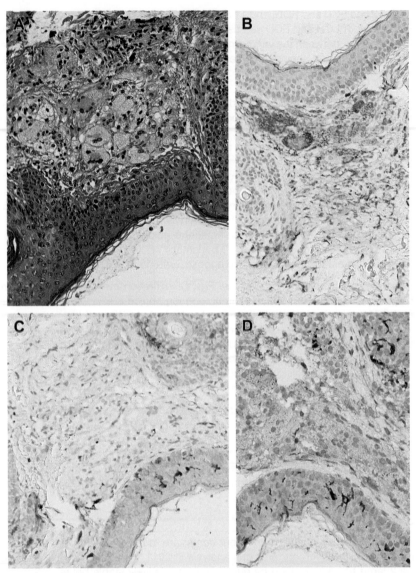

Fig. 1. (*A*) Cutaneous ECD: the papillary dermis is infiltrated by numerous histiocytes with foamy cytoplasm admixed with multinucleate giant Touton cells and a few small lympho-cytes (hematoxylin-eosin, original magnification x100); (*B*) the dermal histiocytes express CD68 (KP1 clone); (*C*) these histiocytes are S100 protein negative, whereas rare dendritic cells in the dermis and Langerhans cells are positive; (*D*) the dermal histiocytes do not express CD1a, because internal control, Langerhans cells are CD1a+ (*B, C* and *D*: immunoperoxidase staining, original magnification x100).

mostly affects the legs, is often mild, and can emerge at any time. Typical skeletal find-ings in cases of ECD are bilateral and symmetric cortical osteosclerosis of the diaph-yseal and metaphyseal regions in the long bones on radiographs or symmetric and excessive labeling of the distal ends of the long bones of the legs, and sometimes

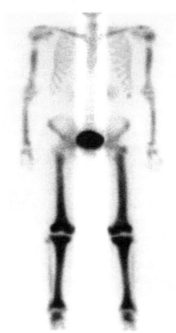

Fig. 2. Symmetric and abnormally increased metaphysodiaphyseal labeling of the long bones, predominantly in the lower limbs, on technetium Tc 99m bone scintigraphy.

the arms, on technetium Tc 99m bone scintigraphy.[5,6] Unlike LCH, the axial skeleton and the mandible are typically not affected in cases of ECD. PET using ^{18}F-labeled fluorodeoxyglucose (PET-CT) has recently been used rather than bone CT scans.[17,18] Bone MRI may be informative in some cases, because unlike radiographs, it may reveal the epiphyseal involvement of the long bones and periostitis.[19] It may also be useful in the rare cases of ECD for which bone CT scans reveal no anomalies.

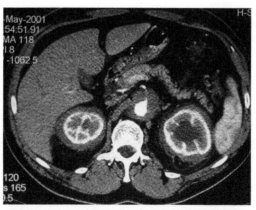

Fig. 3. Contrast-enhanced axial CT scan showing the origin of the superior mesenteric artery, which is stenosed. Note the coated aorta aspect, the symmetric infiltration of the perirenal fat and of the perirenal fascia taking the appearance of hairy kidneys.

Cardiovascular involvement

Recent case reports show how improvements in radiologic imaging techniques have increased the likelihood of detecting cardiovascular involvement. The most frequent cardiovascular manifestations are the involvement of the circumferential periaortic sheathing of the thoracic or abdominal aorta (66% of cases in our series in 2011).[4,5] Serratrice and colleagues[11] coined the term "coated aorta" for cases in which the whole aorta is sheathed (38% of cases in the series we reported in 2006).[20] The peri-arterial infiltration may spread to the main aortic branches, generally with limited clinical consequences apart from renovascular hypertension (21% of our 95 patients), which can be treated by renal artery stenting.[5]

Although myocardium and endocardium may be involved, pericardial involvement is by far the most frequent heart lesion (42% of the 53 patients) and may be complicated by a tamponade.[5,21] Systematic retrospective cardiovascular screening (MRI or heart CT scan) in 2009 revealed abnormal heart imaging results in 70% of 37 patients: 49% showed abnormal infiltration of the right heart, including 30% with pseudotumoral infiltration of the right atrium, and 19% had infiltration of the auriculoventricular sulcus.[22]

Myocardial infarctions secondary to pericoronarial infiltration have been reported in about 15 patients, leading to death in some cases.[5,23,24] Symptomatic heart valve disease (aortic and mitral regurgitations) were reported in 17% of 53 patients studied.[4] Valve replacement was required in 3 patients, including 1 case in our center.[5,25] However, valve replacement should be carefully discussed on a case-by-case basis at a specialist center, because this intervention can be challenging technically due to the overall infiltration of the heart tunics.

Retro-orbital infiltration

One-quarter of the patients in our series developed exophthalmos, often bilateral, because of infiltration of the retro-orbital soft tissues.[26,27] It is massive in rare cases, and may be refractory to conventional therapies and require surgical debulking.

Endocrine involvements

The most frequent endocrine manifestation of ECD is diabetes insipidus caused by infiltration of the pituitary gland (25% of our patients). Pituitary or hypothalamic infiltration with various other endocrine consequences, such as hyperprolactinemia, gonadotropin insufficiency, and abnormally low levels of insulinlike growth factor 1 has been reported in rare cases.[28,29]

We reported 7 cases of adrenal gland enlargement in a series of 22 patients with ECD.[30] In all cases, the diagnosis was radiologic and was confirmed by autopsy in 1 patient. One of these patients had adrenal insufficiency. These investigations indicate that adrenal infiltration is not rare in patients with ECD and may in some cases lead to adrenal insufficiency.

Cutaneomucosal involvements

Xanthelasmas, most frequently on the eyelids or in the periorbital spaces, affected 28% of our 53 patients. Although less frequent, papulonodular lesions,[31] and infiltrations of the vulva and of the clitoris may be observed.[1]

Urologic and nephrologic infiltrations

Approximately 30% of ECD cases present with pseudoretroperitoneal fibrosis, sometimes complicated by bilateral hydronephrosis, which may require ureteral stenting.[32] By contrast with idiopathic retroperitoneal fibrosis, the pelvic ureters are never involved in ECD cases and the inferior vena cava is rarely affected. This fibrosis sheaths the aortic walls completely and circumferentially, whereas in cases of idiopathic retroperitoneal fibrosis, the posterior aortic wall is rarely affected.[5]

Pulmonary involvement
We reported a retrospective study, performed in 2008, of the characteristics of 34 consecutive patients with ECD.[33] High-resolution CT scans of the chest revealed the involvement of lung parenchyma in 53% of the cases, and of the pleura in 41%.[34] The pulmonary lesions predominantly involve the interlobular septa. Pulmonary involvement was not found to be a major prognostic factor in ECD and this finding contrasts with those of previous small case series. A MEDLINE search identified descriptions of pulmonary involvement in 70 (22%) of the 319 patients with ECD reported before November 2008. However, this feature was often incompletely described.

CNS involvement
CNS involvement is a common feature of ECD (15%–25%),[11] and was extensively described in the largest neurologic series, reported in 2006.[35] This multicenter literature review analyzed 66 patients with ECD (including 6 personal cases) with neurologic involvement. The most frequent clinical manifestations were cerebellar and pyramidal syndromes (41% and 45% of cases, respectively); seizures, headaches, neuropsychiatric manifestations or cognitive impairment, sensory disturbances, cranial nerve paralysis, and asymptomatic lesions have also been reported. Neurologic involvement led to severe functional disability in almost all patients. CNS involvement is a major prognostic factor in ECD: our survival analysis in 2011 indicated that it is an independent predictor of death (hazard ratio [HR] = 2.51; 95% confidence interval [CI], 1.28–5.52; P = .006).[4]

We reviewed brain MRI, performed up to 2009, for 33 patients with ECD followed at Pitié-Salpêtrière Hospital. The imaging results were normal for only 3 patients,[36] and at least 2 different anatomic sites were involved in two-thirds of the patients. Lesions of the brain, meninges, facial bones and orbits are frequent in ECD and brain MRI and CT should be used systematically in all patients with ECD, even those who are asymptomatic.

Other infiltrations
Several other organs have been reported to be involved in ECD. In particular, testes, thyroid, and lymph node involvement has been revealed by autopsy.[37] Breast infiltration has also been described in numerous case reports.[38,39]

Trying to Assess Disease Activity
The clinical course of ECD has not been rigorously established, although it seems to be that of a chronic disease. The various organs and systems affected by ECD accumulate lesions that do not generally regress spontaneously. The C-reactive protein (CRP) concentration is increased in more than 80% of cases,[11] but this has little therapeutic impact once the diagnosis is established. Disease activity is mainly evaluated by regular clinical examination and radiologic investigations (about every 6 months). No disease activity score has been established.

Our experience is that PET scanning is particularly valuable for assessing disease activity in cases of ECD.[17] Follow-up PET scans are particularly useful for assessing CNS involvement: PET scanning can reveal early therapeutic responses of CNS lesions, even before MRI shows a decrease in their size. PET scanning can also be used to evaluate the cardiovascular system, and the heart and the entire vascular tree can be studied during a single session. We therefore recommend using PET for assessment of patients with ECD, because this single technique is informative about many of the most relevant lesions encountered in patients with ECD. Furthermore, we found PET investigations particularly valuable in our recent pilot study of use of BRAF inhibitors in patients with ECD.[40]

First-Line Treatment of ECD is Interferon α

The treatments used up to 2005 in cases of ECD included steroids, cytotoxic agents,[41] and double autologous hematopoietic stem cell transplantation.[42,43] It was difficult to assess the efficacy of such treatments because many were used for only a few patients, in combination with other drugs, or the follow-up periods were short. Braiteh and colleagues[44] administered interferon α (IFN-α) to 3 patients with ECD and described rapid, substantial, and long-lasting regression of retro-orbital infiltration and gradual improvement in bone lesions, pain, and diabetes insipidus. However, we found that the efficacy of IFN-α at low doses (3 MU × 3/wk) was different between the 8 patients with ECD treated and according to the site involved in the disease.[14] Symptoms in some cases failed to respond to such low-dose IFN-α, especially in patients with severe multisystem forms of ECD (CNS and cardiovascular involvement).[4] We therefore recommend higher doses, if possible, up to 9 MU × 3/wk, because such doses may be more effective against meningeal infiltrations, suprasellar and retrosellar masses, and pericardial and pseudoatrial infiltrations. Treatment should be long-term, and this may be problematic because of side effects, including depression and fatigue. The effectiveness of IFN-α in cases of pseudodegenerative forms of cerebellar involvement (similar to that observed in LCH) has been disappointing.

Nevertheless, the evidence overall is that IFN-α is a valuable first-line therapy for prolonged treatment of ECD. In a recent survival analysis of our series of 53 patients, we found that treatment with IFN-α or PEGylated IFN-α was a major independent predictor of survival (HR = 0.32; 95% CI, 0.14–0.70; P = .006).[4] Our current attitude is to start treatment with PEGylated forms of IFN-α, because it is generally better tolerated than IFN-α in the long-term.

There were reports in 2010 of the efficacy of imatinib mesylate in histiocytoses,[45] although our preliminary experience with this treatment in 6 patients with ECD was disappointing.[46] Promising results were reported, in the same year, for recombinant human interleukin 1 (IL-1) receptor (anakinra) treatment of 2 patients with ECD; neither of these patients had cardiovascular or CNS involvement.[47] After this report, we administered this treatment to 10 patients with ECD at our institution: overall, the efficacy was poor. Cladribin may be beneficial for treating CNS localizations of the disease refractory to IFN-α,[41] although the outcome was not favorable among the few patients receiving this treatment at our center. The use of infliximab, with some success after 12 to 18 months of treatment, in 2 patients with ECD with cardiac involvement was reported in 2012.[48] Even more encouraging was the demonstration in 2012 of the rapid efficacy of a BRAF inhibitor (vemurafenib) in 3 patients.[40]

BRAF Inhibition May be an Alternative to IFN-α in Patients with ECD Carrying the BRAF^V600E Mutation

The RAS-RAF-MEK-ERK pathway is a cellular signaling pathway, and is involved in diverse tumors.[49] The *BRAF^V600E* mutation has been identified in many human tumors.[50] It is an activating mutation of the proto-oncogene BRAF, and results in an activation of the RAS-ERK pathway, independently of RAS activation. Inhibition of BRAF activation by vemurafenib improves the survival of patients with metastatic melanomas carrying the *BRAF^V600E* mutation.[51] *BRAF^V600E* mutations were detected in patients with LCH in 2010.[52] We therefore tested for this mutation in other types of histiocytosis. We reviewed histology findings for 127 patients with histiocytoses, and screened DNA extracted from paraffin-embedded samples for $BRAF^{V600E}$ mutations by pyrosequencing.[53] The diagnoses corresponding to the samples studied were ECD, LCH, RDD, juvenile xanthogranuloma, histiocytic sarcoma, xanthoma dissemi-natum, interdigitating dendritic cell sarcoma, and necrobiotic xanthogranuloma (n = 46, 39, 23, 12, 3, 2, 1, and 1, respectively). BRAF status was successfully determined in 93 cases, and $BRAF^{V600E}$ mutations were detected in 13 of 24 (54%) ECD samples, 11 of 29 (38%) LCH samples, and none of the other histiocytoses tested. Subse-quently, we reported BRAF mutations in 51% of a series of 37 patients with ECD.[54]

Vemurafenib is a newly approved inhibitor of mutant BRAF, and has some efficacy against both melanoma and hairy-cell leukemia associated with the $BRAF^{V600E}$ muta-tion.[55] We therefore conducted a pilot study of vemurafenib treatment of 3 patients with multisystemic and refractory ECD, and carrying the $BRAF^{V600E}$ mutation; 2 also had skin or lymph node LCH involvement.[40] The patients were followed clinically, bio-logically (CRP values), histologically (skin biopsy), and morphologically (PET, CT, and MRI). Vemurafenib treatment led to substantial and rapid clinical and biologic improvement in all 3 cases. The tumor response was confirmed by PET, CT, or MRI after 1 month of treatment. For 1 patient, the PET response increased between months 1 and 4 of treatment. The treatment remained effective after 9 months of follow-up, although disease activity persisted in 1 patient. These findings lead us to believe that treatment with vemurafenib should be considered for patients with severe and refractory $BRAF^{V600E}$ histiocytoses, particularly when the disease is life-threatening.

Follow-Up

The 2 series we published before the IFN-α era showed the severity of the prognosis of ECD.[5,6] In 2004, 35 (60%) of the 58 patients for whom data were available died, and the mean survival after diagnosis was 19.2 months (range, 0–120 months). However, the most recent data, those from our survival analysis in 2011, show that overall mortality after treatment with IFN-α is now only 26%, and the 5-year survival is 68%.[4]

Pathophysiology

The pathogenesis of ECD was poorly documented, mostly because previous studies included only a few patients. Stoppacciaro and colleagues[56] described an immuno-histochemical study of 3 patients, showing that histiocyte recruitment and accumula-tion in the lesions is regulated by a complex network of cytokines and chemokines. Dagna and colleagues[57] studied both spontaneous and stimulated cytokine produc-tion by mononuclear cells in biopsy fragments from a single patient; these investiga-tors reported the production of tumor necrosis factor α after stimulation, and spontaneous secretion of IL-6 and IL-8, IL-8 being a chemoattractant for polymorpho-nuclear cells and monocytes. Aouba and colleagues[47] reported evidence in 2 patients that targeting the IL-1 pathway might be beneficial. We recently assayed serum samples from 37 patients with ECD for 23 cytokines.[58] We found substantial and systemic immune activation, mainly involving IFN-α, IL-1/IL-1 receptor antagonist, IL-6, IL-12, and monocyte chemotactic protein 1. This finding further confirms that ECD is associated with systemic immune Th-1-oriented perturbation, and provides clues for choosing better-targeted therapeutic agents.

The recent finding of $BRAF^{V600E}$ mutations in more than 50% of ECD cases clearly adds further complexity to the pathophysiology of this disorder: it also provides evidence of clonal proliferation (associated with the $BRAF^{V600E}$ mutation) and of both nonclonal accumulation of histiocytes within the affected tissues (as a consequence of systemic chemokines and proinflammatory cytokines in the circulation).

SUMMARY

ECD is a rare and orphan disease. Despite having been overlooked previously, numerous new cases have been diagnosed more recently. The number of ECD cases reported has increased substantially: more than 300 new cases have been published in the past 10 years. This situation is mainly a result of the generally better awareness among pathologists, radiologists, and clinicians of various aspects of this rare disease. The field has been particularly active in the last few years, with evidence of the efficacy of IFN-α, the description of systemic proinflammatory cytokine signatures, and most recently, reports of the dramatic efficacy of BRAF inhibition in severe, $BRAF^{V600E}$ mutation-associated cases of ECD. Also, BRAF mutations have been found in more than half of the patients with ECD who were tested. Detailed elucidation of the pathogenesis of the disease is likely to lead to the development of better-targeted and more effective therapies.

REFERENCES

1. Chester W. Über Lipoidgranulomatose. Virchows Archiv für Pathologische Anatomie und Physiologie und für Klinische Medizin 1930;279:561–602 [in German].
2. Adam Z, Koukalova R, Sprlakova A, et al. Successful treatment of Erdheim-Chester disease by 2-chlorodeoxyadenosine-based chemotherapy. Two case studies and a literature review. Vnitr Lek 2011;57:576–89 [in Czech].
3. Haroche J, Arnaud L, Amoura Z. Erdheim-Chester disease. Curr Opin Rheumatol 2012;24(1):53–9.
4. Arnaud L, Hervier B, Neel A, et al. CNS involvement and treatment with interferon-alpha are independent prognostic factors in Erdheim-Chester disease: a multicenter survival analysis of 53 patients. Blood 2011;117:2778–82.
5. Haroche J, Amoura Z, Dion E, et al. Cardiovascular involvement, an overlooked feature of Erdheim-Chester disease: report of 6 new cases and a literature review. Medicine (Baltimore) 2004;83:371–92.
6. Veyssier-Belot C, Cacoub P, Caparros-Lefebvre D, et al. Erdheim-Chester disease. Clinical and radiologic characteristics of 59 cases. Medicine (Baltimore) 1996;75:157–69.
7. Brower AC, Worsham GF, Dudley AH. Erdheim-Chester disease: a distinct lipoidosis or part of the spectrum of histiocytosis? Radiology 1984;151:35–8.
8. Tsai JW, Tsou JH, Hung LY, et al. Combined Erdheim-Chester disease and Langerhans cell histiocytosis of skin are both monoclonal: a rare case with human androgen-receptor gene analysis. J Am Acad Dermatol 2010;63:284–91.
9. Wang KH, Cheng CJ, Hu CH, et al. Coexistence of localized Langerhans cell histiocytosis and cutaneous Rosai-Dorfman disease. Br J Dermatol 2002;147:770–4.
10. Balink H, Hemmelder MH, de Graaf W, et al. Scintigraphic diagnosis of Erdheim-Chester disease. J Clin Oncol 2011;29:e470–2.
11. Haroche J, Amoura Z, Wechsler B, et al. Erdheim-Chester disease. Presse Med 2007;36:1663–8 [in French].
12. Andre M, Delevaux I, de Fraissinette B, et al. Two enlarged kidneys: a manifestation of Erdheim-Chester disease. Am J Nephrol 2001;21:315–7.
13. Dion E, Graef C, Haroche J, et al. Imaging of thoracoabdominal involvement in Erdheim-Chester disease. AJR Am J Roentgenol 2004;183:1253–60.

14. Haroche J, Amoura Z, Trad SG, et al. Variability in the efficacy of interferon-alpha in Erdheim-Chester disease by patient and site of involvement: results in eight patients. Arthritis Rheum 2006;54:3330–6.

15. Jeon IS, Lee SS, Lee MK. Chemotherapy and interferon-alpha treatment of Erdheim-Chester disease. Pediatr Blood Cancer 2010;55:745–7.

16. Tran TA, Fabre M, Pariente D, et al. Erdheim-Chester disease in childhood: a challenging diagnosis and treatment. J Pediatr Hematol Oncol 2009;31:782–6.

17. Arnaud L, Malek Z, Archambaud F, et al. 18F-fluorodeoxyglucose-positron emission tomography scanning is more useful in followup than in the initial assessment of patients with Erdheim-Chester disease. Arthritis Rheum 2009;60:3128–38.

18. Stenova E, Steno B, Povinec P, et al. FDG-PET in the Erdheim-Chester disease: its diagnostic and follow-up role. Rheumatol Int 2012;32(3):675–8.

19. Dion E, Graef C, Miquel A, et al. Bone involvement in Erdheim-Chester disease: imaging findings including periostitis and partial epiphyseal involvement. Radiology 2006;238:632–9.

20. Serratrice J, Granel B, De Roux C, et al. "Coated aorta": a new sign of Erdheim-Chester disease. J Rheumatol 2000;27:1550–3.

21. Gupta A, Kelly B, McGuigan JE. Erdheim-Chester disease with prominent pericardial involvement: clinical, radiologic, and histologic findings. Am J Med Sci 2002;324:96–100.

22. Haroche J, Cluzel P, Toledano D, et al. Images in cardiovascular medicine. Cardiac involvement in Erdheim-Chester disease: magnetic resonance and computed tomographic scan imaging in a monocentric series of 37 patients. Circulation 2009;119:e597–8.

23. Fink MG, Levinson DJ, Brown NL, et al. Erdheim-Chester disease. Case report with autopsy findings. Arch Pathol Lab Med 1991;115:619–23.

24. Loeffler AG, Memoli VA. Myocardial involvement in Erdheim-Chester disease. Arch Pathol Lab Med 2004;128:682–5.

25. Kenn W, Stabler A, Zachoval R, et al. Erdheim-Chester disease: a case report and literature overview. Eur Radiol 1999;9:153–8.

26. Alper MG, Zimmerman LE, Piana FG. Orbital manifestations of Erdheim-Chester disease. Trans Am Ophthalmol Soc 1983;81:64–85.

27. Sheidow TG, Nicolle DA, Heathcote JG. Erdheim-Chester disease: two cases of orbital involvement. Eye (Lond) 2000;14(Pt 4):606–12.

28. Khamseh ME, Mollanai S, Hashemi F, et al. Erdheim-Chester syndrome, presenting as hypogonadotropic hypogonadism and diabetes insipidus. J Endocrinol Invest 2002;25:727–9.

29. Tritos NA, Weinrib S, Kaye TB. Endocrine manifestations of Erdheim-Chester disease (a distinct form of histiocytosis). J Intern Med 1998;244:529–35.

30. Haroche J, Amoura Z, Touraine P, et al. Bilateral adrenal infiltration in Erdheim-Chester disease. Report of seven cases and literature review. J Clin Endocrinol Metab 2007;92:2007–12.

31. Opie KM, Kaye J, Vinciullo C. Erdheim-Chester disease. Australas J Dermatol 2003;44:194–8.

32. Droupy S, Attias D, Eschwege P, et al. Bilateral hydronephrosis in a patient with Erdheim-Chester disease. J Urol 1999;162:2084–5.

33. Arnaud L, Pierre I, Beigelman-Aubry C, et al. Pulmonary involvement in Erdheim-Chester disease: a single-center study of thirty-four patients and a review of the literature. Arthritis Rheum 2010;62:3504–12.

34. Brun AL, Touitou-Gottenberg D, Haroche J, et al. Erdheim-Chester disease: CT findings of thoracic involvement. Eur Radiol 2010;20:2579–87.

35. Lachenal F, Cotton F, Desmurs-Clavel H, et al. Neurological manifestations and neuroradiological presentation of Erdheim-Chester disease: report of 6 cases and systematic review of the literature. J Neurol 2006;253:1267–77.

36. Drier A, Haroche J, Savatovsky J, et al. Cerebral, facial, and orbital involvement in Erdheim-Chester disease: CT and MR imaging findings. Radiology 2010;255:586–94.

37. Sheu SY, Wenzel RR, Kersting C, et al. Erdheim-Chester disease: case report with multisystemic manifestations including testes, thyroid, and lymph nodes, and a review of literature. J Clin Pathol 2004;57(11):1225–8.

38. Provenzano E, Barter SJ, Wright PA, et al. Erdheim-Chester disease presenting as bilateral clinically malignant breast masses. Am J Surg Pathol 2010;34(4):584–8.

39. Johnson TR, Lenhard MS, Weidinger M, et al. An unusual breast tumor. Radiologe 2009;49(10):942–5.

40. Haroche J, Cohen-Aubart F, Emile JF, et al. Dramatic efficacy of vemurafenib in both multisystemic and refractory Erdheim-Chester disease and Langerhans cell histiocytosis harbouring the BRAF V600E mutation. Blood 2013;121:1495–500.

41. Myra C, Sloper L, Tighe PJ, et al. Treatment of Erdheim-Chester disease with cladribine: a rational approach. Br J Ophthalmol 2004;88:844–7.

42. Boissel N, Wechsler B, Leblond V. Treatment of refractory Erdheim-Chester disease with double autologous hematopoietic stem-cell transplantation. Ann Intern Med 2001;135:844–5.

43. Gaspar N, Boudou P, Haroche J, et al. High-dose chemotherapy followed by autologous hematopoietic stem cell transplantation for adult histiocytic disorders with central nervous system involvement. Haematologica 2006;91:1121–5.

44. Braiteh F, Boxrud C, Esmaeli B, et al. Successful treatment of Erdheim-Chester disease, a non-Langerhans-cell histiocytosis, with interferon-alpha. Blood 2005;106:2992–4.

45. Janku F, Amin HM, Yang D, et al. Response of histiocytoses to imatinib mesylate: fire to ashes. J Clin Oncol 2010;28:e633–6.

46. Haroche J, Amoura Z, Charlotte F, et al. Imatinib mesylate for platelet-derived growth factor receptor-beta-positive Erdheim-Chester histiocytosis. Blood 2008;111:5413–5.

47. Aouba A, Georgin-Lavialle S, Pagnoux C, et al. Rationale and efficacy of interleukin-1 targeting in Erdheim-Chester disease. Blood 2010;116:4070–6.

48. Dagna L, Corti A, Langheim S, et al. Tumor necrosis factor α as a master regulator of inflammation in Erdheim-Chester disease: rationale for the treatment of patients with infliximab. J Clin Oncol 2012;30(28):e286–90.

49. Beeram M, Patnaik A, Rowinsky EK. Raf: a strategic target for therapeutic development against cancer. J Clin Oncol 2005;23(27):6771–90.

50. Davies H, Bignell GR, Cox C, et al. Mutations of the BRAF gene in human cancer. Nature 2002;417(6892):949–54.

51. Chapman PB, Hauschild A, Robert C, et al. Improved survival with vemurafenib in melanoma with BRAF V600E mutation. N Engl J Med 2011;364(26):2507–16.

52. Badalian-Very G, Vergilio JA, Degar BA, et al. Recurrent BRAF mutations in Langerhans cell histiocytosis. Blood 2010;116(11):1919–23.

53. Haroche J, Charlotte F, Arnaud L, et al. High prevalence of BRAF V600E mutations in Erdheim-Chester disease but not in other non-Langerhans cell histiocytoses. Blood 2012;120(13):2700–3.

54. Emile JF, Charlotte F, Amoura Z, et al. BRAF mutations in Erdheim-Chester disease. J Clin Oncol 2013;31(3):398.

55. Dietrich S, Glimm H, Andrulis M, et al. BRAF inhibition in refractory hairy-cell leukemia. N Engl J Med 2012;366:2038–40.
56. Stoppacciaro A, Ferrarini M, Salmaggi C, et al. Immunohistochemical evidence of a cytokine and chemokine network in three patients with Erdheim-Chester disease: implications for pathogenesis. Arthritis Rheum 2006;54:4018–22.
57. Dagna L, Girlanda S, Langheim S, et al. Erdheim-Chester disease: report on a case and new insights on its immunopathogenesis. Rheumatology (Oxford) 2010;49:1203–6.
58. Arnaud L, Gorochov G, Charlotte F, et al. Systemic perturbation of cytokine and chemokine networks in Erdheim-Chester disease: a single-center series of 37 patients. Blood 2011;117:2783–90.

Whipple's Disease

Sergio Schwartzman, MD[a],*, Monica Schwartzman, BA[b]

KEYWORDS

- Whipple's disease • *Tropheryma whipplei* • Inflammatory arthropathy
- Nervous system disease

KEY POINTS

- Whipple's disease is caused by the bacillus *Tropheryma whipplei*.
- The diagnosis is confirmed by tissue sampling with periodic acid-Schiff staining and/or polymerase chain reaction.
- The clinical manifestations most frequently manifest in the gastrointestinal, musculoskeletal, neurologic, cardiac, and ophthalmic organs, but can affect any site.
- Successful therapy with appropriate antibiotics is potentially curable, but recurrences may occur.

Although it is hypothesized that many rheumatic diseases may be initiated and perhaps maintained by an infectious agent, causative organisms have been rarely delineated as being causative in this group of illnesses. Whipple's disease, an illness caused by *Tropheryma whipplei* and characterized by multivariate clinical manifestations including an inflammatory arthropathy, is one such disease. In the description of the first case of Whipple's disease[1] in a physician who had contracted this disease, by the pathologist George Whipple's, the illness was characterized as an "intestinal lipodystrophy" and, although the focus was on the pathologic manifestations, an infectious cause was in fact considered, as Whipple's noted "a bacillus belonging to the colonic group" in the submucosal layer of the intestine.

Over the last century the etiology of Whipple's disease has been established, and the causative organism has been identified and characterized. However, many questions remain, as it is unknown as to why the clinical spectrum of the disease is so varied and why only a certain number of exposed patients develop the clinical illness. This article reviews the microbiology, pathophysiology, epidemiology, clinical manifestations, diagnostic testing, and treatment of Whipple's disease.

MICROBIOLOGY

George Hoyt Whipple's was the first to consider an infectious cause based on the pathology, which demonstrated a bacillus.[1] However, he was unsure as to whether this

[a] Hospital for Special Surgery, Weill Cornell Medical College, New York, NY, USA; [b] Icahn School of Medicine, Mount Sinai Hospital, New York, NY, USA
* Corresponding author.
E-mail address: SchwartzmanS@HSS.EDU

Rheum Dis Clin N Am 39 (2013) 313–321
http://dx.doi.org/10.1016/j.rdc.2013.03.005
0889-857X/13/$ – see front matter © 2013 Elsevier Inc. All rights reserved.

organism was in fact pathologic or part of the intestinal flora, and did not directly attribute the illness to an infectious cause. It was not until 1949, when the periodic acid-Schiff (PAS) stain revealed that foamy macrophages contained a glycoprotein material and not lipids, that an infectious cause was more concretely suspected.[2] In 1961, Chears and Ashworth[3] definitively identified macrophage-engulfed bacteria on electron microscopy. The PAS-positive bacilli with a classic trilamellar plasma membrane were hypothesized to be causative. The infectious nature of the disease has now been definitively confirmed using cell culture[4] and polymerase chain reaction (PCR) assays.[5,6]

PATHOPHYSIOLOGY

Although there is clearly a direct infectious component to Whipple's disease and, indeed, PCR can identify the characteristic unique bacterial 16S ribosomal RNA in affected tissues, there may be other potential etiologic factors that play a role in the phenotypic expression of this disease. Indeed there are 2 clinical stages of Whipple's disease, separated by a prolonged period of time. The initial manifestations are undoubtedly infectious and are characterized by fever, fatigue, arthralgias, or arthritis, whereas the later manifestation, which includes diarrhea, weight loss, musculoskeletal symptoms, hepatic, cardiac, pulmonary, neurologic, and ophthalmic manifestations, may have an autoimmune component superimposed on an underlying infectious process.

Several autoimmune and genetic abnormalities have been hypothesized to be potentially present in patients with Whipple's disease, with the predominant hypothesis being that immune abnormalities result in an increased risk of developing an infectious process such as Whipple's disease. It is well known that the majority of people exposed to Tropheryma whipplei do not develop this illness. In a study of the prevalence of the organism in saliva and duodenal biopsies and/or gastric juice of asymptomatic healthy carriers, there was evidence of the organism.[7] Between 1.5% and 7% of the general population may be asymptomatic carriers of the organism.[8] T whipplei is a ubiquitous commensal bacterium.

Autoimmune abnormalities have been described in patients with Whipple's disease. Circulating monocytes of patients with active Whipple's disease are endogenously stimulated to express prothrombinase activity.[9,10] A significantly reduced number of mononuclear cells express the complement receptor 3α chain (CD11b). T cells in acute Whipple's disease are activated and exhibit a low CD4/CD8 ratio.[11] Interleukin-16 is a critical cytokine in the pathogenesis of Whipple's disease in that the expression of this cytokine is crucial for the replication of T whipplei in a monocyte/macrophage model, and blocking of this cytokine can result in bacterial clearance.[12] An immune reconstitution syndrome characterized by fever and arthritis/arthralgias has also been described in a minority of patients after antibiotic therapy is instituted.[13] A genetic association with human leukocyte antigen (HLA) B27 has also been hypothesized, though not universally accepted.[14]

It is likely that the immunologic abnormalities in patients with Whipple's disease predispose to the expression of an infectious illness. However, there may be a "reactive" autoimmune type response in the correct genetic host that is responsible for some of the clinical manifestations of this illness.

EPIDEMIOLOGY

Whipple's disease is a rare condition, and little is known about its epidemiology. There is no universally accepted incidence rate,[15] but there have been estimates of a worldwide annual incidence of 12 new cases per year.[16] The incidence may be higher than previously thought owing to the establishment of PCR testing, which has definitively assisted in the diagnosis of this illness.

Whipple's disease tends to present in middle age and is more common in males.[17] As there is often a delay in the diagnosis attributable to nonspecific symptoms at presentation as well as antibiotic use before the expression of the most classic symptoms of the disease, the true age of onset is likely younger.[15] Whipple's disease has been reported in patients from 3 months to 83 years old, and a clinical review of 52 cases by Durand and colleagues[18] found that in such a patient population, the mean age of diagnosis was between 48 and 54 years old.

Whipple's disease affects males more often than females in an 8:1 ratio.[15] However, recent studies have noted an increase in female patients from 13% to 20% compared with earlier data.[16] The gender predisposition of Whipple's disease is largely unexplained. It may be that similarly to ankylosing spondylitis, the disease may be less symptomatic in women. Although there is no evidence supporting a familial prevalence of the disease,[15] genetic causes of disease expression have been proposed. In particular, an X-linked pattern of inheritance of regulatory genes integral in the expression of cytokines has been suggested. In addition, one review noted that 26% of patients with Whipple's disease were positive for HLA B27.[15]

Geographic and ethnic distributions also differ. In 696 cases studied, 55% were from Europe and 38% were from North America, with only a minority of cases in Hispanics, blacks, Indians, and Asians.[11] Farmers and people working outdoors have been noted to be more likely to contract Whipple's disease, suggesting that there may be a zoonotic component of transmission. This concept is particularly attractive, as T whipplei is gram-positive bacterium in the Actinomyces family, a group of bacteria active in decomposition of the soil and organic materials.[19] Although many cases have been noted to occur in rural areas and the disease can occur in local clusters, no environmental factors or habitats have been definitively associated with the disease.[20] The small intestines of a variety of domesticated animals have been tested for the presence of T whipplei. Although none of the samples were positive, the sample size was small and extraintestinal tissue was not sampled, so the presence of T whipplei in animals cannot be excluded. In a study that tested 38 samples of wastewater for DNA specific to T whipplei,[20] 25 of the 38 samples tested positive, supporting the argument that T whipplei may be acquired through the environment.

CLINICAL MANIFESTATIONS

As in other infectious illnesses such as Lyme disease, which have a diverse clinical spectrum including rheumatic manifestations, Whipple's disease tends to have 2 phases: an initial early phase with at times symptoms of infection but frequently including fever, arthritis, and/or arthralgias, followed by a late phase characterized by diarrhea, weight loss, and the potential involvement of almost every other organ system but predominantly affecting the eye, heart, and central nervous system (CNS).

Gastrointestinal

Whipple's disease can affect almost any organ system in the human body. However, this condition, initially termed "intestinal lipodystrophy,"[1] is frequently diagnosed on the basis of 1 of its cardinal symptoms, gastrointestinal involvement.

The mechanism of gastrointestinal manifestations of Whipple's disease is probably from direct infection of macrophages in the small intestine by T whipplei and the consequences of a chronic intestinal infection. The infection appears histologically as foamy, PAS-positive macrophages found throughout the small intestine.[21] The conse-quence of this contagion is the obliteration of the microvilli throughout the small intes-tine as well as lymphatic disruption. The particular localization and the subsequent effects on the surface of the gastrointestinal tract lead to many of the classic symp-toms of Whipple's disease. The duodenum, jejunum, and ileum are almost always affected, although liver, esophagus, stomach, and colon involvement have also been reported.[22] Liver involvement can include granulomas that are negative for PAS staining, perhaps representing an autoimmune rather than a direct infectious origin in this organ.[23]

The diagnosis of Whipple's disease is generally made through endoscopy and a duodenal biopsy that demonstrates the presence of foamy, PAS-positive macro-phages. Endoscopic evaluation reveals the destruction of the small intestinal mucosal architecture that results in pale, yellow lesions with shaggy, erythematous, and erosive mucosa. White-yellow plaques may also be present throughout the small intestine but not necessarily in a uniform pattern.[24] For this reason, it is important to biopsy both the proximal and distal duodenum and jejunum to ensure that the diagnosis is not missed. Although antibiotic therapy may affect the pathologic findings, PAS-positive material in the macrophages can persist for years. An increase in PAS-positive material after prior resolution may be an indication of relapse.[15]

The gastrointestinal symptoms of diarrhea, weight loss, and abdominal pain are the most common symptoms. However, manifestations of hepatosplenomegaly, anorexia, nutritional deficiencies, cachexia, hematochezia, and malabsorption are not uncom-mon findings of this disease. Diarrhea has been described as episodic or continuous, watery or fatty, and often occurs with colicky abdominal pain.[4,12] In one study, occult blood was noted in the stools of up to 20% to 30% of patients with diarrhea.[15] An abdominal mass caused by lymphadenopathy may also be noted. Unfortunately, not all patients with Whipple's disease present with gastrointestinal symptoms. Early on in disease onset, articular symptoms are more common. In a study of 52 patients with Whipple's disease, 35 (67%) showed early articular symptoms before diagnosis, whereas only 8 (15%) had gastrointestinal symptoms.[18] In this same study, before diagnosis 8 of the 52 patients had gastrointestinal manifestations of the disease. By the time of confirmative diagnosis, diarrhea and weight loss were present in 44 (85%) of patients. There are, however, other studies in which gastrointestinal symp-toms of diarrhea and weight loss were almost universally present by the time of diagnosis.[15] A study by Mahnel and Marth[25] of 27 patients with Whipple's disease found that symptoms of arthropathy occurred on average 8 years before the diagnosis of Whipple's disease in a majority of their patients. It is the later, gastrointestinal man-ifestations of the disease that most often lead to the diagnosis. This observation is particularly significant for rheumatologists, as it illustrates that although arthropathy may be a more common presenting symptoms of Whipple's disease, it is the gastro-intestinal symptoms that most often lead to definitive diagnosis.

Whipple's disease has been described in association with *Giardia*. In one study, 53 fixed duodenal biopsy samples from 25 patients with Whipple's disease were tested for the presence of *Giardia* and were compared with 150 duodenal biopsy samples from patients without Whipple's disease.[26] By histologic diagnosis, 3 of the 25 pa-tients with Whipple's disease had histologic evidence of giardiasis, whereas only 1 of the 150 control patients was affected. By PCR, 6 of the patients with Whipple's dis-ease were found to have evidence of *Giardia*, whereas this was found in only 2 of the control patients. A literature review identified 15 other cases of coinfection. There may be a common immune defect, a common source, or, perhaps, infection, with one or-ganism predisposed to infection with the other.

In one study, the gastrointestinal manifestations of Whipple's disease were noted to occur following initiation of immunosuppressive therapy for a presumed autoimmune arthropathy. This finding may lead to earlier identification of the disease, as the gastrointestinal symptoms occurred earlier than they otherwise would have.

Gastrointestinal manifestations of Whipple's disease are varied and may at times be atypical. This organ system tends to be affected later in the disease process, and is a hallmark and, at times, dominant component of this disease. It is important to recognize that there are patients without gastrointestinal manifestations who may have this illness.

Musculoskeletal

Musculoskeletal manifestations of Whipple's disease are very common, probably occurring in more than 80% of patients who have this illness.[17] Involvement of the musculoskeletal system can occur both early and late in the disease. A spectrum of presentations exists. Arthralgias and arthritis both can occur, and these findings usually present 6 to 7 years before a definitive diagnosis of the illness is made.[17] Although any pattern of arthritis can occur, an oligoarticular presentation, usually involving large joints, is most common, and the musculoskeletal symptoms may be migratory. Spondylitis has been described as occurring uncommonly. There may be an acute presentation followed by a more chronic polyarticular disease. As gastrointestinal manifestations present later in disease, frequently the musculoskeletal manifestations precede diarrhea and, as such, Whipple's disease is not usually suspected, given its rarity and the absence of gastrointestinal manifestations. Therefore it is a diagnosis that should at least be considered particularly in male patients with an idiopathic oligoarticular or migratory arthropathy affecting large joints.

Patients are seronegative for other rheumatic illnesses, but radiographic studies may demonstrate joint-space narrowing and ankylosis.[17] The organism has been cultured from synovial fluid[27] and has been detected using PCR amplification in synovial fluid and tissue.[28]

Nervous System

Neurologic manifestations can occur in 10% to 30% of patients with Whipple's disease. These symptoms have been described in both the CNS and peripheral nervous system (PNS). Neurologic involvement in Whipple's disease can present as either focal, isolated symptoms, or in an atypical nonuniform pattern dependent on lesion location. In one small study on postmortem examination of the brain and spinal cord, lesions were found in more than 90% patients.[16] Although most patients who have this disease do not demonstrate clinical evidence of neurologic disease, it seems that *T whipplei* invades the nervous system frequently.

A report of 12 cases of patients with neurologic manifestations of Whipple's disease found that neurologic symptoms in patients with this disease present either alone or with other manifestations of the disease.[29] Clinical patterns and presentations vary depending on the site of infection. For example, if lesions are located in the hemispheres of the brain a patient may display dementia, personality changes, hemiparesis, or seizures. If the lesion is located in the mesencephalon, patients may present with ophthalmoplegia, nystagmus, or Wernicke's encephalopathy. Hypothalamic lesions may lead to insomnia, hypersomnia, polyuria, and/or polydipsia, and hypothalamic-pituitary lesions can result in hypogonadism. Brainstem involvement can occur and is more common than spinal cord involvement. Peripheral nerve involvement has also been noted. Oculomasticatory myorhythmia and oculofacial skeletal myorhythmia do not occur in many other diseases, but have been described in Whipple's disease.

Other manifestations include personality changes, memory loss, psychosyndromes, ataxia, seizure, and hydrocephalus. CNS manifestations in patients with Whipple's disease carry a worse prognosis than those with disease limited to the bowel, and these patients are more likely to relapse.[15,30]

The diagnostic approach to neurologic Whipple's disease includes testing of cerebrospinal fluid (CSF), tissue biopsy, and neuroimaging modalities. Brain magnetic resonance imaging can be used to localize lesions and guide a stereotactic cerebral biopsy with brain computed tomography (CT). On CT, hypodense lesions and edema are characteristic of the disease.[29] PAS-positive perivascular macrophages, PCR-positive CSF or tissue biopsies confirm the diagnosis of neurologic Whipple's disease.

Whipple's disease can present in a myriad of ways in the nervous system. It is important to suspect this condition in any neurologic illnesses, particularly those associated with gastrointestinal symptomatology or other organ involvement. However, it is challenging that the neurologic manifestations of this condition are varied and can exist independently of any other clinical manifestations.

Ocular

Ophthalmic manifestations are uncommon, occurring in 4% to 27% of patients with Whipple's disease.[17] Although the most common ocular manifestation may be uveitis,[31] other manifestations such as keratitis, retinitis, choroiditis, optic neuritis, and orbital inflammatory disease have been described. Indeed, recurrent flares of orbital pseudotumor have been found to indicate relapse of the disease.[32] The diagnostic approach to patients with ophthalmic disease predominantly includes evaluation of vitreous fluid for PAS-positive macrophages and PCR.

Cardiac Manifestations

Although pericarditis has been frequently found in postmortem evaluations of patients with Whipple's disease, this is rarely symptomatic.[33] Endocarditis caused by this organism has been described in what was previously thought to be blood culture–negative endocarditis.[26] Valve replacement has been required in several patients, and PCR analysis of the valve has confirmed evidence of *T whipplei*.

DIAGNOSTIC TESTING

Although the definitive diagnostic approach to Whipple's disease necessitates a tissue diagnosis based on the specific organ involved, there are several useful published paradigms that outline strategies to identify the disease.[8,17] Clearly the disease needs to be suspected and, therefore, as in all rheumatic diseases, a comprehensive history and careful physical examination are the best screening tests.

PCR of stool and saliva may be helpful initial assessments, but a definitive diagnosis requires a targeted evaluation of a clinically involved organ. Therefore, clinically involved organs systems should be evaluated with fluid or tissue sampling for PAS and/or PCR positivity. In patients with gastrointestinal involvement, endoscopy with multiple biopsies of the duodenum and the jejunum should be performed. Patients with arthritis should have synovial fluid and synovial tissue analysis. Those with CNS involvement should have a CSF evaluation and, where appropriate, tissue evaluation of the CNS site of involvement. Those with ocular involvement should have aqueous and/or vitreous fluid evaluation, and those with cardiac disease should have evaluation of appropriate cultures and/or valvular tissue when appropriate. Electron microscopy, immunohistochemical labeling, and culture are available in only limited circumstances.[17]

THERAPY

The therapeutic strategy is to directly target *T whipplei* with appropriate antibiotic therapy, bearing in mind that if there is CNS involvement and/or ocular involvement, antibiotics that penetrate the blood-brain and blood-ocular barrier should be used. CNS Whipple's bears a worse prognosis and therefore should be treated more aggressively.

Various therapies have been recommended, and currently there are several therapeutic strategies. In an interesting prospective randomized study of 40 patients from central Europe with previously untreated Whipple's disease, groups were given daily infusions of either ceftriaxone or meropenem for 14 days, followed by oral trimethoprim-sulfamethoxazole for 12 months. The outcome measured was maintenance of remission for 3 years determined by a composite index. In this study all patients were observed for the entire follow-up period, and all achieved remission.[34] Another therapy proposed for patients without neurologic involvement uses hydroxychloroquine and doxycycline.[17] Interferon-γ has been used in a case report of CNS Whipple's disease.[35]

SUMMARY

Whipple's disease is a relatively new illness that has now been correctly identified as being caused by an infectious organism, *T whipplei*. It can affect any organ system, and the tropisms of this bacillus in an individual patient's organs may define the clinical presentation. The most commonly involved organs are the gastrointestinal, musculoskeletal, neurologic, cardiac, and ophthalmic systems, although all organisms are at risk. It has a predilection to affect males more frequently than females, and tends to strike in middle age. Early and late manifestations of this disease differ, but may overlap. Diagnostic modalities have been devised, but continue to evolve. Therapy can be curative with antibiotics.

The current challenges and future direction of research need to focus on better diagnostic tools such as serum assays for antibodies to *T whipplei* and on more definitive antibiotic regimens to eradicate the organism from an infected host. Overwhelmingly, however, the greatest challenge is to continue to educate physicians as to the nature and characteristics of this illness, as early diagnosis of Whipple's disease will definitively result in a better prognosis and reduced mortality.

REFERENCES

1. Whipple GH. A hitherto undescribed disease characterized anatomically by deposits of fat and fatty acids in the intestinal and mesenteric lymphatic tissues. Bull Johns Hopkins Hosp 1907;18:382–91.
2. Black-Schaffer B. The tinctoral demonstration of a glycoprotein in Whipple's disease. Proc Soc Exp Biol Med 1949;72(1):225–7.
3. Chears WC Jr, Ashworth CT. Electron microscopic study of the intestinal mucosa in Whipple's disease. Demonstration of encapsulated bacilliform bodies in the lesion. Gastroenterology 1961;41:129–38.
4. Raoult D, Birg ML, La Scola B, et al. Cultivation of the bacillus of Whipple's disease. N Engl J Med 2000;342(9):620–5.
5. von Herbay A, Ditton HJ, Maiwald M. Diagnostic application of a polymerase chain reaction assay for the Whipple's disease bacterium to intestinal biopsies. Gastroenterology 1996;110(6):1735–43.
6. Relman DA, Schmidt TM, MacDermott RP, et al. Identification of the uncultured bacillus of Whipple's disease. N Engl J Med 1992;327(5):293–301.

7. Dutly F, Hinrikson HP, Seidel T, et al. *Tropheryma whipplei* DNA in saliva of patients without Whipple's disease. Infection 2000;28(4):219–22.
8. Fenollar F, Puechal X, Raoult D. Whipple's disease. N Engl J Med 2007;356(1):55–66.
9. Ottaway CA, Warren RE, Saibil FG, et al. Monocyte procoagulant activity in Whipple's disease. J Clin Immunol 1984;4(5):348–58.
10. Dobbins WO 3rd. HLA antigens in Whipple's disease. Arthritis Rheum 1987;30(1):102–5.
11. Marth T, Roux M, von Herbay A, et al. Persistent reduction of complement receptor 3 alpha-chain expressing mononuclear blood cells and transient inhibitory serum factors in Whipple's disease. Clin Immunol Immunopathol 1994;72(2):217–26.
12. Desnues B, Raoult D, Mege JL. IL-16 is critical for *Tropheryma whipplei* replication in Whipple's disease. J Immunol 2005;175(7):4575–82.
13. Moos V, Feurle GE, Schinnerling K, et al. Immunopathology of immune reconstitution inflammatory syndrome in Whipple's disease. J Immunol 2013;190(5):2354–61.
14. Feurle GE. Association of Whipple's disease with HLA-B27. Lancet 1985;1(8441):1336.
15. Marth T, Raoult D. Whipple's disease. Lancet 2003;361(9353):239–46.
16. Dutly F, Altwegg M. Whipple's disease and "*Tropheryma whipplei*". Clin Microbiol Rev 2001;14(3):561–83.
17. Puechal X. Whipple's disease. Ann Rheum Dis 2013. [Epub ahead of print].
18. Durand DV, Lecomte C, Cathebras P, et al. Whipple disease. Clinical review of 52 cases. The SNFMI Research Group on Whipple Disease. Societé Nationale Francaise de Médecine Interne. Medicine 1997;76(3):170–84.
19. Schneider T, Moos V, Loddenkemper C, et al. Whipple's disease: new aspects of pathogenesis and treatment. Lancet Infect Dis 2008;8(3):179–90.
20. Maiwald M, Schuhmacher F, Ditton HJ, et al. Environmental occurrence of the Whipple's disease bacterium (*Tropheryma whipplei*). Appl Environ Microbiol 1998;64(2):760–2.
21. Yardley JH, Fleming WH 2nd. Whipple's disease: a note regarding PAS-positive granules in the original case. Bull Johns Hopkins Hosp 1961;109:76–9.
22. Gran JT, Husby G. Joint manifestations in gastrointestinal diseases. 2. Whipple's disease, enteric infections, intestinal bypass operations, gluten-sensitive enteropathy, pseudomembranous colitis and collagenous colitis. Dig Dis 1992;10(5):295–312.
23. Smyth C, Kelleher D, Keeling PW. Hepatic manifestations of gastrointestinal diseases. Inflammatory bowel disease, celiac disease, and Whipple's disease. Clin Liver Dis 2002;6(4):1013–32.
24. Martel W, Hodges FJ. The small intestine in Whipple's disease. Am J Roentgenol Radium Ther Nucl Med 1959;81(4):623–36.
25. Mahnel R, Marth T. Progress, problems, and perspectives in diagnosis and treatment of Whipple's disease. Clin Exp Med 2004;4(1):39–43.
26. Fenollar F, Lepidi H, Raoult D. Whipple's endocarditis: review of the literature and comparisons with Q fever, *Bartonella* infection, and blood culture-positive endocarditis. Clin Infect Dis 2001;33(8):1309–16.
27. Puechal X, Fenollar F, Raoult D. Cultivation of *Tropheryma whipplei* from the synovial fluid in Whipple's arthritis. Arthritis Rheum 2007;56(5):1713–8.
28. O'Duffy JD, Griffing WL, Li CY, et al. Whipple's arthritis: direct detection of *Tropheryma whipplei* in synovial fluid and tissue. Arthritis Rheum 1999;42(4):812–7.

29. Gerard A, Sarrot-Reynauld F, Liozon E, et al. Neurologic presentation of Whipple disease: report of 12 cases and review of the literature. Medicine 2002;81(6): 443–57.
30. von Herbay A, Ditton HJ, Schuhmacher F, et al. Whipple's disease: staging and monitoring by cytology and polymerase chain reaction analysis of cerebrospinal fluid. Gastroenterology 1997;113(2):434–41.
31. Rickman LS, Freeman WR, Green WR, et al. Brief report: uveitis caused by *Tropheryma whipplei* (Whipple's bacillus). N Engl J Med 1995;332(6):363–6.
32. Dearment MC, Woodward TA, Menke DM, et al. Whipple's disease with destructive arthritis, abdominal lymphadenopathy, and central nervous system involvement. J Rheumatol 2003;30(6):1347–50.
33. Maizel H, Ruffin JM, Dobbins WO 3rd. Whipple's disease: a review of 19 patients from one hospital and a review of the literature since 1950. 1970. Medicine 1993; 72(5):343–55.
34. Feurle GE, Junga NS, Marth T. Efficacy of ceftriaxone or meropenem as initial therapies in Whipple's disease. Gastroenterology 2010;138(2):478–86 [quiz: 411–72].
35. Schnider PJ, Reisinger EC, Gerschlager W, et al. Long-term follow-up in cerebral Whipple's disease. Eur J Gastroenterol Hepatol 1996;8(9):899–903.

Amyloidosis: A Clinical Overview

Bouke P.C. Hazenberg, MD, PhD

KEYWORDS

- Systemic amyloidosis • Amyloid fibril • Protein misfolding • Precursor protein
- Typing • Diagnosis • Treatment • Disease monitoring

KEY POINTS

- Amyloidosis is the name for some diseases caused by protein misfolding; 30 different soluble precursor proteins can aggregate and be deposited as insoluble amyloid fibrils.
- Amyloid deposition is localized or systemic; the 4 main types of systemic amyloidosis are AL (light chain), AA (inflammation), ATTR (hereditary and old age), and $A\beta_2M$ (dialysis).
- Clinical management comprises proof of amyloid, systemic evidence, reliable typing, precursor assessment, severity of organ disease, choice of treatment, and planned follow-up.
- The precursor-product concept is the current basis of treatment, thereby aiming to decrease the levels of precursor proteins in serum to normal or undetectable values. Future clinical research will be directed at stopping amyloid deposition and increasing amyloid clearance.
- Protein misfolding is not only a characteristic of amyloidosis; it is also involved in many other disabling cardiac and neurologic degenerative diseases that interfere with healthy aging.

INTRODUCTION

The description of the autopsy of a young man in 1639 by Nicolaes Fonteyn, a Dutch physician and poet who lived in Amsterdam, was probably the first report of a patient with systemic amyloidosis. Since then, lardaceous changes in enlarged organs, such as the liver, spleen, heart, and kidneys, have drawn the attention of pathologists such as Rokitansky. In 1854, Rudolph Virchow was one of the first to use the term amyloid for this amorphous and hyaline change in tissue because of an iodine-staining reaction similar to that of starch (amylon; Greek for origin). Although it is now known that amyloid has nothing to do with starch, the term amyloid is still in use today. Bennhold

Funding Sources: None.
Conflict of Interest: Previous member of the Clinical Advisory Board of Neurochem; Chair of an External Safety Advisory Committee of GSK.
Department of Rheumatology & Clinical Immunology, AA21, University Medical Center Groningen, University of Groningen, PO Box 30.001, 9700 RB Groningen, The Netherlands
E-mail address: b.p.c.hazenberg@umcg.nl

Rheum Dis Clin N Am 39 (2013) 323–345
http://dx.doi.org/10.1016/j.rdc.2013.02.012 rheumatic.theclinics.com
0889-857X/13/$ – see front matter © 2013 Elsevier Inc. All rights reserved.

introduced Congo Red staining in 1922 as a useful method to identify amyloid in tissue specimens. In 1927, Divry and Florkin described the characteristic green birefringence when Congo Red-stained amyloid was viewed under polarized light. In 1959, Cohen and Calkins detected the fibril nature of amyloid when viewed under the electron microscope.[1]

Amyloidosis is the name for 30 protein-folding diseases (**Table 1**), all characterized by extracellular deposition of a specific soluble precursor protein that aggregates in the form of insoluble fibrils. These rigid and unbranching fibrils, approximately 10 nm in diameter, are characterized by a molecular β-pleated sheet structure that is usually composed of peptides arranged in an antiparallel configuration. This structure of the fibrils is responsible for its insolubility, resistance to proteolysis, and binding affinity for Congo Red dye that shows a characteristic green birefringence when viewed under polarized light (**Fig. 1**).[2]

The aim of this article is to present a clinical overview of the different types of amyloidosis, disease manifestations, patient management, diagnosis, imaging techniques, treatment, and follow-up.

AMYLOID STRUCTURE AND PATHOGENESIS

Amyloidoses are protein-misfolding diseases in which small (parts of) proteins of about 10 to 15 kDa acquire an alternative and relatively misfolded state at minimum energy and subsequently aggregate into oligomers and polymers. Three mechanisms seem to operate independently or in combination: the precursor protein may have an intrinsic propensity to misfold that becomes evident with aging (wild-type transthyretin) or as high serum levels (serum amyloid A protein and immunoglobulin free light chains); a hereditary acquired mutated protein (transthyretin); and proteolytic remodeling of the precursor protein (β-amyloid precursor protein). Interaction with the extracellular matrix also seems to be important and may be related to preferential deposition of amyloid in some organs or tissues.[3]

Extracellular deposition of amyloid fibrils in organs and tissues results in tissue infiltration and swelling leading to progressive loss of function of the affected organ. Sometimes toxic effects, believed to be caused by toxic oligomers, have been observed (eg, in cerebral amyloid). These oligomers are nonfibrillar intermediate aggregates that are formed early in the process of fibril formation. Another constituent of all amyloid is serum amyloid P component (SAP), a glycoprotein that belongs to the pentraxin family and binds to all types of amyloid in a calcium-dependent way. SAP is highly protected against proteolysis and thus makes amyloid fibrils resistant to degradation. Apolipoprotein E is also a constituent of amyloid. Glycosaminoglycans (eg, heparan sulfate) are found in all types of amyloid and interact with extracellular matrix components such as laminin, entactin, and collagen IV. This interaction probably constitutes a scaffold that facilitates the initial phase of fibril nucleation and could have a targeting role in the localization of amyloid deposits in tissue.[3]

TYPES OF AMYLOIDOSIS

Deposition of amyloid is localized (ie, fibrils produced in and limited to 1 organ or site of the body) or systemic (ie, fibril deposition in various organs and tissues throughout the body). The current classification of amyloidosis (see **Table 1**) is based on the chemical characterization of the precursor protein.[2,4]

Organ-specific localized amyloidosis can be found in Alzheimer disease (β-protein in the plaques) and diabetes mellitus type 2 (amylin in the islands of Langerhans). The pathogenic role of amyloid deposition in these diseases is unclear.[4] Nodular

Table 1
Amyloid fibril proteins and their precursors in humans

Fibril Protein	Precursor Protein	Systemic or Localized	Acquired or Hereditary	Target Organs
AL	Immunoglobulin light chain	S, L	A	All organs except CNS
AH	Immunoglobulin heavy chain	S, L	A	All organs except CNS
Aβ2M	β2-microglobulin, wild type	S	A	Musculoskeletal system
	β2-microglobulin, variant	S	H	ANS
ATTR	Transthyretin, wild type	S, L	A	Heart mainly in men, tenosynovium
	Transthyretin, variants	S	H	PNS, ANS, heart, eye, leptomeninges
AA	(Apo) serum amyloid A	S	A	All organs except CNS
AApoAI	Apolipoprotein A I, variants	S	H	Heart, liver, kidney, PNS, testis, larynx (C-terminal variants), skin (C-terminal variants)
AApoAII	Apolipoprotein A II, variants	S	H	Kidney
AApoAIV	Apolipoprotein A IV, wild type	S	A	Kidney medulla and systemic
AGel	Gelsolin, variants	S	H	PNS, cornea
ALys	Lysozyme, variants	S	H	Kidney
ALect2	Leukocyte chemotactic factor-2	S	A	Kidney, primarily
AFib	Fibrinogen α, variants	S	H	Kidney, primarily
ACys	Cystatin C, variants	S	H	PNS, skin
ABri	ABriPP, variants	S	H	CNS
ADan[a]	ADanPP, variants	L	H	CNS
Aβ	Aβ protein precursor, wild type	L	A	CNS
	Aβ protein precursor, variant	L	H	CNS
APrP	Prion protein, wild type	L	A	CJD, fatal insomnia
	Prion protein, variants	L	H	CJD, GSS syndrome, fatal insomnia
ACal	(Pro)calcitonin	L	A	C-cell thyroid tumors
AIAPP	Islet amyloid polypeptide[b]	L	A	Islets of Langerhans, insulinomas
AANF	Atrial natriuretic factor	L	A	Cardiac atria
APro	Prolactin	L	A	Pituitary prolactinomas, aging pituitary
AIns	Insulin	L	A	Iatrogenic, local injection
ASPC	Lung surfactant protein	L	A	Lung
AGal7	Galectin 7	L	A	Skin
ACor	Corneodesmin	L	A	Cornified epithelia, hair follicles

(continued on next page)

Table 1
(continued)

Fibril Protein	Precursor Protein	Systemic or Localized	Acquired or Hereditary	Target Organs
AMed	Lactadherin	L	A	Senile aortic, media
AKer	Kerato-epithelin	L	A	Cornea, hereditary
ALac	Lactoferrin	L	A	Cornea
AOaap	Odontogenic ameloblast-associated protein	L	A	Odontogenic tumors
ASem1	Semenogelin 1	L	A	Vesicula seminalis

Abbreviations: ANS, autonomic nervous system; CJD, Creutzfeldt-Jakob disease; CNS, central nervous system; GSS, Gerstmann-Straussler-Scheinker syndrome; PNS, peripheral nervous system.
[a] ADan is the product of the same gene as Abri.
[b] Also called amylin.
Data from Sipe JD, Benson MD, Buxbaum JN, et al. Amyloid fibril protein nomenclature: 2012 recommendations from the Nomenclature Committee of the International Society of Amyloidosis. Amyloid 2012;19:167–70.

localized amyloid is an incidental finding and can be present in the skin (not only nodular but also macular amyloid and lichen amyloidosis), eyelid, conjunctiva, breast, larynx, bronchial tree, lung, and genitourinary tract. In most cases, low numbers of clonal plasma cells can be detected in the biopsy sample. Surgery is usually the treatment of choice. Local recurrence is frequent and can again be treated surgically.[5] Localized nodular skin amyloidosis is sometimes associated with Sjögren disease.[6] In contrast to localized amyloidosis, systemic amyloidosis leads to serious signs and symptoms caused by progressive disease in organs and tissues. There are many types of systemic amyloidosis (see **Table 1**), but 4 types are seen most frequently: AL, AA, ATTR, and $A\beta_2M$ amyloidosis.[4]

AL amyloidosis is the most common type. This disease is caused by a clonal plasma cell dyscrasia; it often occurs as low-grade clonal disease, sometimes multiple myeloma, and rarely non-Hodgkin lymphoma or Waldenström disease. The precursor of this type of amyloid is either lambda or kappa immunoglobulin free light chain. Clinical manifestations are diverse, such as cardiomyopathy, nephrotic syndrome, renal failure, hepatomegaly, splenomegaly, orthostatic hypotension, diarrhea, intestinal

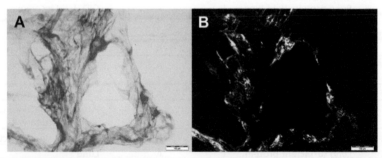

Fig. 1. A sample of abdominal subcutaneous fat aspirate containing amyloid deposits, stained with Congo Red. (*A*) Viewed in normal light, amyloid is stained red. Bar length is 100 µm. (*B*) Viewed in polarized light, amyloid shows apple-green birefringence (*collagen is bluish-gray*).

pseudoobstruction, peripheral neuropathy, autonomic neuropathy, arthropathy, carpal tunnel syndrome (CTS), bleeding, adrenal dysfunction, goiter, pulmonary problems, weight loss, fatigue, malaise, and glossomegaly.[7]

The second most common type is AA amyloidosis. This disease is caused by long-standing inflammation, such as rheumatoid arthritis, inflammatory bowel disease, chronic infections (eg, tuberculosis, osteomyelitis, leprosy), and hereditary autoinflammatory diseases (eg, familial Mediterranean fever, also called FMF). The precursor of this type is the HDL3-associated apolipoprotein serum amyloid A protein (SAA), an acute phase reactant. Signs of kidney disease, such as proteinuria (progressing to nephrotic syndrome) and loss of renal function (progressing to renal failure), are observed most frequently (in about 90% of cases), followed at a distance by autonomic neuropathy, bowel involvement, splenomegaly, hepatomegaly, goiter, and cardiomyopathy.[8,9]

The third most common type is ATTR amyloidosis. The familial form of this disease is caused by many autosomal dominantly inherited point mutations of the precursor protein transthyretin (TTR). Transthyretin is an acronym for the transport protein of thyroid hormone and retinol-binding protein. About 100 of these TTR mutations have been described, but most common is the TTR-Met30 mutation. Clinical manifestations are predominantly peripheral and autonomic neuropathy, but also cardiomyopathy, renal failure, and eye involvement (vitreous opacities) are frequently observed. Sometimes a severe cardiomyopathy is the initial presentation of the disease.[10] There is also a nonfamilial acquired form of ATTR amyloidosis. In this disease of old-aged men (rarely women), nonmutated (wild-type) TTR can also act as an amyloid precursor by a still unknown mechanism. This wild-type ATTR amyloidosis (formerly called senile systemic amyloidosis) is characterized by a slowly progressive cardiomyopathy, frequently associated with CTS, but without other neuropathy.[11]

The fourth type is $A\beta_2M$ amyloidosis. This disease is caused by end-stage renal disease in which highly increased serum levels of β_2-microglobulin persist for years because β_2-microglobulin is not effectively cleared by dialysis. The disease is characterized by high serum levels of β_2-microglobulin and posttranslational modifications to be deposited as amyloid fibrils in predominantly osteoarticular tissues. CTS and shoulder pain are among the first manifestations, followed by large periarticular cysts and sometimes by pathologic fractures, or a destructive spondylarthropathy.[12,13] Recently, a hereditary $A\beta_2M$ amyloidosis has been described, characterized by autonomic neuropathy and slowly progressive gastrointestinal symptoms.[14]

Other types of systemic amyloidosis are rare.[15] However, in patients without a family history of amyloid disease, a hereditary type of amyloidosis may be present.[16] In patients with almost exclusive kidney disease, other types should be considered, such as fibrinogen α,[17] lysozyme,[18] apolipoprotein A I, apolipoprotein A II, apolipoprotein A IV, and the recently described leukocyte chemotactic factor-2.[19] In patients with almost exclusive cardiac or neuropathic disease, the apolipoprotein A I type should not be overlooked. In patients with hepatic amyloid, the lysozyme and apolipoprotein A I type can be present. Apolipoprotein A I can be present in the skin and larynx. Gelsolin is typically found in lattice corneal dystrophy.[20]

EPIDEMIOLOGY

Even in developed countries, few incidence data have been collected systematically.[21] The data from 1 study about the incidence of AL amyloidosis in Olmsted County, Minnesota, are still used. In this study, the overall age-adjusted and sex-adjusted 95% confidence interval was 5.1 to 12.8 per million patients per year.[22] In a recent Swedish study, the estimated incidence of AL amyloidosis was 3.2 per million per year and AA amyloidosis 2.0 per million per year.[23] The median age for AL and AA amyloidosis is between 55 and 60 years.[24] The prognosis of untreated patients is poor, as noticed in older studies; median survival was 6 to 12 months for AL amyloidosis and 3 to 4 years for AA amyloidosis.[24] The estimated median survival of untreated patients with hereditary ATTR amyloidosis is almost 10 years, although some patients may survive up to 15 years. An estimate of mortality is that 0.5 to 1.0 per 1000 persons die in the United Kingdom because of AL amyloidosis.[25] In most studies of patients with the AL type, the proportion of men is somewhat higher (about 1.1–1.3) than women. The reverse (more women than men) is observed for AA amyloidosis because of the high proportion of patients (mainly women) with underlying rheumatoid arthritis. In developing countries, the prevalence of AA amyloidosis is higher than AL amyloidosis because of the higher prevalence of associated underlying infectious diseases.

PATIENT MANAGEMENT

A stepwise approach is useful for the clinical management of a patient with systemic amyloidosis (**Box 1**).[26] If amyloidosis is suspected, the first step is to obtain histologic proof of amyloid, followed by a search for evidence of systemic amyloid deposition in the patient. The next 2 steps are to determine the type of amyloid with confidence followed by detection and (in AA and AL) quantification of the precursor protein in the blood. A thoughtful clinical evaluation should lead to useful knowledge on the severity of organ involvement, associated risks, prognosis, and an overview of all treatment options. The most effective treatment of the underlying precursor-producing process with acceptable risks and side effects should then be discussed with the patient. In the final step, a proactive plan is made to evaluate the chosen treatment during follow-up. In this plan, the effects of treatment must be monitored by assessing serum precursor levels and the amyloid load of the body. Although the amyloid load of the body cannot be measured directly, it is indirectly reflected by the function and size of affected organs and by specific imaging techniques.

DETECTION OF AMYLOID

Detection of amyloid should start with a reasonable clinical suspicion of amyloidosis. Clinical suspicion may increase on finding unexplained signs such as proteinuria, organomegaly (liver, spleen, or tongue), right-sided cardiac failure and/or biventricular hypertrophic cardiac walls, orthostatic hypotension, peripheral axonal polyneuropathy or autonomic neuropathy (especially the combination of the 2), and malabsorption.[4]

Box 1
Clinical management of a patient with systemic amyloidosis

Definite proof of amyloid in tissue

Convincing evidence for systemic amyloid deposition

Unequivocal characterization of the type of amyloid

Detection and/or quantification of the serum precursor protein

Assessment of clinical severity of organ and tissue involvement

Balanced choice of the most effective treatment with lowest risks

Planned monitoring of the effect of treatment during follow-up

Sometimes, however, an alert pathologist performs a Congo Red stain after finding eosinophilic material in a tissue biopsy even without any clinical suspicion of amyloid. In that situation, the clinician has to deal with amyloid as a new and unsuspected finding.

Amyloid is a tissue-based diagnosis. Therefore, the diagnosis of amyloid is based on detecting its presence in tissue. The presence of amyloid is proved by a tissue specimen showing positive for Congo Red stain and the characteristic apple-green birefringence in polarized light (see **Fig. 1**). Subcutaneous abdominal fat tissue is easily accessible for this purpose and a video of such a fat aspiration procedure is available on the Web site at www.amyloid.nl.[27] Ample fat tissue can also be obtained by a simple surgical procedure.[28] Fat tissue stained with Congo Red has high sensitivity for AL, AA, and hereditary ATTR (up to 90%) and high specificity (almost 100%) if stained properly and viewed by experienced observers using a high-quality microscope with a good light source.[29] Sensitivity of rectum tissue for these types is about 80% and about 60% for bone marrow in AL. Although a biopsy of the affected organ (eg, kidney, liver, or heart) has the highest sensitivity (about 100%), it is recommended to start with a biopsy of a clinically uninvolved site, such as fat tissue, rectum, bone marrow, salivary gland, or gingiva, to avoid a biopsy of a vital organ and the associated risk of serious bleeding. In wild-type ATTR amyloidosis, the sensitivity of fat tissue analysis is a bit lower, about 73%.[30]

New staining methods for amyloid have been developed, such as luminescent conjugated oligothiophenes (LCOs). The first results showed that these molecules seem to bind to amyloid with higher sensitivity and greater selectivity than Congo Red, as determined by fluorescence microscopy and light polarization microscopy. Spectral profiles of tissue samples from 96 patients identified 3 nonoverlapping classes, which were found to match AA, AL, and ATTR types.[31] If these promising data can be confirmed by other investigators, this new staining technique might lead to improved detection of amyloid.

If amyloid has been found in a site specific for localized amyloidosis (genitourinary tract, eyelid, conjunctiva, larynx, and so forth.) it is recommended to screen for amyloid in another site of the body, such as fat tissue, rectum, bone marrow, or salivary glands, before diagnosing localized amyloidosis. Systemic amyloidosis is diagnosed if amyloid is present in 2 different sites of the body. There is consensus that systemic amyloidosis is also present if amyloid has been detected in only 1 site of the body in combination with a classic picture of amyloidosis (**Table 2**) at an alternate site.[32]

TYPING OF AMYLOID WITH CONFIDENCE

After detection of amyloid, the specific type of amyloid should be characterized with confidence. In most cases the type of amyloid can be assumed because of the medical history and clinical picture. Nevertheless, even in patients with strong clinical evidence for a particular type of amyloid, it is still necessary to search for solid evidence of the specific type of amyloid involved because incorrect typing of amyloid can have severe clinical consequences. The prognosis and treatment modalities differ enormously among the 4 main types of systemic amyloidosis.

The usual method of typing amyloid is by immunohistochemistry of a biopsy sample using specific antibodies. In AA amyloidosis, this technique is sufficient provided sensitive and specific monoclonal antibodies are used. However, immunohistochemistry is less reliable in ATTR amyloidosis and is frequently even useless to demonstrate AL amyloidosis.[33,34] The absence of a positive family history does not exclude ATTR

Table 2 Organ involvement: positive biopsy at an alternate site[a] and a positive organ criterion	
Organ	**Criterion**
Kidney	24-h urine protein >0.5 g/d, predominantly albumin
Heart	Echo: mean wall thickness >12 mm, no other cardiac cause
Liver	Total liver span >15 cm in the absence of heart failure or alkaline phosphatase >1.5 times institutional upper limit of normal
Nerve	Peripheral: clinical; symmetric lower extremity sensorimotor peripheral neuropathy Autonomic: gastric-emptying disorder, pseudoobstruction, voiding dysfunction not related to direct organ infiltration
Gastrointestinal tract	Direct biopsy verification with symptoms
Lung	Direct biopsy verification with symptoms Interstitial radiographic pattern
Soft tissue	Tongue enlargement, clinical Arthropathy Claudication, presumed vascular amyloid Skin Myopathy by biopsy or pseudohypertrophy Lymph node (may be localized) Carpal tunnel syndrome

[a] Alternate sites available to confirm the histologic diagnosis of amyloidosis: fine-needle abdominal fat aspirate and/or biopsy of the minor salivary glands, rectum, or gingiva.

Data from Gertz MA, Comenzo R, Falk RH, et al. Definition of organ involvement and treatment response in immunoglobulin light chain amyloidosis (AL): a consensus opinion from the 10th International Symposium on Amyloid and Amyloidosis, Tours, France, 18–22 April 2004. Am J Med 2005;79:319–28.

amyloidosis, as demonstrated by several sporadic cases.[16] Therefore, a TTR mutation has to be confirmed by DNA analysis in ATTR amyloidosis. The exception to this rule is wild-type ATTR amyloidosis in which, by definition, a TTR mutation is absent.

In patients with AL amyloidosis, an underlying monoclonal plasma cell dyscrasia with overproduction of either lambda or kappa light chains can usually be detected by investigating bone marrow (clonal dominance by immunophenotyping of plasma cells), urine (Bence Jones proteins, immunofixation of concentrated urine), and blood (M-protein, immunofixation, and, most important of all, by the free light chain assay). Detection of a monoclonal gammopathy of undetermined significance does not exclude other types than AL amyloidosis. The clinical pictures of ATTR amyloidosis and AL amyloidosis are sometimes quite similar, for example, in cases with polyneuropathy, autonomic neuropathy, cardiomyopathy, or CTS. If such a clinical picture is present, it is not sufficient to detect the presence of a plasma cell dyscrasia; it is also necessary to exclude a TTR mutation before reliably concluding AL amyloidosis.[16] In elderly men, the choice between wild-type ATTR and AL amyloidosis may be hard to make if a slightly increased serum free light chain is detected in a patient with cardiomyopathy as the sole disease manifestation.

New proteomics techniques have been developed to chemically analyze the protein composition of tissues. The application of proteomics seems to be a promising tool for reliable typing of amyloid.[35–39] These techniques, with high sensitivity and high specificity, are especially helpful to distinguish between AL and ATTR amyloid. One of these elegant techniques combines specific sampling by laser microdissection with the analytical power of proteomic analysis based on tandem mass spectrometry.[37]

However, currently these sophisticated, expensive, and time-consuming techniques are only available in highly specialized centers, so for the time being immunohisto-chemistry remains the standard procedure for typing of amyloid.[40]

DISEASE MANIFESTATIONS

Although amyloidosis must have been present for a long time (often more than a year, looking back to the start of the first symptoms), the disease goes unnoticed until alarming symptoms appear relatively late in its course. Nonspecific complaints such as fatigue and weight loss gradually appear and can be debilitating, but are often noticed only after disease progression leads to more specific signs, such as edema, dyspnea, bleeding, or orthostatic hypotension. A limited overview of the diverse disease manifestations of the main types of amyloidosis[4,7–10,24] is presented in this section.

Renal disease is often seen in both AL and AA amyloidosis (in about 70%–90% of cases) and rarely in ATTR amyloidosis. Sometimes the presentation is unremark-able as asymptomatic proteinuria, but often it appears dramatically as frank nephrotic syndrome or severe renal failure. The insidious nature of amyloidosis keeps the disease unnoticed for a while until edema appears as a first sign of the disease.

Edema, however, is also a presenting sign of cardiac disease. Signs and symptoms of right-sided heart failure (edema, increased jugular venous pressure, third heart sound, and hepatomegaly) are often seen. The clinical picture is that of a constrictive cardiomyopathy, initially affecting the inflow of the heart more than the outflow. The ejection fraction and cardiac size on the chest radiograph usually remain in the normal range for a long time. Hypotension is often a prominent feature. Rapidly progressive cardiac involvement is frequently part of the clinical picture of AL amyloidosis (in about 40%–60% of cases), whereas slowly progressive cardiomyopathy is usually seen in ATTR amyloidosis. Cardiomyopathy is infrequent (about 5% of cases) in AA amyloid-osis. A characteristic low-voltage pattern or a pseudoanteroseptal infarction pattern is sometimes visible on the electrocardiogram. The combination of a low-voltage pattern and thickened ventricular walls (left and right) on cardiac ultrasonography is pathogno-monic for an infiltrative cardiomyopathy such as amyloidosis. Accumulation of amyloid in the coronary arteries may lead to (often atypical) angina or infarction. Ventricular tachycardia is a frequent and dangerous complication of AL amyloidosis. Conduction disturbances are often seen in ATTR amyloidosis and can necessitate insertion of a pacemaker in the long term. Increased serum N-terminal pro-brain natriuretic peptide (NT-proBNP) and troponin-T concentrations can reveal asymptomatic cardiac involvement and help to assess associated risks before the start of any treatment.[41] Midregional proadrenomedullin (MR-proADM) seems to be a new and powerful prog-nostic marker in AL amyloidosis, which may not only reflect cardiac dysfunction but also widespread systemic disease, and can be combined with troponin-T to detect patients at risk of early death.[42]

Hepatomegaly is rare in AA amyloidosis and is not seen in ATTR amyloidosis. It is sometimes a presenting feature of AL amyloidosis, and the characteristic biochemical profile of intrahepatic cholestasis shows an increase in γ-glutamine transpeptidase, followed by alkaline phosphatase and the bilirubin concentration. It is not always easy to distinguish amyloid hepatomegaly from liver enlargement secondary to right-sided cardiac failure. Splenomegaly is seen in about 5% of patients with AL amyloid-osis and hyposplenism (identified by Howell-Jolly bodies or target cells) is present in about 25%. Malabsorption, pseudoobstruction, ulceration, and gastrointestinal bleeding are infrequent but severe manifestations of bowel involvement. Gastroparesis, constipation, and diarrhea are more common and seem to be caused by autonomic neuropathy. Sometimes the clinical picture is worsened by bacterial overgrowth.

Peripheral sensory polyneuropathy, with ascending symptoms of numbness, paresthesia, and pain, is frequently observed in AL and ATTR amyloidosis but is extremely rare in AA amyloidosis. Autonomic neuropathy is seen in all types of amyloidosis but is most frequent and severe in AL and ATTR amyloidosis; it can lead to orthostatic hypotension, impotence, bladder voiding disturbances, early sensation of fullness, nausea, vomiting, diarrhea, and constipation.

Although CTS is a neuropathy of the median nerve and can therefore be part of a generalized polyneuropathy, it is usually caused by entrapment caused by synovial thickening through amyloid. CTS can be a manifestation of amyloid arthropathy (with the characteristic shoulder-pad sign and pseudoarthritis of the small hand joints and wrists) in AL and $A\beta_2M$ amyloidosis. CTS is sometimes seen in wild-type ATTR amyloidosis. A diversity of other manifestations may be present in AL amyloidosis, such as waxy skin and skin nodules, easy bruising (vascular wall fragility), periorbital purpura (raccoon eyes), coagulation abnormalities caused by Factor X deficiency (as a result of increased removal by binding to amyloid), macroglossia (in about 20% of cases) with indentations and submandibular swelling, dystrophic nails, taste disturbance, hoarseness, jaw claudication, musculopathy (pseudohypertrophy or muscular dystrophy), bladder bleeding, lymphadenopathy, subclinical hypothyroidism, and hypoadrenalism. Pulmonary amyloidosis is characterized by a reticulonodular pattern on the chest radiograph and is rare. Pleural amyloidosis goes often undetected, but becomes visible as rapidly progressive, relatively large, and diuretics-resistant pleural effusions, usually during concomitant cardiac failure. Vitreous opacities may be present, but only in ATTR amyloidosis in some of the TTR mutations. Central nervous system involvement is unusual. Meningeal amyloidosis is only seen in some mutations in ATTR amyloidosis. Involvement of the pituitary gland has been described, but is rare.[43–45] Ischemic stroke may be seen and is often caused by an embolism derived from the affected heart.[46]

IMAGING OF AMYLOIDOSIS

Amyloidoses are difficult diseases to diagnose. Their insidious appearance, the diverse ways they present to many medical specialists, the often severely affected organ function at diagnosis and the dangerous combinations of vital organs affected all demand that the treating physician obtains a clear overview of the amyloid disease. The clinician needs relevant information about the function and size of affected vital organs. This information is essential both for diagnosis and for disease monitoring during follow-up. Blood tests can be used to assess organ function, whereas imaging can be used to assess size and function of organs. Ultrasonography of the abdomen, heart, and musculoskeletal system, magnetic resonance imaging (MRI) of the heart, bone scintigraphy, and SAP scintigraphy are all useful imaging techniques in selected cases.

Ultrasonography, computed tomography (CT), and MRI are well-known techniques to evaluate the size of the kidneys, liver, and spleen. Musculoskeletal ultrasonography is useful in $A\beta_2M$ amyloidosis.[47] Cardiac ultrasonography is the method of choice to quickly investigate the presence of myocardial sparkling, restriction to diastolic filling, ejection fraction, and the thickness of the interventricular septum, left ventricular posterior wall, and right ventricular wall. MRI of the heart can show global gadolinium late enhancement in a subendocardial distribution that is highly sensitive and specific for the identification of cardiac involvement.[48] [^{123}I]metaiodobenzylguanidine may help to detect cardiac sympathetic denervation.[49] Aprotinin scintigraphy has been used successfully for the identification of cardiac involvement in AL amyloidosis.[50] A disadvantage of this tracer, however, is the potential infectious risk, because it is a polypeptide derived from bovine lung tissue. Technetium Tc 99m pyrophosphate and diphosphonate sometimes bind to amyloid and have been used as imaging agents in amyloidosis, especially for detecting cardiac involvement in ATTR amyloidosis (**Fig. 2**).[51,52] A similar tracer (3,3-diphosphono-1,2-propanodicarboxylic acid) has also been shown to be useful for this purpose.[53,54]

SAP scintigraphy was developed in London by Hawkins and colleagues[55] to detect and identify the distribution of amyloid in systemic amyloidosis. SAP binds in a calcium-dependent way to all amyloid deposits. Scintigraphy with ^{123}I-labeled SAP shows

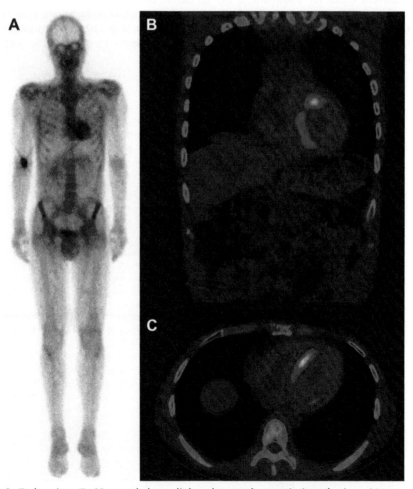

Fig. 2. Technetium Tc 99m-methylene diphosphonate bone scintigraphy in a 31-year-old man with ATTR amyloidosis. (A) Total body scan with increased cardiac uptake and soft tissue uptake. The skeletal uptake is relatively diminished. (B) Coronal and (C) transverse single photon emission-computed tomography/CT images of the heart showing increased uptake in the ventricular walls.

specific uptake in the liver, spleen, kidneys, adrenals, bone marrow, and joints (**Fig. 3**).[55–57] The heart cannot be visualized with this technique. Sensitivity of the SAP scan for AL and AA amyloidosis is about 90%, but it is only 48% for hereditary ATTR amyloidosis. Specificity is about 90%. SAP is isolated and purified from serum of healthy donors and the potential infectious risk is probably the major reason why this useful technique is currently being used only in the United Kingdom and The Netherlands. Measurement of ^{123}I SAP retention in the body after 24 or 48 hours provides a rough quantitative estimate of the amyloid load in the patient.[58,59] Recently, an amyloid fibril–specific monoclonal antibody, 11-1F4, has shown promising results in detecting AL amyloidosis when used as a tracer in positron emission tomography/CT.[60]

TREATMENT

The current basis for treatment is the so-called precursor-product concept. The central idea of this concept is that further growth of amyloid deposits will stop when the supply of necessary precursors is stopped. Thus, it is important to diagnose amyloidosis early and start treatment as early as possible to stabilize the disease and prevent ongoing progression.

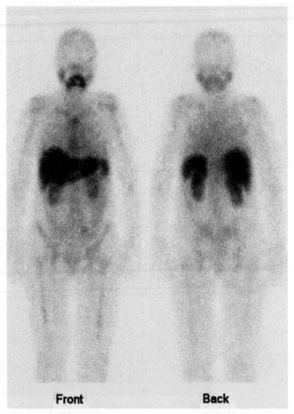

Front   **Back**

Fig. 3. Total body SAP scintigraphy (anterior and posterior images) of a 60-year-old woman with systemic amyloidosis (probably AL type) with increased uptake (++) in the liver, spleen, and kidneys and (+) bone marrow. Minor nonspecific uptake can be seen in the parotid glands, nasopharynx and stomach.

Treatment for AA amyloidosis is aimed at decreasing SAA serum levels to normal basal values (<3 mg/L).[8] If this level can be reached and maintained at less than 10 mg/L, the 10-year survival rate increases to 90%; when the SAA levels are more than 10 mg/L, this figure is less than 40%.[61] The only way to achieve a normal basal serum value of SAA is by complete suppression or eradication of the underlying chronic inflammatory disease. This can be realized in patients with infectious diseases such as tuberculosis, leprosy, recurrent pulmonary infections, and osteomyelitis through eradication of the infection by antibiotic treatment sometimes combined with surgery. The treatment of chronic inflammatory diseases such as rheumatoid arthritis, ankylosing spondylitis, psoriatic arthritis, and Crohn disease has improved dramatically in the last decades. Because of the introduction of more effective antiinflammatory drugs such as methotrexate and biologics, especially those directed against tumor necrosis factor (TNF) and interleukin-1 (IL-1), effective suppression of SAA to low or even normal serum concentrations has become a realistic goal. In addition, the autoinflammatory diseases such as FMF, TNF-receptor associated periodic syndromes, the hyper-IgD syndrome, and cryopyrin-associated periodic syndromes often respond well to some of these biologics, especially anakinra, which is directed against IL-1.[62] A promising new biologic is tocilizumab, an anti-IL6 receptor antibody that directly suppresses the production of C-reactive protein and SAA by the liver.[63]

Treatment for AL amyloidosis is aimed at eradicating the underlying plasma cell dyscrasia by chemotherapy, and return the abnormally increased level of kappa or lambda free light chain in the blood to the normal range.[64] High-dose melphalan (HDM) followed by autologous stem cell transplantation (ASCT) in eligible patients has shown considerable benefits.[65] Median survival in this low-risk group, the ones illegible for ASCT, was 4.6 years. However, 1 randomized clinical trial questioned the favorable results of HDM followed by ASCT.[66] Meanwhile, many more studies of novel drugs, such as thalidomide, bortezomib, lenalidomide, pomalidomide, and MLN9708, have shown clear effects, often with the best effects in combination with dexamethasone.[67] In a review by Gatt and Palladini,[67] a state-of-the-art treatment schedule is presented for low-risk, intermediate-risk and high-risk patients. The survival of responding patients has increased and recent reports of patient cohorts on long-term survival are encouraging. However, early deaths due to advanced, irreversible cardiac dysfunction at presentation remain a huge unsolved problem. Median survival of such untreated patients with advanced cardiac involvement is 3 to 6 months and does not really change with treatment. The debate concerning the most effective and least dangerous treatment regimens will probably continue for the next few years. The concept of striving for normalization of the free light chain involved is still unchallenged and this normalization seems to result in actual regression of the amount of amyloid in tissue, as has been shown in fat tissue.[68]

Until recently, the only treatment for patients with hereditary ATTR amyloidosis was liver transplantation with the aim of removing the source of 99% of the mutated TTR in the circulation.[69] However, this approach is not always successful because ATTR amyloid sometimes progresses in the heart after liver transplantation (**Fig. 4**). For this reason, patients with late disease onset (often men with cardiomyopathy) and non–TTR-Met30 mutations are less suitable for liver transplantation.[69,70] The amyloid fibril composition also seems to predict progressive cardiomyopathy after liver transplantation.[71] The 10-year survival of the TTR-Met30 patients after liver transplantation is currently about 85%.[69]

In $A\beta_2M$ amyloidosis, high-flux membranes and adsorption columns have been studied in hemodialysis in an attempt to lower the β_2M serum concentrations. Kidney

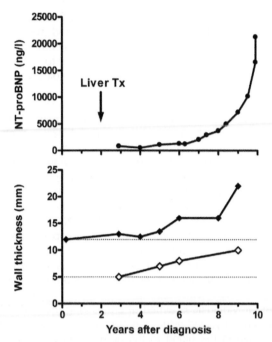

Fig. 4. A 51-year-old woman with hereditary ATTR amyloidosis who received a liver transplant (Liver Tx) 2 years after diagnosis. Progressive cardiomyopathy reflected by an increase of NT-proBNP (*black circles*), mean left ventricular wall size (*black diamonds*), and right ventricular wall size (*white diamonds*). The dotted lines represent the upper limits of the right ventricular wall diameter (5 mm) and left ventricular wall diameter (12 mm).

transplantation, however, remains the treatment of choice. After transplantation, the amyloidosis seems to stabilize; the β_2M serum levels decrease to normal, bone pain and stiffness decrease, the cystic lesions do not increase further in size, but regression of amyloid deposits has not been reported.[72]

Apart from treating the underlying precursor-producing process, it is also important to provide supportive treatment for decreased organ function caused by amyloid deposition. Involvement of more than 1 vital organ frequently results in a mixture of serious problems. It is often difficult and sometimes impossible to find an acceptable solution for all problems. To get the best results of supportive treatment for the individual patient with amyloidosis, it is necessary that all medical specialists involved collaborate closely and that 1 specialist coordinates the collective efforts.

DISEASE MONITORING

Maintaining a good overview of the effect of treatment is important for such an intangible disease as systemic amyloidosis. The accumulation of amyloid is expected to stop after successful elimination of the precursor supply and the tissue itself tries to remove amyloid. Repeated measurements are useful to monitor the effect (or lack of effect) of treatment. Two different processes need to be monitored (**Box 2**).

The first process is that of the underlying production of the precursor proteins SAA, free kappa or lambda light chain, and (mutated) TTR in AA, AL, and ATTR amyloidosis, respectively. After successful treatment, the SAA levels should decrease and remain

---

Box 2
Monitoring of systemic amyloidosis during follow-up using a set of core data. Not all items are always indicated; the choice depends on type of amyloid and patient characteristics

Frequent (3–6 times per year):
Precursor	SAA and CRP (AA)
	Kappa or lambda free light chain, M-protein, Bence Jones in urine (AL)
Serum	Urea, creatinine, albumin
	Total bilirubin, alkaline phosphatase, gamma glutamyl transpeptidase
	N-terminal pro-brain natriuretic peptide, troponin-T
Urine	Endogenous creatinine clearance
	Protein/24 h, protein/creatinine ratio

Infrequent (once per year, two years, or if indicated):
Precursor	Bone marrow biopsy (AL) to verify complete response or suspicion of relapse
Imaging	Echocardiography (ventricular wall thicknesses, ejection fraction)
	Abdominal echography (sizes of liver, spleen, and kidneys)
	Diphosphonate scintigraphy (ATTR)
	SAP scintigraphy (AA and AL)
Function	ECG, Holter monitoring for 24 h
Tissue	Amyloid grade (or amyloid protein concentration) in subcutaneous fat tissue

---

at less than 3 mg/L continuously, the free kappa and lambda levels and the kappa/lambda ratio should definitely decrease within the reference ranges, and mutant TTR should no longer be detectable in the blood.

The second process is that of amyloid accumulation, the so-called clinical amyloid load. Quantitative clinical abnormalities are available for monitoring this clinical amyloid load, such as serum albumin, alkaline phosphatase, bilirubin, NT-proBNP, troponin, creatinine clearance, proteinuria, ventricular wall thickness, ejection fraction, conduction and rhythm, heart rate variability, Ewing battery results of autonomic function, and the sizes of enlarged organs, such as the liver, spleen, and kidneys. Imaging techniques and subcutaneous fat tissue samples can be used for monitoring (**Fig. 5**). At a consensus meeting in Tours in 2004, a set of response criteria for systemic AL amyloidosis was accepted by the international amyloidosis community,[32] with the addition of some modifications after the last consensus meeting in Groningen in 2012.[67]

CURRENT PERSPECTIVES

The precursor-product concept helps in understanding why the current treatment aimed at normalization of the precursor protein is important to prevent further accumulation of amyloid. New developments in this area include antisense[73] and RNAi[74] treatment. Both treatments suppress TTR production by the liver resulting in low TTR serum concentrations. Most of the current research, however, has changed its focus to the development of new drugs to stabilize precursor proteins, interfere with amyloid deposition, or stimulate amyloid removal.

New drugs are under investigation for ATTR amyloidosis, such as diflunisal and tafamidis, that stabilize the conformation of TTR in the circulation and interfere with deposition of amyloid. Both diflunisal and tafamidis stabilize the TTR tetramer in blood in vitro and inhibit the tetramer in breaking up into amyloidogenic dimers and monomers.[75] A clinical trial of tafamidis has recently been published and shows an inhibitory effect on the progression of polyneuropathy in patients with ATTR amyloidosis.[76] A clinical trial of diflunisal comprising 130 patients was completed at the end of 2012, so the results are expected soon.[77] A study of doxycyclin in combination with

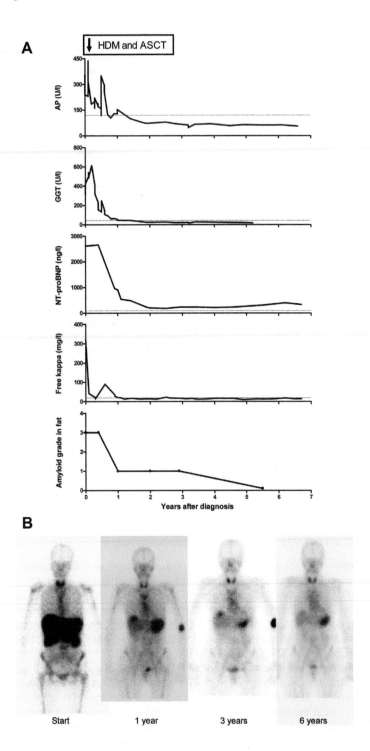

tauroursodeoxycholic acid, a biliary acid, in mice showed that this combination was capable of stimulating removal of ATTR amyloid deposits.[78] A phase II study of this drug combination has been started in patients with ATTR amyloidosis.[79]

Eprodisate, another promising drug, has shown an inhibitory effect on the progression of kidney disease in patients with AA amyloidosis in a first clinical trial.[80] This drug interferes with the binding of SAA to glycosaminoglycans in tissue.[81] Although the magnitude of the clinical effects of tafamidis in ATTR amyloidosis and eprodisate in AA amyloidosis is moderate, the real relevance of both studies is that they show proof of concept that interference with the formation and deposition of amyloid is a realistic goal. Epigallocatechin-3-gallate (EGCG), a green tea extract, seems to have an inhibitory effect on the formation of AL and ATTR amyloid.[82–84] A clinical trial has started to evaluate a possible role of EGCG in promoting regression of residual cardiac damage in patients with AL amyloidosis who have successfully completed chemotherapy.[67]

An interesting development is the combined use of a drug called CPHPC and anti-SAP antibodies. CPHPC (the abbreviation of (R)-1-[6-[(R)-2-carboxy-pyrrolidin-1-yl]-6-oxo-hexanoyl]pyrrolidine-2-carboxylic acid) is a drug that effectively depletes SAP from the circulation.[85] This mechanism possibly stops accumulation of amyloid and may be useful for all types of systemic amyloidosis, although fibrinogen-derived amyloidosis seems to respond best.[86] Vaccination against amyloid has been attempted in the past with poor results. Early vaccination research was primarily focused on the induction of antibodies against conformational epitopes that were believed to be present in all types of amyloid.[87] The Royal Free group in London recently demonstrated that CPHPC followed by anti-SAP antibodies resulted in a quick removal of almost all AA amyloid from the tissues in mice with AA amyloidosis.[88] If this dramatic effect on amyloid can be replicated in humans, it may lead to a major change in the prognosis for patients with all types of systemic amyloidosis.

HEALTHY AGING AND PROTEIN MISFOLDING

Autopsy data suggest that supercentenarians (110 years or older) die in about 70% of cases from ATTR amyloidosis-related causes.[89] Neurodegenerative diseases such as Alzheimer disease, Parkinson disease, amyotrophic lateral sclerosis, and Huntington disease, in all of which protein misfolding is a prominent feature, emerge with aging. The induction of aggregation involves a crystallizationlike seeding mechanism by which a specific protein is structurally corrupted by its misfolded conformer.[90] Seeding is also described in other forms of amyloidosis and, although the clinical consequences do not seem to be prominent, this prionlike behavior is an aspect of these

◄──

Fig. 5. A 62-year-old woman with systemic AL kappa amyloidosis associated with multiple myeloma. She was treated with HDM followed by ASCT. (A) Follow-up of serum concentrations of alkaline phosphatase (AP), γ-glutamyl transpeptidase (GGT), NT-proBNP, and the kappa free light chain. The bottom part shows the semiquantitative grading of amyloid in fat tissue (ranging from 0 to 4+). Dotted lines display the upper limit of the reference control values. (B) Follow-up of SAP scintigraphy (anterior view) at the start of treatment and 1, 3, and 6 years thereafter. At the start, intensive uptake in an enlarged liver (+++), spleen (+++) and in bone marrow (++) is visible. After 1 year, diminished bone marrow and splenic uptake (+) is visible and the liver uptake has become normal except for a small upper segment of the right lobe. After 3 and 6 years, some splenic uptake persists (+), the localized liver uptake diminishes slowly, and the bone marrow uptake has disappeared. Some nonspecific uptake or excretion can be seen in thyroid, stomach, and bladder (and minimal extravasation of blood or tracer at the injection site near the left elbow after 1 and 3 years).

protein-misfolding diseases that certainly deserves serious attention.[91,92] In common cardiac diseases, such as pathologic cardiac hypertrophy and dilated and ischemic cardiomyopathies, misfolded proteins have a direct causative role.[93] Protein misfolding is not only a characteristic of some obscure amyloid diseases but is a much broader phenomenon that is involved in many other degenerative diseases closely associated with aging.[94] Therefore, a better understanding of the nature and pathogenesis of all types of amyloidosis may also increase our knowledge of these common and disabling degenerative diseases that interfere so much with healthy aging.

ACHIEVEMENTS

The amyloidoses are fascinating representatives of a new disease category of protein-misfolding diseases. Hundred years ago it was a mystery why so different diseases as multiple myeloma and tuberculosis could end up with organs massively filled with apparently similar amyloid. Often, however, amyloidosis appeared in a patient without any clear cause, and was therefore thought to be primary. Occasionally the disease was found in succeeding generations of a family. But diagnostic possibilities improved steadily. The iodine sulphuric staining test was replaced by metachromatic stains, such as Congo red, in order to better identify amyloid in tissue. It was the introduction of biopsies that enabled clinicians to diagnose amyloid during life, although biopsies were used restrictively until the mid twentieth century. But the major breakthrough came with the work of Pras in 1968, who succeeded in isolating amyloid fibrils by extraction with distilled water.[95] Since that time the amyloid protein became accessible for chemical analysis. The amyloid proteins were chemically characterized, amyloid precursor proteins were detected in blood, and many DNA mutations were connected to familial types of amyloidosis.

The current classification of amyloidosis is in a way a monument of the recent analytical and clinical research. Nowadays a patient suffering from systemic amyloidosis can be diagnosed and typed rapidly with minimal discomfort. The patient undergoes a clinical assessment consisting of blood analyses, function tests, and imaging techniques that yields a quick overview of the severity of organ disease and associated risks. Treatment possibilities range widely from several biologic modifiers, novel cytostatic drugs, or drugs specifically designed for amyloidosis to transplantation of liver or bone marrow. Monitoring the effects of treatment during follow-up has improved and enables the clinician to assess early whether or not the amyloidosis responds to the chosen treatment.

CURRENT CHALLENGES

Despite these favorable developments, however, the prognosis remains grim for many patients suffering from systemic amyloidosis. The reasons are manifold, but the current main challenges are lack of awareness and loss of precious time in waiting for - often ineffective - precursor elimination.

Lack of awareness leads to late detection and far advanced disease at presentation, often severe cardiac disease or multi-organ disease. Doctors should think of amyloidosis - or their computers should suggest it - if key symptoms for the diagnosis are present. This is especially true if more symptoms than one are present. Typical key symptoms are right sided cardiac failure, proteinuria or renal failure, organ swelling (of tongue, myocardium, liver, or spleen), polyneuropathy, or autonomic neuropathy that are all unaccounted for. In many such cases looking for an elevated serum free light chain and performing an abdominal fat aspiration may speed up the diagnosis by months.

Waiting until the precursor has decreased to normal levels is sometimes impossible, because the disease progresses meanwhile. Many patients with severe cardiac AL amyloidosis have not had any profit of improved treatment, because they die from disease progression in the first months after diagnosis. And even sometimes the amyloidosis progresses despite successful reduction or even elimination of the precursor. This is frequently observed in some types of ATTR amyloidosis after liver transplantation, because wild-type TTR becomes deposited in the heart instead of mutant TTR. There is a need for reliable methods to measure the actual production and deposition of amyloid. And treatment tools need to be developed that stop amyloid deposition immediately after detection as well as additional tools that effectively help to remove amyloid from the body. So, although much has been achieved in the last fifty years, there is much left for fundamental and clinical researchers to improve the prospects of patients suffering from these deadly, but also fascinating amyloid diseases.

ACKNOWLEDGMENTS

I would like to thank Johan Bijzet BSc and Andor Glaudemans MD for their kind support in obtaining material for the figures.

REFERENCES

1. Kyle RA. Amyloidosis: a convoluted story. Br J Haematol 2001;114:529–38.
2. Sipe JD, Benson MD, Buxbaum JN, et al. Amyloid fibril protein nomenclature: 2012 recommendations from the Nomenclature Committee of the International Society of Amyloidosis. Amyloid 2012;19:167–70.
3. Merlini G, Bellotti V. Molecular mechanisms of amyloidosis. N Engl J Med 2003; 349:583–96.
4. Falk RH, Comenzo RL, Skinner M. The systemic amyloidoses. N Engl J Med 1997; 337:898–909.
5. Westermark P. Localized AL amyloidosis: a suicidal neoplasm? Ups J Med Sci 2012;117:244–50.
6. Meijer JM, Schönland SO, Palladini G, et al. Sjögren's syndrome and localized nodular cutaneous amyloidosis: coincidence or a distinct clinical entity? Arthritis Rheum 2008;58:1992–9.
7. Kyle RA, Gertz MA. Primary systemic amyloidosis: clinical and laboratory features in 474 cases. Semin Hematol 1995;32:45–59.
8. Lachmann HJ, Goodman HJ, Gilbertson JA, et al. Natural history and outcome in systemic AA amyloidosis. N Engl J Med 2007;356:2361–71.
9. Hazenberg BP, van Rijswijk MH. Clinical and therapeutic aspects of AA amyloidosis. Baillieres Clin Rheumatol 1994;8:661–90.
10. Connors LH, Lim A, Prokaeva T, et al. Tabulation of human transthyretin (TTR) variants, 2003. Amyloid 2003;10:160–84.
11. Dungu JN, Anderson LJ, Whelan CJ, et al. Cardiac transthyretin amyloidosis. Heart 2012;98:1546–54.
12. Drüeke TB, Massy ZA. Beta2-microglobulin. Semin Dial 2009;22:378–80.
13. Heegaard NH. Beta(2)-microglobulin: from physiology to amyloidosis. Amyloid 2009;16:151–73.
14. Valleix S, Gillmore JD, Bridoux F, et al. Hereditary systemic amyloidosis due to Asp76Asn variant β2-microglobulin. N Engl J Med 2012;366:2276–83.
15. Benson MD. Ostertag revisited: the inherited systemic amyloidoses without neuropathy. Amyloid 2005;12:75–87.

16. Lachmann HJ, Booth DR, Booth SE, et al. Misdiagnosis of hereditary amyloidosis as AL (primary) amyloidosis. N Engl J Med 2002;346:1786–91.

17. Gillmore JD, Lachmann HJ, Rowczenio D, et al. Diagnosis, pathogenesis, treatment, and prognosis of hereditary fibrinogen A alpha-chain amyloidosis. J Am Soc Nephrol 2009;20:444–51.

18. Sattianayagam PT, Gibbs SD, Rowczenio D, et al. Hereditary lysozyme amyloidosis – phenotypic heterogeneity and the role of solid organ transplantation. J Intern Med 2012;272:36–44.

19. Larsen CP, Walker PD, Weiss DT, et al. Prevalence and morphology of leukocyte chemotactic factor 2-associated amyloid in renal biopsies. Kidney Int 2010;77:816–9.

20. Kiuru S. Gelsolin-related familial amyloidosis, Finnish type (FAF), and its variants found worldwide. Amyloid 1998;5:55–66.

21. Simms RW, Prout MN, Cohen AS. The epidemiology of AL and AA amyloidosis. Baillieres Clin Rheumatol 1994;8:627–34.

22. Kyle RA, Linos A, Beard CM, et al. Incidence and natural history of primary systemic amyloidosis in Olmsted County, Minnesota, 1950 through 1989. Blood 1992;79:1817–22.

23. Hemminki K, Li X, Försti A, et al. Incidence and survival in non-hereditary amyloidosis in Sweden. BMC Public Health 2012;12:974.

24. Janssen S, van Rijswijk MH, Meijer S, et al. Systemic amyloidosis: a clinical survey of 144 cases. Neth J Med 1986;29:376–85.

25. Pepys MB. Pathogenesis, diagnosis and treatment of systemic amyloidosis. Philos Trans R Soc Lond B Biol Sci 2001;356:203–10.

26. Hazenberg BP, van Gameren II, Bijzet J, et al. Diagnostic and therapeutic approach of systemic amyloidosis. Neth J Med 2004;62:121–8.

27. Bijzet J, van Gameren II, Hazenberg BP. Fat tissue analysis in the management of patients with systemic amyloidosis. In: Picken MM, Dogan A, Herrera GA, editors. Amyloid and related disorders: surgical pathology and clinical correlations. New York: Humana Press; 2012. p. 191–207.

28. Westermark P. Subcutaneous adipose tissue biopsy for amyloid protein studies. Methods Mol Biol 2012;849:363–71.

29. van Gameren II, Hazenberg BP, Bijzet J, et al. Diagnostic accuracy of subcutaneous abdominal fat tissue aspiration for detecting systemic amyloidosis and its utility in clinical practice. Arthritis Rheum 2006;54:2015–21.

30. Ikeda S, Sekijima Y, Tojo K, et al. Diagnostic value of abdominal wall fat pad biopsy in senile systemic amyloidosis. Amyloid 2011;18:211–5.

31. Nilsson KP, Ikenberg K, Åslund A, et al. Structural typing of systemic amyloidoses by luminescent-conjugated polymer spectroscopy. Am J Pathol 2010;176:563–74.

32. Gertz MA, Comenzo R, Falk RH, et al. Definition of organ involvement and treatment response in immunoglobulin light chain amyloidosis (AL): a consensus opinion from the 10th International Symposium on Amyloid and Amyloidosis, Tours, France, 18-22 April 2004. Am J Med 2005;79:319–28.

33. Kebbel A, Rocken C. Immunohistochemical classification of amyloid in surgical pathology revisited. Am J Surg Pathol 2006;30:673–83.

34. Satoskar AA, Efebera Y, Hasan A, et al. Strong transthyretin immunostaining: potential pitfall in cardiac amyloid typing. Am J Surg Pathol 2011;35:1685–90.

35. Murphy CL, Wang S, Williams T, et al. Characterization of systemic amyloid deposits by mass spectrometry. Methods Enzymol 2006;412:48–62.

36. Lavatelli F, Perlman DH, Spencer B, et al. Amyloidogenic and associated proteins in systemic amyloidosis proteome of adipose tissue. Mol Cell Proteomics 2008;7:1570–83.

37. Vrana JA, Gamez JD, Madden BJ, et al. Classification of amyloidosis by laser microdissection and mass spectrometry-based proteomic analysis in clinical biopsy specimens. Blood 2009;114:4957–9.
38. Lavatelli F, Vrana JA. Proteomic typing of amyloid deposits in systemic amyloidoses. Amyloid 2011;18:177–82.
39. Brambilla F, Lavatelli F, Di Silvestre D, et al. Reliable typing of systemic amyloidoses through proteomic analysis of subcutaneous adipose tissue. Blood 2012; 119:1844–7.
40. Picken MM. Amyloidosis-where are we now and where are we heading? Arch Pathol Lab Med 2010;134:545–51.
41. Dispenzieri A, Gertz MA, Kyle RA, et al. Serum cardiac troponins and N-terminal pro-brain natriuretic peptide: a staging system for primary systemic amyloidosis. J Clin Oncol 2004;22:3751–7.
42. Palladini G, Barassi A, Perlini S, et al. Midregional proadrenomedullin (MR-proADM) is a powerful predictor of early death in AL amyloidosis. Amyloid 2011; 18:216–21.
43. Ozdemir D, Dagdelen S, Erbas T, et al. Amyloid goiter and hypopituitarism in a patient with systemic amyloidosis. Amyloid 2011;18:32–4.
44. Ishihara T, Nagasawa T, Yokota T, et al. Amyloid protein of vessels in leptomeninges, cortices, choroid plexuses, and pituitary glands from patients with systemic amyloidosis. Hum Pathol 1989;20:891–5.
45. Erdkamp FL, Gans RO, Hoorntje SJ. Endocrine organ failure due to systemic AA-amyloidosis. Neth J Med 1991;38:24–8.
46. Zubkov AY, Rabinstein AA, Dispenzieri A, et al. Primary systemic amyloidosis with ischemic stroke as a presenting complication. Neurology 2007;69:1136–41.
47. Kay J, Benson CB, Lester S, et al. Utility of high-resolution ultrasound for the diagnosis of dialysis-related amyloidosis. Arthritis Rheum 1992;35:926–32.
48. Dubrey SW, Hawkins PN, Falk RH. Amyloid diseases of the heart: assessment, diagnosis, and referral. Heart 2011;97:75–84.
49. Noordzij W, Glaudemans AW, van Rheenen RW, et al. Iodine-123 labelled meta-iodobenzylguanidine for the evaluation of cardiac sympathetic denervation in early stage amyloidosis. Eur J Nucl Med Mol Imaging 2012;39:1609–17.
50. Aprile C, Marinone G, Saponaro R, et al. Cardiac and pleuropulmonary AL amyloid imaging with technetium-99m labelled aprotinin. Eur J Nucl Med 1995; 22:1393–401.
51. Janssen S, Piers DA, van Rijswijk MH, et al. Soft-tissue uptake of 99mTc-diphosphonate and 99mTc-pyrophosphate in amyloidosis. Eur J Nucl Med 1990; 16:663–70.
52. Wechalekar K, Ng FS, Poole-Wilson PA, et al. Cardiac amyloidosis diagnosed incidentally by bone scintigraphy. J Nucl Cardiol 2007;14:750–3.
53. Rapezzi C, Quarta CC, Guidalotti PL, et al. Role of (99m)Tc-DPD scintigraphy in diagnosis and prognosis of hereditary transthyretin-related cardiac amyloidosis. JACC Cardiovasc Imaging 2011;4:659–70.
54. Kristen AV, Haufe S, Schonland SO, et al. Skeletal scintigraphy indicates disease severity of cardiac involvement in patients with senile systemic amyloidosis. Int J Cardiol 2011. http://dx.doi.org/10.1016/j.ijcard.2011.06.123.
55. Hawkins PN, Lavender JP, Pepys MB. Evaluation of systemic amyloidosis by scintigraphy with ^{123}I-labeled serum amyloid P component. N Engl J Med 1990;323: 508–13.
56. Jager PL, Hazenberg BP, Franssen EJ, et al. Kinetic studies with iodine-123-labeled serum amyloid P component in patients with systemic AA

and AL amyloidosis and assessment of clinical value. J Nucl Med 1998;39: 699–706.

57. Hazenberg BP, van Rijswijk MH, Piers DA, et al. Diagnostic performance of ^{123}I-labeled serum amyloid P component scintigraphy in patients with amyloidosis. Am J Med 2006;119:355.e15–24.

58. Hawkins PN, Richardson S, MacSweeney JE, et al. Scintigraphic quantification and serial monitoring of human visceral amyloid deposits provide evidence for turnover and regression. Q J Med 1993;86:365–74.

59. Hazenberg BP, van Rijswijk MH, Lub-de Hooge MN, et al. Diagnostic performance and prognostic value of extravascular retention of ^{123}I-labeled serum amyloid P component in systemic amyloidosis. J Nucl Med 2007;48:865–72.

60. Wall JS, Kennel SJ, Stuckey AC, et al. Radioimmunodetection of amyloid deposits in patients with AL amyloidosis. Blood 2010;116:2241–4.

61. Gillmore JD, Lovat LB, Persey MR, et al. Amyloid load and clinical outcome in AA amyloidosis in relation to circulating concentration of serum amyloid A protein. Lancet 2001;358:24–9.

62. Caorsi R, Federici S, Gattorno M. Biologic drugs in autoinflammatory syndromes. Autoimmun Rev 2012;12:81–6.

63. Hakala M, Immonen K, Korpela M, et al. Good medium-term efficacy of tocilizumab in DMARD and anti-TNF-α therapy resistant reactive amyloidosis. Ann Rheum Dis 2013;72:464–5.

64. Gertz MA, Lacy MQ, Dispenzieri A, et al. Effect of haematological response on outcome of patients undergoing transplantation for primary amyloidosis: importance of achieving a complete response. Haematologica 2007;92: 1415–8.

65. Skinner M, Sanchorawala V, Seldin DC, et al. High-dose melphalan and autologous stem-cell transplantation in patients with AL amyloidosis: an 8-year study. Ann Intern Med 2004;140:85–93.

66. Jaccard A, Moreau P, Leblond V, et al. High-dose melphalan versus melphalan plus dexamethasone for AL amyloidosis. N Engl J Med 2007;357:1083–93.

67. Gatt ME, Palladini G. Light chain amyloidosis 2012: a new era. Br J Haematol 2013;160:582–98.

68. van Gameren II, van Rijswijk MH, Bijzet J, et al. Histological regression of amyloid in AL amyloidosis is exclusively seen in patients with a complete response of serum free light chain. Haematologica 2009;94:1094–100.

69. Wilczek HE, Larsson M, Ericzon BG, et al. Long-term data from the Familial Amyloidotic Polyneuropathy World Transplant Registry (FAPWTR). Amyloid 2011; 18(Suppl 1):193–5.

70. Okamoto S, Zhao Y, Lindqvist P, et al. Development of cardiomyopathy after liver transplantation in Swedish hereditary transthyretin amyloidosis (ATTR) patients. Amyloid 2011;18:200–5.

71. Gustafsson S, Ihse E, Henein MY, et al. Amyloid fibril composition as a predictor of development of cardiomyopathy after liver transplantation for hereditary transthyretin amyloidosis. Transplantation 2012;93:1017–23.

72. Yamamoto S, Gejyo F. Historical background and clinical treatment of dialysis-related amyloidosis. Biochim Biophys Acta 2005;1753:4–10.

73. Ackermann EJ, Guo S, Booten S, et al. Clinical development of an antisense therapy for the treatment of transthyretin-associated polyneuropathy. Amyloid 2012;19(Suppl 1):43–4.

74. Barros SA, Gollob JA. Safety profile of RNAi nanomedicines. Adv Drug Deliv Rev 2012;64:1730–7.

75. Hammarstrom P, Wiseman RL, Powers ET, et al. Prevention of transthyretin amyloid disease by changing protein misfolding energetics. Science 2003;299:713–7.
76. Coelho T, Maia LF, Martins da Silva A, et al. Tafamidis for transthyretin familial amyloid polyneuropathy: a randomized, controlled trial. Neurology 2012;79:785–92.
77. Berk JL, Suhr OB, Sekijima Y, et al. The diflunisal trial: study accrual and drug tolerance. Amyloid 2012;19(Suppl 1):37–8.
78. Cardoso I, Martins D, Ribeiro T, et al. Synergy of combined doxycycline/TUDCA treatment in lowering Transthyretin deposition and associated biomarkers: studies in FAP mouse models. J Transl Med 2010;8:74.
79. Obici L, Cortese A, Lozza A, et al. Doxycycline plus tauroursodeoxycholic acid for transthyretin amyloidosis: a phase II study. Amyloid 2012;19(Suppl 1):34–6.
80. Dember LM, Hawkins PN, Hazenberg BP, et al. Eprodisate for the treatment of AA amyloidosis. N Engl J Med 2007;356:2349–60.
81. Inoue S, Hultin PG, Szarek WA, et al. Effect of poly(vinylsulfonate) on murine AA amyloid: a high-resolution ultrastructural study. Lab Invest 1996;74:1081–90.
82. Hunstein W. Epigallocathechin-3-gallate in AL amyloidosis: a new therapeutic option? Blood 2007;110:2216.
83. Mereles D, Buss SJ, Hardt SE, et al. Effects of the main green tea polyphenol epigallocatechin-3-gallate on cardiac involvement in patients with AL amyloidosis. Clin Res Cardiol 2010;99:483–90.
84. Kristen AV, Lehrke S, Buss S, et al. Green tea halts progression of cardiac transthyretin amyloidosis: an observational report. Clin Res Cardiol 2012;101:805–13.
85. Pepys MB, Herbert J, Hutchingson WL, et al. Targeted pharmacological depletion of serum amyloid P component for treatment of human amyloidosis. Nature 2002;417:254–9.
86. Gillmore JD, Tennent GA, Hutchinson WL, et al. Sustained pharmacological depletion of serum amyloid P component in patients with systemic amyloidosis. Br J Haematol 2010;148:760–7.
87. Hrncic R, Wall J, Wolfenbarger DA, et al. Antibody-mediated resolution of light chain-associated amyloid deposits. Am J Pathol 2000;157:1239–46.
88. Bodin K, Ellmerich S, Kahan MC, et al. Antibodies to human serum amyloid P component eliminate visceral amyloid deposits. Nature 2010;468:93–7.
89. Coles LS, Young RD. Supercentenarians and transthyretin amyloidosis: the next frontier of human life extension. Prev Med 2012;54(Suppl):S9–11.
90. Walker LC, LeVine H 3rd. Corruption and spread of pathogenic proteins in neurodegenerative diseases. J Biol Chem 2012;287:33109–15.
91. Westermark GT, Westermark P. Prion-like aggregates: infectious agents in human disease. Trends Mol Med 2010;16:501–7.
92. Solomon A, Richey T, Murphy CL, et al. Amyloidogenic potential of foie gras. Proc Natl Acad Sci U S A 2007;104:10998–1001.
93. Willis MS, Patterson C. Proteotoxicity and cardiac dysfunction – Alzheimer's disease of the heart? N Engl J Med 2013;368:455–64.
94. Schnabel J. Protein folding: the dark side of proteins. Nature 2010;464:828–9.
95. Pras M, Schubert M, Zucker-Franklin D, et al. The characterization of soluble amyloid prepared in water. J Clin Invest 1968;47:924–33.

Localized Cutaneous Fibrosing Disorders

Aaliya Yaqub, MD[a], Lorinda Chung, MD, MS[a],
Kerri E. Rieger, MD, PhD[b], David F. Fiorentino, MD, PhD[c],*

KEYWORDS

- Localized scleroderma • Morphea • Cutaneous fibrosis • Scleredema
- Scleromyxedema • Nephrogenic systemic fibrosis
- Chronic graft-versus-host disease

KEY POINTS

- Localized cutaneous fibrosing disorders are a heterogeneous group of diseases that must be differentiated from systemic sclerosis to provide the patient with accurate prognostic information and treatment.
- Identifying and diagnosing a particular cutaneous sclerosing disorder requires integration of key clinical and histopathologic features.
- Although considered "localized" disorders to differentiate them from systemic sclerosis, these diseases can be associated with significant systemic organ involvement and may even lead to death.
- Current therapies for localized fibrosing diseases are not satisfactory and may require a better understanding of disease pathophysiology.

INTRODUCTION

Although systemic sclerosis (SSc) is often considered the cardinal disease that causes cutaneous sclerosis, there are many other cutaneous fibrosing disorders that can be confused with SSc. Many of these disorders either are completely localized to the skin and adjacent structures or they have systemic implications that are different from those seen in SSc. Thus, it is imperative that these entities be recognized by the clinician to provide the patient with correct prognostic and treatment information. This article reviews the main types of cutaneous fibrosing disorders including morphea,

Funding Sources: Dr Chung is funded by the Scleroderma Research Foundation.
Conflicts of Interest: The authors declare no conflicts of interest.
[a] Division of Immunology and Rheumatology, Stanford University School of Medicine, 300 Pasteur Drive, Stanford, CA 94305, USA; [b] Department of Pathology, Stanford Medical Center, Stanford University School of Medicine, H2110, 300 Pasteur Drive, Stanford, CA 94305, USA; [c] Department of Dermatology, Stanford University School of Medicine, 450 Broadway, C-234, Redwood City, CA 94063, USA
* Corresponding author.
E-mail address: fiorentino@stanford.edu

scleredema, scleromyxedema, drug-induced cutaneous fibrosing reactions, nephro-genic systemic fibrosis (NSF), eosinophilic fasciitis, and chronic graft-versus-host disease (cGVHD) (**Box 1**). These distinct entities as well as important features of their etiology, clinical presentation, differential diagnosis, histopathology, and treatment are the focus of this review.

MORPHEA
Background

Morphea (localized scleroderma [LS]) is a form of pathologic sclerosis that is typically limited to the skin and underlying structures. In contrast to SSc, there are typically no sclerodactyly or nailfold capillary abnormalities, and morphea is much less frequently associated with Raynaud phenomenon. In general, morphea affects only the skin, although involvement of the subcutaneous fat, fascia, and even muscle and bone can be seen in some variants. In addition, rarely there can be associated central nervous system involvement when it presents on the face and head. Several studies have suggested that morphea can also be associated with arthralgias, ocular involve-ment (usually as aforementioned central nervous system manifestation), and gastroin-testinal symptoms stemming from esophageal dysmotility and reflux.[1,2]

The pathogenesis of morphea is unclear, but it is characterized by excess collagen deposition caused by both excess production and decreased degradation.[3] The exact initiating events are unclear, although infection, trauma, radiation, or medications have all been implicated. *Borrelia* organisms have been linked to LS in Europe but not in the United States, and thus their role remains unclear. In morphea skin there is upregula-tion of various adhesion molecules, as well as release of key cytokines such as trans-forming growth factor β (TGF-β), as well as platelet-derived growth factor, connective tissue growth factor, and interleukins 4, 6, and 8.

Epidemiology

Morphea is rare, with an estimated incidence ranging between 0.4 and 2.7 per 100,000 people based on very few epidemiologic studies.[4,5] It most frequently affects whites, but may occur in all races.[3,6] There is a female predominance at a ratio of 2.4:1 to 4.2:1.[6,7] Disease prevalence is equally distributed between adults and children; however, plaque-variant morphea comprises most adult cases, whereas linear mor-phea is the most common variant in children.[8]

Classification and Subtypes

Morphea (or LS) can present in a variety of clinical phenotypes, but there is no uniformly accepted classification scheme. In 1995, Peterson and colleagues[9] proposed

---

Box 1
Cutaneous fibrosing disorders

- Localized scleroderma (morphea)
- Drug-induced cutaneous reactions
- Scleredema
- Scleromyxedema
- Nephrogenic systemic fibrosis
- Chronic graft-versus-host disease

a classification scheme that distinguishes plaque, generalized, deep, bullous, and linear types as the 5 main subtypes of LS. This classification scheme has been widely accepted, but has some drawbacks. For instance, it does not take into account that children may present with more than 1 subtype of morphea, or that bullous lesions might appear in all different LS subtypes. In 2006, Laxer and Zulian[10] proposed an alternative classification scheme to overcome these weaknesses, but in 2009 a German group of experts proposed a final classification that considers the depth and extent of fibrosis and refers to the treatment of the respective subtypes (**Table 1**).[11]

The classic plaque type of morphea is the most frequent subtype, especially in adults. Initially it can present as oval-shaped lesions surrounded by an erythematous border (appears as a "lilac ring"), which then later become sclerotic in the center (**Fig. 1**).[12] However, some morphea lesions can present purely as pink or hyperpigmented macules and patches that never become indurated. These lesions are often called superficial morphea (see later discussion). Morphea lesions are typically found on the trunk and area between the hip and inguinal regions, although the breasts and extremities are commonly involved. In general, the hands, feet, and head are spared. Guttate morphea is a rare subtype that presents with multiple small sclerotic lesions, yellow or white in color with a shiny surface. These lesions may be confused with extragenital lichen sclerosis clinically and histopathologically (**Fig. 2**).

Idiopathic atrophaderma of Pierini and Pasini (IAPP) is a form of dermal atrophy that manifests as single or multiple sharply demarcated, round to oval, hyperpigmented to erythematous, nonindurated depressed papules and plaques. It is relatively poorly described in the literature, but is known to have a predilection for the trunk (particularly the back) and occurs predominantly in young healthy women in their teens and second decade.[13,14] The patches seen in IAPP are marked by a slight depression of the skin with an abrupt edge ("cliff-drop border").[15] The precise classification of IAPP has been long debated. Some consider it a variant of LS or morphea, as presented in the German classification (see **Table 1**), but others disagree with this classification because there are certain features to suggest that IAPP and morphea are separate entities. IAPP lacks sclerosis as a feature, and lesions commonly merge over time, creating a moth-eaten appearance (Swiss cheese–like appearance) not consistent with typical morphea. The more recently described term superficial morphea has become a more accepted way to describe IAPP given its lack of sclerosis and its hypopigmented or hyperpigmented appearance (**Fig. 3**).[16,17]

Generalized LS is a more severe subtype of LS, as it is characterized by 4 or more indurated plaques greater than 3 cm in diameter involving 2 or more anatomic

Table 1	
Classification of localized scleroderma	
Limited type	Morphea (plaque type of localized scleroderma)
	Guttate morphea
	Atrophoderma idiopathica of Pierini and Pasini (superficial morphea)
	Generalized localized scleroderma
Generalized type	Disabling pansclerotic morphea
	Eosinophilic fasciitis (Shulman syndrome)
	Linear localized scleroderma of the extremities
Linear type	Linear localized scleroderma "en coup de sabre"
	Progressive facial hemiatrophy (Parry-Romberg syndrome)
Deep type	Deep morphea

From Kreuter A. Localized scleroderma. Dermatol Ther 2012;25:137; with permission.

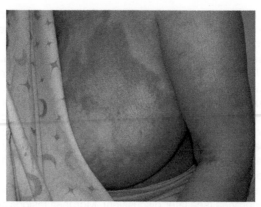

Fig. 1. Morphea, plaque type. Shown is an indurated oval plaque with a lilac colored border and a yellow, indurated center.

sites (head and neck, each extremity, anterior trunk, and posterior trunk) according to Laxer and Zulian.[10] These plaques are often symmetric and can coalesce over time.

Disabling pansclerotic morphea is a very rare and severe variant of LS that predominantly occurs in children, leading to rapidly progressive and extensive involvement of skin, subcutaneous fat, fascia, muscle, and even bone. Pansclerotic refers to involvement of all layers of the skin, not necessarily implying total body involvement. It can lead to severe contractures, musculoskeletal atrophy, poorly healing ulcerations, and skin necrosis.[18]

Eosinophilic fasciitis (Shulman syndrome) is another rare form of LS characterized by symmetric, often painful swelling, and induration and thickening of the skin and soft tissue. After some time lesions may become more indurated and fibrotic, leading to a peau d'orange–like appearance. The onset is often abrupt and can be triggered by intense physical activity or mechanical trauma. Clinically, eosinophilic fasciitis exclusively affects the extremities but, in contrast to SSc, typically spares the hands

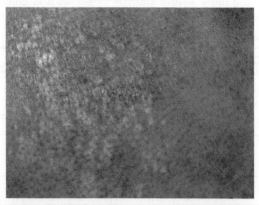

Fig. 2. Morphea, guttate and superficial type. Shown is a classic lesion with lichen sclerosus et atrophicus overlap, consisting of atrophic, hypopigmented macules with areas of follicular plugging (*black dots*).

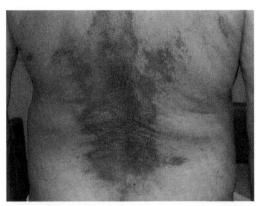

Fig. 3. Morphea, superficial type. This patient has large truncal hyperpigmented patches on the back without any induration.

and feet. If only the deep tissues are involved, the overlying skin can feel soft, but deep palpation reveals very firm tissue beneath. A helpful clinical sign is to have the patient raise the arms above the head and to look for longitudinal furrowing, which represents sparing of deep sclerosis in the area of the veins (so-called groove sign). Diagnosis is based on characteristic skin abnormalities, thickened fascia, and perivascular inflammatory infiltrates composed of lymphocytes and/or eosinophils.[19] A peripheral eosinophilia is frequently seen but is not mandatory in making the diagnosis.

Linear LS is the most common LS subtype in children, and is characterized by band-like lesions arranged longitudinally on the extremities. In mild disease the lesions can heal with some hyperpigmentation, but in more severe disease linear LS can lead to flexion contractures, muscle atrophy, severe growth retardation, myositis, and arthritis. The most well-recognized linear subtype is "en coup de sabre," which affects the frontoparietal region of the head, usually ranging from the eyebrows to the hair-bearing scalp where it can cause scarring alopecia. This subtype can also affect the central nervous system, causing seizures and headache or ophthalmologic findings such as uveitis. Many have suggested that progressive facial hemiatrophy (Parry-Romberg syndrome) and en coup de sabre are actually the same entity.[20,21] Progressive hemifacial atropy is a rare condition marked by unilateral facial atrophy affecting the skin, subcutaneous tissue, muscles, and potentially even bone. Sometimes skin fibrosis is absent in this subtype, which typically affects children and adolescents. It coincides simultaneously up to 40% of the time with linear LS en coup de sabre.[20]

The deep subtype of LS, deep morphea, is the rarest variant, accounting for fewer than 5% of all cases of LS. In deep morphea, the deeper connective tissue layers including fat, fascia, and muscle tend to be affected by fibrosis. The lesions are typically symmetric and are located on the extremities. This subtype may occur in childhood.

The histology of morphea depends on the clinical subtype, as changes can be seen in the epidermis, dermis, and subcutaneous fat. Early lesions show thickened collagen bundles in the reticular dermis and dense inflammatory infiltrates around blood vessels and adnexa (**Fig. 4**). Later stages contain tightly packed collagen fibers with absent or atrophic sweat glands, while the subcutaneous fat may be either absent or "trapped" more superficially in the lower reticular dermis.

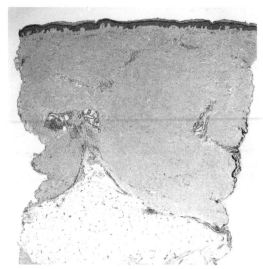

Fig. 4. Morphea, skin biopsy. There is a superficial and deep perivascular inflammatory cell infiltrate with dense, pink dermal collagen and attenuated spaces between collagen bundles (hematoxylin and eosin stain, original magnification ×100).

ENVIRONMENTALLY TRIGGERED SCLERODERMA-LIKE DISORDERS

Although the etiology of scleroderma-like disorders (SLD) remains unknown, 4 factors have been linked to the development of sclerodermoid reactions: trauma, radiation, medications, and other chemical exposures.

Trauma

In a large retrospective study examining 750 children with morphea-like lesions, approximately 9% of patients reported some type of mechanical trauma (including insect bites and vaccination) to the affected area before disease onset.[6] In the literature there are 8 cases reported of sclerodermoid reactions after vaccination, and several vaccines are implicated, including the measles/mumps/rubella, hepatitis B, and tetanus vaccines.[22] Different theories for the pathogenesis of these cutaneous reactions have been postulated, including hypersensitivity to the vehicle or preservative in the vaccine as well as trauma from the injection itself. Local sclerodermoid injection-site reactions have also been reported, most commonly with vitamin K, as well as with other less commonly reported injectable agents such as progesterone and vitamin B_{12}.[23]

Medications and Chemicals

Several medications have been linked to the development of morphea-like lesions, including bisoprolol, bleomycin, peplomycin, D-penicillamine, bromocriptine, pentazocine, balicatib, and L-5-hydroxytryptophane in combination with carbidopa (**Box 2**).[24] However, medication-induced lesions mimicking morphea are a rare occurrence, and the literature is derived from case reports. The pathogenesis of these drug-induced reactions is not completely understood, but a profibrotic effect caused by collagen synthesis and fibroblast growth has been described for bleomycin,[25] peplomycin,[26] and dopaminergic drugs.[27] D-Penicillamine has been known to interfere with collagen and elastin maturation and synthesis, and possibly with regulatory T cells.[28]

Box 2	
Medications and chemicals associated with SLD	
Medications	Bisoprolol
	Bleomycin
	Peplomycin
	D-Penicillamine
	Bromocriptine
	L-5-Hydroxytryptophane
	Carbidopa
	Pentazocine
	Balicatib
Chemicals	Vinyl chloride monomers
	Benzene
	Trichloroethylene
	Toluene
	Naphthalene
Pesticides	Malathion
	Diniconazole

In a recent clinical trial testing the cathepsin K (catK) inhibitor, balicatib, for the treatment of osteoporosis, 9 of 709 treated patients developed morphea-like skin changes, whereas there were no reports of cutaneous reactions in the placebo group.[29] The skin fibrosis in these patients is thought to have been due to the inhibition of matrix-degrading functions of catK in the skin, therefore skin fibrosis may be a class effect of catK inhibitors.

Occupational exposure to various chemical and physical agents has been associated with the development of scleroderma-like cutaneous disorders. The literature on such associations is sparse, with most of the knowledge arising from individual case reports, but historically organic solvents and compounds such as vinyl chloride monomers, benzene, trichloroethylene, toluene, and naphthalene have been associated with the development of SLD.[30] The link between these compounds and SLD has been described in 2 case-control studies.[31,32]

Many studies also highlight the toxicity of pesticides, and the relationship between exposure to pesticides and the development of cutaneous sclerotic diseases.[33] A recent case series reports development of a scleroderma-like cutaneous sclerosis in children exposed to pesticides containing malathion and diniconazole.[30] Unfortunately, the mechanism of action of these pesticides and others remains unclear.

Radiation

Postirradiation morphea-like reactions are a potential complication after radiation therapy, particularly in cancer treatment. Women receiving radiation for the treatment of breast cancer are particularly at risk, with manifestations in other parts of the body being much rarer.[34] The incidence of postirradiation morphea-like lesions has been reported to be approximately 1 in 500 irradiated patients.[35,36] Onset of the cutaneous lesion typically occurs within a year of radiation, although latencies of up to 32 years have been described.[37] Radiation-induced morphea-like lesions have to be differentiated from chronic radiodermatitis, bacterial cellulitis, or recurrence of an inflammatory type of cancer.[38] Therefore, a diagnosis of postirradiation morphea must be confirmed by histologic examination whereby an inflammatory and a sclerosing phase can be seen. The inflammatory changes are characterized by superficial and deep perivascular and interstitial lymphoplasmacytic infiltrate, and the sclerosing changes are marked by thickening of collagen bundles in the reticular dermis.[39] Radiation is thought to cause localized sclerodermoid reactions by affecting a clonal fibroblast population, causing selective local immune alteration and altering endothelial cells.[35]

Treatment

Topical therapies for morphea include corticosteroids, calcipotriol, and calcineurin inhibitors such as tacrolimus or pimecrolimus.[40] Systemic corticosteroids tend to be used in linear, generalized, or deep forms of morphea. Methotrexate has the best evidence for efficacy as a disease-modifying agent, alone or in combination with corticosteroids.[12] Mycophenolate mofetil has also been suggested as an effective therapy for methotrexate-resistant disease.[41] Several other systemics have been reported in cases of morphea, including infliximab, bosentan, antimalarial drugs, imatinib, extracorporeal photopheresis, cyclosporine, and penicillin, but their efficacy has yet to be confirmed in large studies.[12] Ultraviolet (UV) light therapy has antifibrotic and anti-inflammatory activity, and case series totaling more than 100 patients have reported effective outcomes primarily for UVA and UVA-1 therapy; UVA (rather than UVB) has been used most often, as UVA penetrates more deeply into the dermis.[40] However, because UV light does not penetrate deeper than the dermis, it is not effective for deeper forms of scleroderma involving the fat, muscle, or bone.

SCLEREDEMA

Scleredema is primarily a disorder of mucin deposition in the dermis, although there is some abnormality in collagen deposition as well. Patients present with asymptomatic, poorly defined areas of woody skin induration that may have a peau d'orange appearance, with lesions primarily found on the neck, upper back, shoulders, and arms (**Fig. 5**).[42] Patients typically complain of restriction of motion of the neck and head. In contrast to SSc, the hands and feet are not involved. The lesions can develop abruptly, and diagnosis is based on the pattern and type of skin involvement. Systemic involvement is rare, but esophageal and cardiac dysfunction has been reported.[43] Skin biopsies demonstrate broad collagen bundles with increased mucin deposition in the dermis (**Fig. 6**).

There are 3 scleredema subtypes (**Table 2**). Type I, scleredema of Buschke or scleredema adultorum, is the most prevalent type. Most cases occur in individuals younger

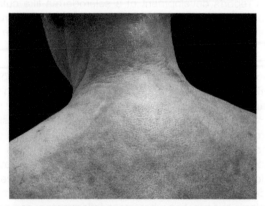

Fig. 5. Scleredema. Infiltrated, slightly erythematous plaques and papules on the upper back giving a peau d'orange-like appearance due to severe involvement of the superficial dermis.

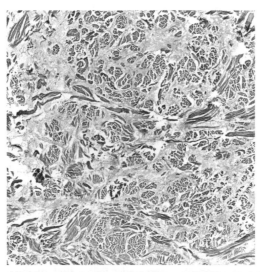

Fig. 6. Scleredema, skin biopsy. The collagen bundles are slightly expanded, with increased space between the bundles that is filled by mucin (*stained blue*) (hematoxylin and eosin with colloidal iron stain, original magnification ×200).

than 20 years, and there is a female predominance of 2 to 1.[43] The condition is typically preceded by a febrile illness with many implicated viral and bacterial causes described, including influenza, measles, mumps, varicella, and streptococcal infections. This form often has a rapid onset but a benign course, with resolution of symptoms occurring over 6 months to 2 years. Type II scleredema is associated with the development of paraproteins, most commonly hypergammaglobulinemia involving immunoglobulin G (IgG) κ. In 25% to 45% of patients, there is progression to multiple myeloma.[44] These patients usually have a chronic, progressive course. Type III scleredema, or scleredema diabeticorum, is associated with poorly controlled type 1 or 2 diabetes. Patients who are obese, older than 40 years, male, and have severe vascular complications of their diabetes are more likely to be affected.[43] It is thought that poor glucose control leads to glycosylation of collagen, resulting in abnormal deposition of collagen in the dermis.

Treatment of scleredema is generally very difficult. Many types of immunosuppressive agents have been tried, with little success. Phototherapy has produced

Table 2
Subtypes of scleredema

Subtype	Clinical Associations
I (Scleredema of Buschke/Scleredema adultorum)	Age <20 y Female predominance Preceding febrile illness
II	Hypergammaglobulinemia (immunoglobulin G, immunoglobulin A) Progression to multiple myeloma in 25%–45%
III (Scleredema diabeticorum)	Poorly controlled diabetes Male predominance

inconsistent results, although more recent reports suggest that perhaps UVA-1 therapy may be of benefit.[45] There are case reports of radiation, including electron-beam radiation, being successful.[46] Recently, both tamoxifen and colchicine have been reported to have benefit.[47] Physical therapy, especially of the neck and shoulders, may be of benefit given the generally restrictive nature of this disorder.

SCLEROMYXEDEMA

Scleromyxedema, a form of the more generalized class of diseases known as lichen myxedematosus, is a rare disorder that usually affects middle-aged adults between 30 and 80 years old.[45] It affects men and women equally. Scleromyxedema has both papular and sclerodermatous involvement and is a disorder of mucin deposition, fibroblast proliferation, and fibrosis. The 4 typical diagnostic findings in scleromyxedema are a generalized papular and sclerodermoid eruption, a monoclonal gammopathy, the absence of a thyroid disorder, and a skin biopsy with the microscopic triad of mucin deposition, fibroblast proliferation, and fibrosis (**Box 3**).

A paraproteinemia, typically an IgG λ, is observed in more than 80% of patients with this disorder.[43] Multiple myeloma can develop in 10% of cases.[43] In general the course of skin disease does not necessarily follow that of the gammopathy. The etiology of this disease is obscure, but involves increased production of hyaluronic acid from dermal fibroblasts. Some studies have shown that serum from scleromyxedema patients can activate fibroblasts to proliferate and to produce increased glycosaminoglycans.[45]

Clinically, patients present with 2- to 3-mm, diffuse, waxy papules that tend to be predominantly located on the face, neck, forearms, and hands, but sparing the palms (**Fig. 7**).[48] The lesions tend not to itch, and the papules can sometimes be linear or coalesce into more sclerodermatous plaques. Diffuse infiltration of the face and glabella can occur, giving rise to so-called leonine facies. The proximal interphalangeal joints can have papules with raised borders and a central depression (doughnut sign).[48] Hair loss in the eyebrow, axilla, and groin can be seen. Patients often have stiffness of the mouth, hands, and extremities. Biopsies from affected skin demonstrate a perivascular infiltrate of mononuclear cells as well as a proliferation of spindle-shaped fibroblasts with at least mildly increased dermal mucin deposition (**Fig. 8**).

Extracutaneous involvement is common, and cannot always be explained by diffuse mucin deposition (**Box 4**).[48] The most common symptom is dysphagia, resulting in hoarseness or aspiration. Neurologic involvement can occur in 10% to 15% of scleromyxedema cases and can include carpal tunnel syndrome, headache, peripheral neuropathy, dysarthria, and cognitive involvement. A rare and sometimes fatal neurologic manifestation of scleromyxedema, termed the dermato-neuro syndrome, consists of fever, convulsions, and coma, often preceded by an influenza-like prodrome.[49] A myopathy can occur, which clinically can resemble inflammatory myopathies with

---

Box 3
Diagnostic findings in scleromyxedema

Generalized papular and sclerodermoid eruption

Monoclonal gammopathy (IgG)

Absence of thyroid disease

Skin biopsy with microscopic triad of mucin deposition, fibroblast proliferation, fibrosis

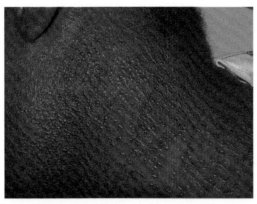

Fig. 7. Scleromyxedema. Diffuse and uniform configuration of 2–3 mm firm, slightly hyperpigmented papules on the head and neck.

proximal weakness, interstitial infiltrates on muscle biopsy, elevated muscle enzymes, and electromyogram changes suggestive of inflammatory myopathy. A destructive polyarthritis can occur, which can result in contractures. Pulmonary, cardiac, and renal systems can all be rarely involved. The disease tends to be progressive and chronic, with rare remissions.

The differential diagnosis for scleromyxedema includes NSF, scleredema, diffuse morphea, SSc and other depositional disorders such as myxedema, amyloidosis, and leprosy. Keys to differentiating scleromyxedema from morphea, SSc, and scleredema are that the latter disorders generally do not produce papules. NSF typically spares the face, unlike scleromyxedema.

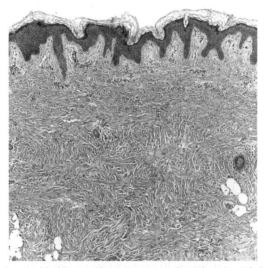

Fig. 8. Scleromyxedema, skin biopsy. There is a normal epidermis with both a perivascular and interstitial infiltrate of cells, with a slight increase in vascular spaces in the papillary dermis. There is increased mucin deposition manifested in this stain as an increase in white space between the pink collagen bundles (hematoxylin and eosin stain, original magnification ×100).

Box 4
Extracutaneous involvement in scleromyxedema

Multiple myeloma

Dysphagia

Neurologic features (seizures, carpal tunnel syndrome, cognitive)

Inflammatory myopathy

Arthralgia/arthritis

Pulmonary (dyspnea, restrictive or obstructive disease)

Cardiac (hypertension, atherosclerosis, myocardial infarction)

Renal failure

Treatment of scleromyxedema includes topical therapy (corticosteroids and UV therapy), which is of limited benefit. Melphalan, cyclophosphamide, and other chemotherapies have been described to be effective, although their use can lead to significant side effects including sepsis and secondary malignancies.[45] There are reports of success with plasma exchange. Recently, many reports of successful therapy with intravenous immunoglobulin or thalidomide suggest that these therapies might be of general clinical benefit.[50,51]

NEPHROGENIC SYSTEMIC FIBROSIS

This disorder, first known as nephrogenic fibrosing dermopathy, was first described in 2001 as a fibrosing skin disorder occurring exclusively in patients with renal impairment.[52] In general, most NSF patients are on dialysis while a smaller number have chronic renal insufficiency; a final small group consists of patients following kidney transplant.[53] This disorder is highly associated with the use of gadolinium-containing contrast agents, although some cases have occurred without history of this exposure, so it is not a strict requirement for the diagnosis.[54] If there is a history of exposure, NSF typically presents 2 to 10 weeks (median 5 weeks) following gadolinium exposure. Deposits of gadolinium can be detected in involved skin, but the precise mechanism of skin fibrosis is not known.[53] It is thought that CD34$^+$ cells contribute to this phenotype.

There is no gender predilection, and patients tend to be middle-aged, although children and the elderly can be affected. Although there is no gender of racial predisposition, the disease is mostly reported in the United States and parts of Europe.[53] Patients present initially with limb edema (usually on the legs) accompanied by infiltrative, erythematous papules and plaques overlying areas of deep fibrosis (**Fig. 9**). There is often a deep, woody induration of the affected areas that can mimic eosinophilic fasciitis, which can result in pain and limb contractures. Yellow scleral plaques can occur (**Box 5**).[53]

NSF is also associated with fibrotic damage to internal viscera such as the esophagus, lungs, heart, skeletal muscle, and kidneys (prompting a change in name from nephrogenic fibrosing dermopathy to nephrogenic systemic fibrosis). In some cases NSF can result in death.

Biopsies from NSF are often indistinguishable from those of scleromyxedema, showing a dermal proliferation of CD34$^+$ cells and variable mucin deposition (**Fig. 10**). Often the process involves the fat, unlike scleromyxedema.

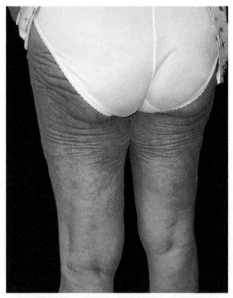

Fig. 9. Nephrogenic systemic fibrosis. Diffuse, ill-defined woody plaques on the legs and buttocks with extensive folding of the skin giving a wrinkled appearance.

In general, treatment of NSF using topical corticosteroids, immunosuppressive therapy, and plasmapheresis has been ineffective.[53] Several studies have described anecdotal treatments that may improve NSF, including UVA exposure, pentoxifylline, sodium thiosulfate, photopheresis, and rapamycin; however, these studies suffered from small numbers and lack of controls.[53] Recently, successful therapy with imatinib mesylate has been demonstrated, although this improvement is characterized by relapse following drug discontinuation.[55] Rarely patients can benefit from improvement in their renal function, and there are cases of renal transplantation resulting in improvement of the skin fibrosis.[56]

CHRONIC GRAFT-VERSUS-HOST DISEASE

Approximately 70% of patients who receive an allogeneic bone marrow transplant will eventually be diagnosed with cGVHD, a multisystem disorder that can affect any organ, although the skin is commonly affected. The skin manifestations of cGVHD

Box 5
Clinical features associated with NSF

- NSF is a fibrosing skin disorder occurring exclusively in patients with renal impairment.
- NSF is highly associated with the use of gadolinium-containing contrast agents, and typically presents 2 to 10 weeks after exposure.
- Cutaneous features include limb edema accompanied by infiltrative, erythematous papules and plaques overlying areas of deep fibrosis, and woody induration of affected areas.
- Extracutaneous features can include limb contractures associated with pain, yellow scleral plaques, and fibrotic damage to the esophagus, lungs, heart, skeletal muscle, and kidneys.

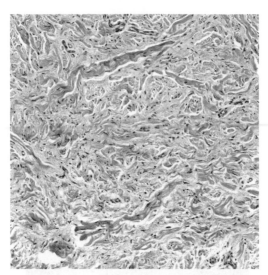

Fig. 10. Nephrogenic systemic fibrosis, skin biopsy. Some of the collagen bundles are expanded and eosinophilic, with an increase in interstitial cellularity as well as mucin (seen as *white spaces*) (hematoxylin and eosin, original magnification ×200).

can be variable, and approximately 15% of patients can be affected with scleroderm-atous changes of the skin.[57] As with LS, cGVHD can present differently depending on the depth of skin disease. Involvement of the papillary dermis results in thin, white atrophic papules and plaques, whereas involvement of the reticular dermis results in sclerotic plaques, often hidebound, which can affect the trunk or extremities. Contractures can develop, and epidermal atrophy can result in ulcerations, especially on the legs and pretibial regions. Involvement of the fat and subcutaneous tissue is insidious and results in a firm, nodular texture, and the overlying skin can have a "cellu-lite" appearance with or without hyperpigmentation. Involvement of the deeper tissues can mimic eosinophilic fasciitis, with a groove sign and deep woody induration.

Extracutaneous signs include muscle weakness, pain, and cramping. Mucosal disease commonly occurs, in the form of sensitivity, inflammation, or ulceration. Virtu-ally any organ system can be involved in cGVHD, so the clinician must have a high index of suspicion for systemic disease in a patient presenting with cutaneous lesions.

Histopathology of cGVHD reflects the clinical involvement. Sclerotic involvement of the papillary dermis demonstrates atrophy, hyperkeratosis, follicular plugging, and a pale, homogenized appearance of the collagen. If the process is deeper, dermal fibrosis with thickened collagen bundles and loss of periadnexal fat involvement is seen, which may be indistinguishable from idiopathic morphea/scleroderma. Sometimes both epidermal involvement (in the form of keratinocyte injury) and dermal sclerosis can be seen in the same biopsy (**Fig. 11**). Subcutaneous and fascial involvement accordingly reveals changes in the fat septae and fascia, including thickening, edema, and fibrosis, with variable infiltration of lymphocytes, histiocytes, and eosinophils.

One can differentiate cGVHD from SSc primarily because cGVHD involves the trunk and extremities (rather than starting with the hands), and is more patchy in its distribu-tion than SSc. It can be difficult to differentiate from LS, but mucosal involvement and a history of bone marrow transplant favor cGVHD.

Treatment for sclerotic cGVHD often includes phototherapy, especially psoralen-UVA and UVA-1.[58] Systemic immunosuppressants have not been proved to be

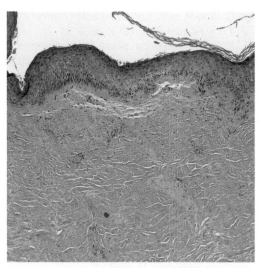

Fig. 11. Chronic graft-versus-host-disease, skin biopsy. The epidermis is slightly thickened and displays features of interface dermatitis as manifested by pigment deposition in the superficial dermis. There is a mild perivascular inflammatory cell infiltrate in the papillary dermis, as well as tightly packed, thickened eosinophilic collagen bundles (hematoxylin and eosin stain, original magnification ×100).

effective, and in fact 2 randomized trials have shown poorer outcomes in patients treated with both systemic corticosteroids and mycophenolate mofetil.[58] Extracorporeal photopheresis has demonstrated efficacy in case reviews but not in a randomized controlled trial, and is limited by time and expense. Mammalian target of rapamycin inhibitors (such as everolimus or sirolimus) have demonstrated benefit in approximately 75% of patients in retrospective analyses.[58] Small case series have recently demonstrated benefits with imatinib, and a pilot clinical trial is under way to test this more formally.[59–61]

SUMMARY

Several disorders can mimic SSc because of the clinical findings of cutaneous induration and fibrotic changes. In general, these are uncommon diseases that can sometimes be recognized and differentiated from one another by a careful history and clinical examination, although usually a clinicopathologic correlation is required to make the diagnosis. These disorders might be localized to the skin, but often have unique systemic implications that justify a careful search for the correct diagnosis. In general, management of these diseases is challenging, owing to both a lack of understanding of disease pathogenesis and a lack of evidence-based data regarding therapy. The recent work carried out to develop validated outcome markers for some of these diseases paves the way for clinical trials of new and old medications for the management of these diseases.

REFERENCES

1. Dehen L, Roujeau JC, Cosnes A, et al. Internal involvement in localized scleroderma. Medicine 1994;73(5):241–5.

2. Zulian F, Vallongo C, Woo P, et al. Localized scleroderma in childhood is not just a skin disease. Arthritis Rheum 2005;52(9):2873–81.

3. Fett N, Werth VP. Update on morphea: part I. Epidemiology, clinical presentation, and pathogenesis. J Am Acad Dermatol 2011;64(2):217–28 [quiz: 229–30].

4. Peterson LS, Nelson AM, Su WP, et al. The epidemiology of morphea (localized scleroderma) in Olmsted County 1960-1993. J Rheumatol 1997;24(1):73–80.

5. Murray KJ, Laxer RM. Scleroderma in children and adolescents. Rheum Dis Clin North Am 2002;28(3):603–24.

6. Zulian F, Athreya BH, Laxer R, et al. Juvenile localized scleroderma: clinical and epidemiological features in 750 children. An international study. Rheumatology (Oxford) 2006;45(5):614–20.

7. Christen-Zaech S, Hakim MD, Afsar FS, et al. Pediatric morphea (localized scleroderma): review of 136 patients. J Am Acad Dermatol 2008;59(3):385–96.

8. Leitenberger JJ, Cayce RL, Haley RW, et al. Distinct autoimmune syndromes in morphea: a review of 245 adult and pediatric cases. Arch Dermatol 2009; 145(5):545–50.

9. Peterson LS, Nelson AM, Su WP. Classification of morphea (localized scleroderma). Mayo Clin Proc 1995;70(11):1068–76.

10. Laxer RM, Zulian F. Localized scleroderma. Curr Opin Rheumatol 2006;18(6): 606–13.

11. Kreuter A, Krieg T, Worm M, et al. AWMF Guideline no. 013/066. Diagnosis and therapy of circumscribed scleroderma. J Dtsch Dermatol Ges 2009;7(Suppl 6): S1–14 [in German].

12. Kreuter A. Localized scleroderma. Dermatol Ther 2012;25(2):135–47.

13. Buechner SA, Rufli T. Atrophoderma of Pasini and Pierini. Clinical and histopathologic findings and antibodies to *Borrelia burgdorferi* in thirty-four patients. J Am Acad Dermatol 1994;30(3):441–6.

14. Saleh Z, Abbas O, Dahdah MJ, et al. Atrophoderma of Pasini and Pierini: a clinical and histopathological study. J Cutan Pathol 2008;35(12):1108–14.

15. Murphy PK, Hymes SR, Fenske NA. Concomitant unilateral idiopathic atrophoderma of Pasini and Pierini (IAPP) and morphea. Observations supporting IAPP as a variant of morphea. Int J Dermatol 1990;29(4):281–3.

16. Jacobson L, Palazij R, Jaworsky C. Superficial morphea. J Am Acad Dermatol 2003;49(2):323–5.

17. Jablonska S, Blaszczyk M. Is superficial morphea synonymous with atrophoderma Pasini-Pierini? J Am Acad Dermatol 2004;50(6):979–80 [author reply: 980].

18. Tekin NS, Altinyazar HC, Tekin IO, et al. Disabling pansclerotic morphoea: a case report. Int J Clin Pract 2010;64(1):99–101.

19. Lebeaux D, Sene D. Eosinophilic fasciitis (Shulman disease). Best Pract Res Clin Rheumatol 2012;26(4):449–58.

20. Orozco-Covarrubias L, Guzman-Meza A, Ridaura-Sanz C, et al. Scleroderma 'en coup de sabre' and progressive facial hemiatrophy. Is it possible to differentiate them? J Eur Acad Dermatol Venereol 2002;16(4):361–6.

21. Blaszczyk M, Krolicki L, Krasu M, et al. Progressive facial hemiatrophy: central nervous system involvement and relationship with scleroderma en coup de sabre. J Rheumatol 2003;30(9):1997–2004.

22. Torrelo A, Suarez J, Colmenero I, et al. Deep morphea after vaccination in two young children. Pediatr Dermatol 2006;23(5):484–7.

23. Ho J, Rothchild YH, Sengelmann R. Vitamin B12-associated localized scleroderma and its treatment. Dermatol Surg 2004;30(9):1252–5.

24. Peroni A, Zini A, Braga V, et al. Drug-induced morphea: report of a case induced by balicatib and review of the literature. J Am Acad Dermatol 2008;59(1):125–9.
25. Haustein UF, Haupt B. Drug-induced scleroderma and sclerodermiform conditions. Clin Dermatol 1998;16(3):353–66.
26. Asano Y, Ihn H, Shikada J, et al. A case of peplomycin-induced scleroderma. Br J Dermatol 2004;150(6):1213–4.
27. Kvernmo T, Hartter S, Burger E. A review of the receptor-binding and pharmacokinetic properties of dopamine agonists. Clin Ther 2006;28(8):1065–78.
28. Liddle BJ. Development of morphoea in rheumatoid arthritis treated with penicillamine. Ann Rheum Dis 1989;48(11):963–4.
29. Runger TM, Adami S, Benhamou CL, et al. Morphea-like skin reactions in patients treated with the cathepsin K inhibitor balicatib. J Am Acad Dermatol 2012;66(3): e89–96.
30. Sozeri B, Gulez N, Aksu G, et al. Pesticide-induced scleroderma and early intensive immunosuppressive treatment. Arch Environ Occup Health 2012;67(1):43–7.
31. Bovenzi M, Barbone F, Pisa FE, et al. A case-control study of occupational exposures and systemic sclerosis. Int Arch Occup Environ Health 2004;77(1):10–6.
32. Nietert PJ, Sutherland SE, Silver RM, et al. Is occupational organic solvent exposure a risk factor for scleroderma? Arthritis Rheum 1998;41(6):1111–8.
33. Stinco G, Piccirillo F, de Francesco V, et al. Scleroderma-like lesions and Parkinson's disease: possible links with exposure to pesticides. Eur J Dermatol 2007; 17(3):256–7.
34. Herrmann T, Gunther C, Csere P. Localized morphea—a rare but significant secondary complication following breast cancer radiotherapy. Case report and review of the literature on radiation reaction among patients with scleroderma/ morphea. Strahlenther Onkol 2009;185(9):603–7.
35. Davis DA, Cohen PR, McNeese MD, et al. Localized scleroderma in breast cancer patients treated with supervoltage external beam radiation: radiation port scleroderma. J Am Acad Dermatol 1996;35(6):923–7.
36. Bleasel NR, Stapleton KM, Commens C, et al. Radiation-induced localized scleroderma in breast cancer patients. Australas J Dermatol 1999;40(2):99–102.
37. Schaffer JV, Carroll C, Dvoretsky I, et al. Postirradiation morphea of the breast presentation of two cases and review of the literature. Dermatology 2000; 200(1):67–71.
38. Cheah NL, Wong DW, Chetiyawardana AD. Radiation-induced morphea of the breast: a case report. J Med Case Rep 2008;2:136.
39. Laetsch B, Hofer T, Lombriser N, et al. Irradiation-induced morphea: x-rays as triggers of autoimmunity. Dermatology 2011;223(1):9–12.
40. Zwischenberger BA, Jacobe HT. A systematic review of morphea treatments and therapeutic algorithm. J Am Acad Dermatol 2011;65(5):925–41.
41. Martini G, Ramanan AV, Falcini F, et al. Successful treatment of severe or methotrexate-resistant juvenile localized scleroderma with mycophenolate mofetil. Rheumatology 2009;48(11):1410–3.
42. Meguerditchian C, Jacquet P, Beliard S, et al. Scleredema adultorum of Buschke: an under recognized skin complication of diabetes. Diabetes Metab 2006; 32(5 Pt 1):481–4.
43. Beers WH, Ince A, Moore TL. Scleredema adultorum of Buschke: a case report and review of the literature. Semin Arthritis Rheum 2006;35(6):355–9.
44. Dziadzio M, Anastassiades CP, Hawkins PN, et al. From scleredema to AL amyloidosis: disease progression or coincidence? Review of the literature. Clin Rheumatol 2006;25(1):3–15.

45. Nashel J, Steen V. Scleroderma mimics. Curr Rheumatol Rep 2012;14(1):39–46.
46. Konemann S, Hesselmann S, Bolling T, et al. Radiotherapy of benign diseases—scleredema adultorum Buschke. Strahlenther Onkol 2004;180(12):811–4.
47. Alsaeedi SH, Lee P. Treatment of scleredema diabeticorum with tamoxifen. J Rheumatol 2010;37(12):2636–7.
48. Jackson EM, English JC 3rd. Diffuse cutaneous mucinoses. Dermatol Clin 2002; 20(3):493–501.
49. Fleming KE, Virmani D, Sutton E, et al. Scleromyxedema and the dermato-neuro syndrome: case report and review of the literature. J Cutan Pathol 2012;39(5): 508–17.
50. Sroa N, Campbell S, Bechtel M. Intravenous immunoglobulin therapy for scleromyxedema: a case report and review of literature. J Drugs Dermatol 2010;9(3): 263–5.
51. Efthimiou P, Blanco M. Intravenous gammaglobulin and thalidomide may be an effective therapeutic combination in refractory scleromyxedema: case report and discussion of the literature. Semin Arthritis Rheum 2008;38(3):188–94.
52. Cowper SE, Robin HS, Steinberg SM, et al. Scleromyxoedema-like cutaneous diseases in renal-dialysis patients. Lancet 2000;356(9234):1000–1.
53. Bernstein EJ, Schmidt-Lauber C, Kay J. Nephrogenic systemic fibrosis: a systemic fibrosing disease resulting from gadolinium exposure. Best practice & research. Clinical rheumatology 2012;26(4):489–503.
54. Girardi M, Kay J, Elston DM, et al. Nephrogenic systemic fibrosis: clinicopathological definition and workup recommendations. J Am Acad Dermatol 2011; 65(6):1095–1106.e7.
55. Kay J, High WA. Imatinib mesylate treatment of nephrogenic systemic fibrosis. Arthritis Rheum 2008;58(8):2543–8.
56. Cuffy MC, Singh M, Formica R, et al. Renal transplantation for nephrogenic systemic fibrosis: a case report and review of the literature. Nephrol Dial Transplant 2011;26(3):1099–101.
57. Hymes SR, Alousi AM, Cowen EW. Graft-versus-host disease: part I. Pathogenesis and clinical manifestations of graft-versus-host disease. J Am Acad Dermatol 2012;66(4):515.e1–18 [quiz: 533–4].
58. Hymes SR, Alousi AM, Cowen EW. Graft-versus-host disease: part II. Management of cutaneous graft-versus-host disease. J Am Acad Dermatol 2012;66(4): 535.e1–16 [quiz: 551–2].
59. Chen GL, Arai S, Flowers ME, et al. A phase 1 study of imatinib for corticosteroid-dependent/refractory chronic graft-versus-host disease: response does not correlate with anti-PDGFRA antibodies. Blood 2011;118(15):4070–8.
60. Magro L, Mohty M, Catteau B, et al. Imatinib mesylate as salvage therapy for refractory sclerotic chronic graft-versus-host disease. Blood 2009;114(3):719–22.
61. Olivieri A, Locatelli F, Zecca M, et al. Imatinib for refractory chronic graft-versus-host disease with fibrotic features. Blood 2009;114(3):709–18.

Retroperitoneal Fibrosis

Paul J. Scheel Jr, MD*, Nancy Feeley, CRNP

KEYWORDS

- Retroperitoneal fibrosis • Chronic periaortitis • Review • Management

KEY POINTS

- Retroperitoneal fibrosis (RPF) is a fibroinflammatory disorder of unknown etiology that surrounds the infrarenal aorta and may progress to surrounding structures.
- A lack of standardized definition of disease, small numbers of patients, and differing end points in research publications has limited our efficiency in understanding the optimum treatment.
- There are currently 5 different diseases that lead to infrarenal periaortitis: inflammatory abdominal aortic aneurysm, perianeurysmal retroperitoneal fibrosis, RPF, Erdheim-Chester disease, and immunoglobulin G4–related disease.
- Management includes alleviation of urinary obstruction and Immunosuppressive therapy.

INTRODUCTION

Retroperitoneal fibrosis (RPF) is a condition characterized by the presence of inflammation and fibrosis in the retroperitoneal space. Unfortunately, no standard definition exists that clearly defines the criteria that must be present for the diagnosis of RPF. It is this ambiguity that has made formal investigation into this disease challenging and comparison of multiple different reports vulnerable to misinterpretation. As a starting point, most agree that a pathologic specimen obtained anywhere in the retroperitoneum indicating fibrosis is not sufficient for the diagnosis of RPF. Rather, the salient feature that must be present is the radiographic finding of periaortitis. There are currently 5 different diseases that lead to infrarenal periaortitis: inflammatory abdominal aortic aneurysm (IAAA), perianeurysmal retroperitoneal fibrosis, RPF, Erdheim-Chester disease (ECD), and immunoglobulin G4 (IgG4)-related disease. In most reports IAAA, perianeurysmal retroperitoneal fibrosis, and RPF have been lumped together for the purposes of analysis. ECD, while sharing some similar radiographic features, has a distinct histologic and clinical presentation. IgG4-related disease was not recognized as a possible isolated condition until 2003. It is unclear how many, if any, of these patients were included in analyses of patients with RPF.

Division of Nephrology, The Johns Hopkins University School of Medicine, 1830 East Monument Street, Room 416, Baltimore, MD 21205, USA
* Corresponding author.
E-mail address: Pscheel1@jhmi.edu

Rheum Dis Clin N Am 39 (2013) 365–381
http://dx.doi.org/10.1016/j.rdc.2013.02.004
0889-857X/13/$ – see front matter © 2013 Elsevier Inc. All rights reserved.
rheumatic.theclinics.com

Because no standard definition exists, it is important to establish the definition to be used when reviewing the literature on RPF. The following must be present:

1. A soft-tissue density surrounding the infrarenal aorta or iliac vessels by contrast-enhanced computed tomography (CT) or magnetic resonance imaging (MRI).
2. Absence of a biopsy in the retroperitoneum that is positive for malignancy.
3. Absence of a systemic, multicentric, fibrosis processing such as IgG4-related disease.

RPF begins with clinical symptoms of flank pain and unexplained weight loss. Radiographically, fibrosis starts to surround the infrarenal aorta, and progresses inferiorly toward the iliac bifurcation and laterally toward the renal hilum and surrounding structures, ultimately leading to ureteral obstruction and acute renal failure. Historically, treatment has focused on relieving the obstruction with percutaneous or cystoscopic assisted placement of ureteral stents followed by more definitive resolution of ureteric obstruction with open or laparoscopic ureterolysis, with or without omental wrapping.

Over the past several years, case reports and small series have documented successful, nonsurgical management with the use of various immunosuppressive agents including prednisone, cyclosporine, methotrexate, azathioprine, cyclophosphamide, mycophenolate mofetil (MMF), infliximab, rituximab, colchicine, and the selective estrogen receptor antagonist tamoxifen.[1–10] Management therefore has shifted from primarily a surgical approach to a therapy aimed at modulation of the immune system.

This review focuses on the recent advances in the classification, epidemiology, pathophysiology, pathology, imaging, and treatment of these disease states.

DEMOGRAPHICS

Patients with RPF present to medical attention in the fifth, sixth, and seventh decades of life with a mean age of 54 years.[11] There is a slight male to female predominance with ratios ranging from 1:1 to 3:1, depending on the report.[11–14] All races appear to be affected equally. Few epidemiologic studies exist that accurately characterize the incidence and prevalence of the disease. One report from the Netherlands suggests an incidence of 0.10 per 100,000 individuals.[15]

RISK FACTORS

The proposed risk factors for RPF are listed in **Box 1**. Multiple agents have been suggested as possible etiologic factors in RPF. Of the suggested pharmacologic agents, methysergide and ergotamine are the best studied and documented. A frequently used medication to treat migraine headaches, methysergide is a serotonin antagonist. Increased circulating levels of endogenous serotonin have been suggested to lead to endocardial, pulmonary, and retroperitoneal fibrosis. RPF has been ascribed to methysergide in up to 12% of cases in older series; however, the present-day incidence is much lower, secondary to infrequent use of this medication.[16] Ergotamine-derived agents stimulate serotonergic receptors, causing proliferation of myofibroblasts and increased fibrotic deposition.[17] Although alternative agents have been found to treat migraine headaches, ergot derivatives are still used to treat Parkinsonism (pergolide, cabergoline, and bromocriptine) and the use of these agents should be specifically noted in the history.

Other medications that have been associated with RPF include β-blockers, methyldopa, phenacetin, and hydralazine.[18–23] These associations have been presented in

---

Box 1
Reported risk factors for retroperitoneal fibrosis

- Radiation
- Exposure to asbestos
- Malignancy
- Tuberculosis
- Medications:
  - Methysergide
  - Ergotamine
  - Hydralazine
  - Methyldopa
  - Phenacetin
  - β-Blockers

---

isolated case reports and have failed to document a cause-and-effect relationship. In a recent report the authors were unable to find any association with the use of any of these medications.[14]

Asbestos exposure has also been found to be associated with RPF in male workers in Finland. In workers with heavy exposure to asbestos, it is postulated that asbestos fibers are transported to the retroperitoneal space via lymphatic drainage from the gastrointestinal tract or via lymphatic drainage from the lung. This theory is supported by findings of asbestos bodies in retroperitoneal organs such as the kidneys and adrenal glands. Uibu and colleagues[15] performed a case-control study of 43 patients with RPF in Finland, and found a 9-fold increased risk for RPF in association with more than 10 fiber-years of asbestos exposure. Smaller series have documented the coexistence of RPF with pleural plaques in male workers with asbestos exposure, but fail to provide evidence for a cause-and-effect relationship.[24,25] In those patients with RPF and pleural plaques, the mean time from first occupational exposure until the patient was diagnosed with RPF was 30 years.[25] The authors have added a detailed occupational exposure questionnaire as part of their initial evaluation. In the most recent report, 18% of their patients had some possible exposure to asbestos, but none of these patients had pulmonary findings of asbestos exposure on high-resolution CT.[14]

External-beam radiation is a well-described risk factor for fibrotic reactions in multiple different anatomic locations. The exact mechanism(s) remains an intense area of investigation. Irradiation has been shown to lead to premature terminal differentiation of fibroblasts, which results in increased collagen production.[26] In the authors' current population of a 140 patients with RPF, only 2 patients have had a history of radiation; 1 for a spinal cord tumor and a second on brachytherapy for prostate cancer (Scheel, unpublished data, 2013). In these cases it is unclear whether the radiation caused the fibrosis or was just of historical interest. From a therapeutic perspective, these patients' response to therapy was no different from the rest of the cohort.

Malignancy is often listed as a risk factor or a secondary form of RPF. In reality, these patients have a malignancy metastatic to the retroperitoneal space with a surrounding inflammatory and fibrotic reaction. A thorough physical examination with age-appropriate cancer screening is required for all patients presenting with newly diagnosed RPF. Patients with a history of or known malignancy outside of the retroperitoneum, or patients who present with atypical clinical or radiographic findings, should undergo a biopsy before consideration of treatment. The most common cancers found in the retroperitoneal space are lymphomas, cancers of the genitourinary tract, and breast cancer.[27]

GENETICS

Limited information is available on whether genetic or epigenetic factors predispose to the development of RPF. Three case reports exist that describe RPF in twins or siblings. Unfortunately, all of these reports were published before the common use of cross-sectional imaging or the application of immunofluorescence to pathologic material staining specifically for IgG4. Goldstein reported on 2 siblings ages 6 and 9 years who developed ureteral obstruction secondary to "RPF."[28] The diagnosis was made by intravenous pyelography (IVP), and at the time of surgery periureteral masses were found with a pathologic appearance suggestive of RPF. Because RPF is unusual in children, and given that RPF does not typically present as retroperitoneal masses, it is possible that this actually represents a report of IgG4-related disease that can present with masses and in this age group. Phyllis and colleagues[29] described 3 siblings in their 20s with RPF, all of whom were diagnosed by IVP. All 3 presented with acute onset of pain, weight loss, anemia, and the presence of autoantibodies. Of note, all were found to be sickle-trait positive. Duffy and colleagues[30] reported on twins in their 60s diagnosed with RPF and ureteral obstruction 2 years apart. Both patients presented with elevated erythrocyte sedimentation rate (ESR) and medial deviation of the ureter.

In the absence of modern series describing a familial component in RPF, investigators have focused on genetic susceptibility factors, namely human leukocyte antigen (HLA) serotypes. Martorana and colleagues[31] performed a case-control study on 39 patients with RPF and 350 controls. For their study group they batched patients with RPF, IAAA and perianeurysmal fibrosis. HLA DRB1*03 was found in 48.5% of the patients with periaortitis and only 16% of controls. HLA B*08 was found in 17.9% of patients with chronic periaortitis (CP) and only 6.78% of controls. Both of these differences were highly statistically significant. This small study needs to be confirmed by larger studies that include correlation with pathologic specimens, with each group of patients with CP studied independently.

PRESENTING SIGNS AND SYMPTOMS

The most common presenting signs and symptoms for RPF are shown in **Table 1**. Pain is the most common presenting symptom.[27,32,33] The pain is typically described as

Table 1
Symptoms on presentation with retroperitoneal fibrosis

Symptoms	% of Patients	References
Pain	86–100	11,32,33
Hypertension	40–57	11,33
Fatigue	25–52.9	11,27,32
Weight loss	40–50	11,27,33
Hydrocele	17–29	11,33
Deep venous thrombosis/pulmonary embolism	6–14	11,27

deep within the abdomen, affecting one or both flanks and radiating to the inguinal area. The pain is noncolicky and is unaffected by movement, defecation, or voiding. Significant fatigue is present in the majority of patients. Males commonly have scrotal pain secondary to associated hydroceles. Significant unexplained weight loss occurs in up to 50% of diagnosed cases, leading to investigation into an undiagnosed malignancy.[27,32] New onset or worsening of essential hypertension can occur if the renal vessels are extrinsically compressed or if the patient develops acute kidney injury (AKI) secondary to ureteral obstruction. Lower extremity edema may occur secondary to caval compression and obstruction of venous outflow from the lower extremities. In the authors' experience, 5% to 10% of patients who present for evaluation have been diagnosed with a lower extremity deep venous thrombosis or pulmonary embolus. Signs and symptoms of lower extremity or mesenteric arterial insufficiency may be present, depending on involvement of the superior mesenteric, inferior mesenteric, or iliac vessels.

Vaglio and colleagues[34] have reported a strong association between the presence of periaortitis and coexisting rheumatic diseases, including inflammatory and noninflammatory arthritis.

Although a review of IgG4-related disease is beyond the scope of this article, it is noteworthy that contrary to RPF, it is reported that IgG4 disease presents in a subacute fashion.[35] Most patients are not constitutionally ill; fevers and elevations of inflammatory markers are rare.[35] The disease is often diagnosed incidentally on imaging or unexpectedly in pathologic specimens.[35] Although many organs can be affected, submandibular glands, parotid glands, pancreas, and aorta are most common. Unlike patients with RPF, patients with IgG4-related disease have a history of chronic allergic conditions such as eczema and asthma.[8]

Lymphadenopathy can be seen in both IgG4-related disease and RPF, but is more common and more significant in the former. Both disease processes can cause thyroid involvement either through direct deposition of IgG4 or via the production of antithyroid antibodies.

LABORATORY FEATURES

A significant normochromic normocytic anemia occurs in 25% to 50% or patients at the time of presentation.[11,13] Fifty percent to 100% of patients will have an elevated ESR or C-reactive protein.[11,13,27,36] Twenty-five percent to 60% of patients with RPF will be positive for antinuclear antibodies.[11,36] Vaglio and colleagues[37] also reported the presence of other autoantibodies in patients with RPF. In a 2006 study they reported that 31% of patients with RPF have the presence of antithyroid antibodies, 14% have documented anti–smooth-muscle antibodies, 14% have rheumatoid factor, and 10% are positive for perinuclear or cytoplasmic antineutrophil cytoplasmic antibodies (ANCA).

In patients with suspected IgG4-related disease, IgG4 levels are elevated in 70% of patients with biopsy-proven IgG4-related disease.[35] Anemia is not a common feature, nor is elevated markers of inflammation.[35] IgG4-related disease commonly causes a tubular interstitial nephritis, therefore urine protein may be elevated. Eosinophilia is common in IgG4-related disease and is rare in RPF.[35,38]

PATHOPHYSIOLOGY

As mentioned previously, there is no formal agreement on the clinical definition of RPF. It is therefore not surprising that several different proposed mechanisms exist to explain the evolution of this disease process. Unfortunately no animal model has been developed to further study this family of diseases, thus making elucidation of these mechanisms protracted. There are currently 3 different hypotheses proposed to explain the pathogenesis of RPF. The first model is based on the finding that many patients with RPF have a significant burden of atherosclerosis in the abdominal aorta. The incidence of this finding varies by series. Other patients present with no evidence of an atherosclerotic burden, and alternative explanations have been proposed. Each may correctly explain a subset of patients with RPF, or components of each may uniformly apply to the broader heterogeneous population currently labeled as RPF.

Atherosclerosis Model

This model was originally proposed in the mid-1980s by Michinson and Parums,[39] who noticed that the affected sections of aorta had a heavy atherosclerotic burden. Microscopically it was noted that the inflammatory reaction to the atherosclerosis was not limited to the intimal layer but expanded to the media and adventitial layers. These investigators postulated that this "breach" into the media allowed lipid-laden macrophages to present oxidized low-density lipoprotein (LDL) and ceroid as antigens to T and B cells, thus initiating an immune reaction. This inflammatory reaction progressed to the adventitial layer and periaortic space, leading to the periaortitis and fibrosis.

These same investigators were able to subsequently demonstrate that in patients with periaortitis, IgG could be shown to be in close apposition to extracellular ceroid.[40] In addition, they were able to show that ceroid-laden macrophages could be found in the adventitia and regional lymph nodes and that T and B cells found in the aorta media demonstrated markers of activation and proliferation. Finally, there was evidence of elevated serum immunoglobulin M and IgG antibodies to oxidized LDL and ceroid in patients with CP but not in a control population.[41]

Autoimmune Model

The evidence that RPF represents an autoimmune disease is broad but circumstantial. Ormond[42] noted that the periaortic vessels in 2 of his patients resembled the vasculitis seen in polyarteritis nodosa. Similar findings of vasculitis of the vasa vasorum of the aorta have been documented by other investigators.[43] Using flow cytometry, Moroni and colleagues[44] reported that in patients with RPF there were increased numbers of circulating endothelial cells and that these cells were of microvascular origin. Similar findings were not found in patients with atherosclerosis or in healthy controls. These circulating endothelial cells returned to normal levels with suppression of the immune system. Martorana and colleagues[31] discovered the presence of the HLA DRB1*03 allele in patients with RPF. This allele has also shown to be present in high numbers in other autoimmune diseases, namely type 1 diabetes mellitus, myasthenia gravis, and systemic lupus erythematosus (SLE).[45] Patients with RPF have been documented to present with various other autoantibodies.[37] There are also case reports of patients presenting with both RPF and with autoimmune diseases such as seropositive inflammatory arthritis, ankylosing spondylitis, SLE, and ANCA-associated vasculitis.[34,36,46–48]

IgG4-Related Disease

Since 2003 the IgG4 molecule has been associated or labeled as being responsible for human disease in nearly every major organ system.[49–62] The IgG4 molecule typically represents less than 5% of circulating immunoglobulins in healthy individuals.[5] In IgG4-related disease it is postulated that some inciting event, perhaps autoimmunity, stimulates T-helper 2 (Th2)-positive cells, leading to an inflammatory response via the transcription of inflammatory interleukins, namely interleukin (IL)-4, IL-5, IL-10, and IL-13.[35] A second proposed event is the activation of T-regulatory (Treg) cells. Treg cells are believed to contribute to the inflammatory reaction leading to the production of IL-10, with a subsequent increase in B cells producing IgG4 and transforming growth factor β (TGF-β).[4,63] TGF-β is thought to have significant responsibility for the fibrosis seen in this disease. Once produced, it is unclear whether IgG4 represents a tissue-destructive antibody or merely is overexpressed in response to an unclear stimulus.

Recent reviews have suggested that idiopathic RPF can now be ascribed to and categorized under the IgG4-related umbrella.[35] Unfortunately, the evidence to support this hypothesis is lacking or based on studies involving small groups of patients, not all of whom even had periaortitis. In the best characterized study, Zen and colleagues[64] reported on 17 patients with "retroperitoneal fibrosis." Only 14 of these patients had periaortitis, and 3 had evidence of extraretroperitoneal disease such as autoimmune pancreatitis. Eight of these 14 patients met the criteria for IgG4-related disease via increased numbers of IgG4 plasma cells in the inflammatory lesion. Based on this study, Stone and colleagues[35] stated that "55% of all RPF is caused by IgG4-related disease." Additional biopsy studies will need to be performed in patients with RPF to clarify the role of IgG4 in this disease process.

PATHOLOGY

RPF is described grossly as a gray-white hard material covering the infrarenal aorta, extending in a caudal direction to the iliac bifurcation and involving the proximal iliac vessels.[42] On rare occasions this process has been shown to progress cephalad to involve the renal vessels, but no further. Over time this process proceeds laterally to surround and compress the vena cava, leading to compression and occasional thrombosis with subsequent collateral formation. As lateral extension continues, the ureters are drawn into this inflammatory process and are displaced in a medial direction.

Microscopically there is a fibroinflammatory infiltrate. The fibrotic material is composed of spindle cells and bands of fibers that stain positive for α type I collagen antibody.

The inflammatory infiltrate is composed of CD3, CD4, and CD8 T lymphocytes, CD20 B lymphocytes, macrophages, and CD138 plasma cells.[65] These inflammatory cells may be found surrounding and infiltrating the adventitial layer of small vessels with occasional necrosis, mimicking a small-vessel vasculitis. Dispersed throughout the fibrotic material is a looser aggregate of lymphocytes, macrophages, and eosinophils.

Aortic-wall histology shows atherosclerotic changes to the intima and thinning of the media, with significant adventitial inflammation.

In those patients who have greater than 50% of plasma cells positive for IgG4 (ie, IgG4-related disease), there are reports of lymphoid follicle formation and significant eosinophilic infiltrate.[35] In addition, as this infiltrate progresses laterally the ureter is not only surrounded but infiltrated through the outer layers while the endothelium is spared.[35] In those cases where the entire aorta was available for microscopic examination the intima was not significantly affected by atherosclerotic plaque, the media was normal, and, as in IgG4-negative patients, there was significant inflammation in the adventitial layer.[35]

IMAGING

Imaging studies are essential in the diagnosis and chronic management of patients with RPF. Historically, IVP or retrograde urograms were the gold standard for diagnosing RPF. The triad of hydronephrosis, medial deviation, and extrinsic compression of the ureters was all that was needed to make the diagnosis. Nowadays cross-sectional imaging with either contrast CT or MRI has replaced these antiquated and less sensitive imaging techniques.

Contrast-enhanced CT is the preferred method of imaging in the authors' center. CT images show a rim of soft-tissue density surrounding the aorta, possibly extending from the renal vessels to the proximal iliac arteries (**Fig. 1**). Typically arterial-phase, venous-phase and delayed (urogram) images are obtained if renal function permits. Arterial-phase imaging allows for excellent definition of the aorta, abdominal branches, and iliac vessels. The luminal size of the aorta can be accurately measured, and the presence or absence of aneurismal dilation allows for rapid classification. Narrowing of the renal, iliac, or mesenteric vessels may provide the clinician with valuable information pertaining to clinical symptoms of worsening or new-onset hypertension, postprandial abdominal pain, or symptoms of claudication. Arterial-phase imaging also allows for definition of crisp margins between the aorta and the soft-tissue density surrounding the aorta, allowing for accurate measurements of the size of the soft-tissue mass.

Venous-phase imaging provides information on the presence or absence of caval narrowing or thrombosis, or the presence, size, and location of venous collaterals. Venous-phase imaging may also provide clarity on the burden of mass that surrounds the iliac vessels.

Urogram images are helpful in defining the extent and location of ureteral compression and possible obstruction. Use of urogram images may obviate nuclear imaging when attempting to define the extent of ureteral compression and obstruction. If patients have bilateral indwelling ureteral stents, the authors omit this phase of imaging because it provides no useful information.

Although obtaining all 3 phases of the CT imaging provides valuable information, it also increases both the dose of radiation exposure and cost. A patient's history of irradiation has to be taken into account when deciding on an imaging strategy.

Additional findings on abdominal/pelvic CT in patients with RPF may include regional adenopathy. Absence of an infrarenal perirenal soft-tissue mass or the

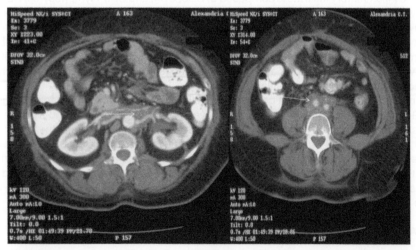

Fig. 1. Computed tomography (CT) scan of abdomen and pelvis with intravenous contrast. Arrows indicate soft-tissue density surrounding renal arteries, aorta, and iliac arteries.

presence of other abdominal/pelvic masses should raise significant doubt regarding the diagnosis of RPF, and strong consideration should be given to biopsy.

ECD is a rare form of non–Langerhans cell histiocytosis and is reviewed elsewhere in this issue. ECD is frequently misdiagnosed as RPF, as the periaortic soft-tissue mass may be identical to that seen in RPF. The distinguishing feature on CT is the presence of bilateral perirenal soft-tissue inflammation or soft-tissue mass (**Fig. 2**). Presence of this perirenal soft-tissue mass is not consistent with RPF, and evaluation for ECD should be pursued. The authors proceed with a Tc-99 bone scan, which is positive in more than 90% of cases of ECD. This scan shows significant uptake in long bones, usually of the lower extremity.

The use of MRI is an acceptable alternative to CT for the diagnosis of RPF. MRI allows for the avoidance of ionizing radiation, the risk of dye-induced kidney injury, and systemic allergic reaction to contrast dye. MRI is more costly, can be difficult to perform in those with claustrophobia, has significantly longer scan times, and, depending on the center, may have less expertise readily available for diagnostic review with the clinician. RPF is hypodense on T1-weighted images, and on T2-weighted images its intensity is high in the early or active stages of disease and low in late stages. Mirault and colleagues[66] recently documented some important MRI differences between idiopathic RPF and retroperitoneal fibrosis from an underlying malignancy (m-RPF). Important differences included: extension of fibrosis above the renal arteries and below aortic bifurcation was more common in m-RPF than in RPF (47% vs 0%; $P = .001$); extension of fibrosis behind the aorta was greater in RPF than in m-RPF (5 vs 2 mm; $P = .03$); and medial deviation of ureters was less common in m-RPF than in RPF (24% vs 83%; $P \leq .001$).

[18]F-fluorodeoxyglucose positron emission tomography (FDG PET) scans show avid uptake of ^{18}F-FDG in the periaortic soft-tissue density in patients with RPF. Increased activity in multiple locations would argue against RPF and in favor of a multisystem disease such as IgG4-related disease, ECD, or a malignancy. Some have used PET

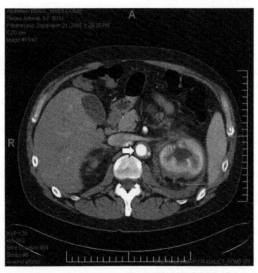

Fig. 2. CT scan of abdomen with intravenous contrast. Large arrow indicates soft-tissue density surrounding infrarenal aorta. Small arrow indicates histiocytic infiltrate surrounding left kidney.

scanning to determine whether the residual soft-density tissue rind following therapy continues to have active inflammation as a marker of the need for ongoing chemotherapy.[67,68] Given the high cost of PET scans and frequent denials by third-party payers, the authors rely on other clinical indicators of disease activity, namely anemia and inflammatory markers such as ESR and CRP.

Radioisotopic Mag-3 scans are a valuable tool in both the initial evaluation and chronic management decisions in patients with RPF and urinary obstruction. Communication with the radiologist is important when ordering these studies. Unlike perfusion scans used to diagnose renal artery stenosis, in RPF the clinician is most interested in the excretion phase of these studies. For these studies to be useful the patient must have a glomerular filtration rate (GFR) adequate enough to excrete the isotope from the renal parenchyma into the collecting system. Although no formal GFR cutoff is agreed upon, the authors have found these studies to be of little use when the GFR is less than 25 mL/min. When ordering these studies, the protocol is to also request the addition of furosemide to be given intravenously during the diuresis phase of the study. Finally, the radiologist is requested to calculate an excretion half-time ($T_{1/2}$) from each renal unit. $T_{1/2}$ differ slightly according to the protocol used, and normative values differ from center to center. In general, a normal $T_{1/2}$ would be less than 10 minutes. A partial obstruction is suspected with a $T_{1/2}$ between 11 and 20 minutes, and a $T_{1/2}$ of greater than 20 minutes is consistent with a complete obstruction.

TREATMENT

Although controversy remains regarding the appropriate classification and pathophysiology of RPF, it is clear that inflammation progressing to fibrosis is a common pathologic finding of the diseases currently under the umbrella of RPF. In addition, if left untreated this fibroinflammatory process will lead to ureteral obstruction, with possible loss of one or both renal units. Therefore, the goals of therapy are to halt inflammation, reverse fibrosis, and implement measures to protect the kidney from chronic injury from ureteral obstruction.

There is no one immunosuppression protocol that has been shown to be superior to other treatment options. The difficulty in interpreting the existing literature lies in the fact that all studies have involved small numbers of patients with varying forms of RPF. Each has had different inclusion criteria and primary end points. To date there is only one randomized controlled trial (RCT), and several prospective case series.[14,69,70] The remainder are retrospective series or isolated case reports. The immunosuppressive therapies that have the most data include corticosteroids, tamoxifen, and MMF.

It is well known that corticosteroids have potent anti-inflammatory effects, and are used to treat inflammatory conditions multiple causes in nearly every organ of. Corticosteroids have also been found to have limited antifibrotic properties. For instance, in nonviral autoimmune hepatic fibrosis, prednisone has been shown to induce clinical remission and improved histology.[71] High-dose steroids are also used to treat pulmonary fibrosis, with response rates of 10% to 40%.[71]

In treating RPF most reports use corticosteroids, alone or in combination with other agents. Prednisone is inexpensive and readily available, and its rapid onset of action attenuates the inflammatory response. Patients typically subjectively feel better, have increased hemoglobin concentrations, and have decreased markers of inflammation within the first 4 to 6 weeks of treatment.[69,70] The most appropriate dose of steroids for this condition has not been determined.

The only RCT for the treatment of RPF was conducted by Vaglio and colleagues.[69] In this trial, 36 patients with RPF were randomized to steroids alone or steroids plus tamoxifen. At the start of treatment all patients received 1 mg/kg/d of prednisone. After 1 month or when patients achieved a clinical remission, they were randomized to a prednisone taper over 7 months or 7 months of tamoxifen. For the purposes of this study, remission was defined as symptomatic improvement and normalization of ESR/CRP. Six percent of patients in the steroid arm relapsed during the trial while 39% of patients in the tamoxifen arm relapsed during therapy. Following discontinuation of therapy, the steroid group had an 11.8% relapse rate and the tamoxifen arm had an 18.2% relapse rate. There was no difference in time to removal of the ureteral stent(s) in those patients who were obstructed, and there was a greater reduction in the periaortic mass in the steroid arm. Despite this being a well-designed and well-executed study, the number of patients was small, and the relapse rates during and following therapy were high.

Multiple case reports have documented successful management of RPF with tamoxifen.[10,72–74] Recently, van Bommel and colleagues[70] reported on a prospective case series of 55 patients with RPF treated with monotherapy consisting of tamoxifen, 20 mg administered orally twice daily. The primary end point was a composite of 3 secondary end points: subjective clinical improvement by 6 weeks; stable or decreasing periaortic mass by 4 months and definite decreasing mass by 8 months; and resolution of ureteric obstruction sufficient enough to allow for stent removal. Sixty-five percent of patients met the composite end point. The most common side effects were hot flashes, fatigue, and loss of libido in men. Thirty-two percent of those who achieved the composite end point relapsed at a median of 26 months following completion of therapy. Although a majority of patients reached the composite end point, 35% did not. Combined with a 32% relapse rate in those who initially responded, this finding raises some concern for the routine use of this protocol.

The third drug that has been shown to be effective in a prospective series is MMF combined with low-dose prednisone. MMF is an inosine monophosphate dehydrogenase inhibitor that interrupts the response of B and T cells. In addition to those immunologic properties, MMF has been shown to reverse fibrosis in laboratory animals. In cell cultures of pulmonary fibroblasts, the addition of MMF led to the reduction in type I collagen and to increased production of collagenase I.[71] In other animal models, MMF has been shown to decrease myofibroblast infiltration and collagen III deposition in a rat remnant kidney model of chronic kidney disease, and to reduce renal fibrosis in an ischemia reperfusion model of AKI.[75,76]

Scheel and colleagues[14] reported a prospective case series of 28 patients with RPF treated with MMF and low-dose steroids. The treatment consisted of 40 mg oral prednisone administered for 30 days with a 10-mg taper each month combined with MMF at a dose of 1000 mg administered orally twice daily. The MMF was continued for 6 months following resolution of ureteric obstruction. For patients without ureteric obstruction, the drug was continued for 6 months following a 25% greater reduction of periaortic mass and complete resolution of symptoms. Patients were treated for a mean of 29.3 months. Systemic symptoms resolved in all patients, as did normalization of inflammatory markers. Eighty-nine percent of patients had a greater than 25% reduction in the periaortic mass. Eighty-six percent of patients with obstruction had successful removal of the ureteral stent. It is interesting that both patients who failed therapy in this series were African American. In the transplant literature it is customary to increase the dose of MMF to 1500 mg twice daily, because of the more rapid metabolism of this drug in African Americans. It is possible that both of these patients failed to improve secondary to underdosing of MMF. Only 7% of patients in this series relapsed. Patients in this report were treated for a significantly longer period of time than in the reports of Vaglio and Van Bommel. This factor may explain the higher response rate and lower relapse rate.

In addition to steroids, MMF, and tamoxifen, case reports and small retrospective series have documented the success with several other immunosuppressant agents including cyclosporine, methotrexate, azathioprine, cyclophosphamide, and colchicines.[2–5,9] Recently there have also been 2 case reports describing the successful use of the newer biological agents infliximab and rituximab in patients with RPF who have failed other oral immunosuppressant agents.[7,0]

Surgical mobilization of the entrapped ureters with or without corticosteroids had been the mainstay for the treatment of RPF since its description by Ormond[77] in 1948. Indications for surgical intervention in patients with primary or secondary RPF had traditionally included radiographic evidence of obstruction and deteriorating renal function. With the recent paradigm shift toward medical therapy, the indications for surgery have changed, with many using surgery as a second-line option after failed medical therapy, or in those with a contraindication or unwillingness to proceed with prolonged immunosuppression.

Physicians treating patients with RPF will also need to have a working knowledge of the management of ureteral obstruction. Although a detailed review of this topic is beyond the scope of this article, the treating physician should understand the types of stents available, their complications, and timing of exchange.

Internal ureteral stents are typically placed through a cystoscope, and have the advantage of not having any external hardware. Urine from the renal pelvis flows through and around these stents. In patients with significant extrinsic compression, these stents may not allow for successful decompression of the obstructed kidney. Recent data have indicated that for extrinsic compression of the ureters from retroperitoneal and pelvic malignancies, metallic stents have an improved patency rate.[78] Data on using these stents in patients with RPF is lacking. Complications of these stents are primarily infection and pain that is worse with voiding. These stents also become encrusted with calcium and other minerals, a process that not only limits patency but increases the risk of removal and exchange. The authors' protocol calls for stent exchange every 3 months until removal.

Nephroureteral stents (NUS) are placed percutaneously. The stent passes through the skin with continuation through the renal pelvis, where side holes exist, and down the ureter into the urinary bladder. These stents may be the first stents to be placed when the patient is diagnosed, especially if there is evidence of extensive ureteral compression. The advantage of NUS over internal stents is that the kidney can be drained externally into a urinary bag or antegrade through the ureter. When deciding if the ureter is patent enough for internal stents, the external portion of the NUS is clamped and a trial of antegrade flow is attempted. If successful, an internal stent can be placed via a guide wire over the NUS at the 3-month exchange.

Percutaneous nephrostomy (PCN) tubes are reserved for patients with severe extrinsic compression of the ureter where the ureter will not permit safe passage of an internal stent or NUS. Patients with PCN tubes should be periodically reassessed for conversion to internal stents.

When attempts are made to permanently remove these devices based on reduction of periaortic mass and lack of ureteral compression by imaging, the authors recommend removing only one side at a time in those with bilateral stents. Following removal, patients are assessed for increased pain and decreased urine output. At 48 hours, blood is obtained for analysis of creatinine and potassium. If there is no indication of obstruction, a Mag-3 nuclear scan is performed at 14 days. If excretion is normal, one proceeds with removal of the contralateral side. At this 14-day stage a partial obstruction may exist, owing to ureteral edema associated with prolonged intubation. If a partial obstruction is demonstrated at 14 days, the procedure is repeated in 2 weeks. If the partial obstruction still exists, the ureteral stent is replaced.

LONG-TERM FOLLOW-UP

As already mentioned, RPF has been reported to recur at high rates.[69,70] After discontinuation of therapy, patients with RPF must be followed for life. Following discontinuation of immunosuppression, the authors obtain monthly laboratory data assessing for renal function, anemia, and evidence of inflammation for the first 6 months, and quarterly thereafter. Patients are instructed to call immediately if they experience any unexplained weight loss or recurrent pain.

SUMMARY

RPF is a fibroinflammatory disorder of unknown etiology that surrounds the infrarenal aorta and may progress to surrounding structures. Unfortunately, despite a recent surge in the number of publications on this topic, little progress has been made in our understanding of the classification, pathophysiology, and, most importantly, the most appropriate treatment for this disease. A lack of standardized definition of disease, small numbers of patients, and differing end points in research publications has limited our efficiency in understanding the optimum treatment. Future studies should strive to develop common definitions of this disease, as has been done for other rheumatic conditions, and an emphasis should be placed on multicenter, randomized trials in an attempt to define the most effective treatment.

REFERENCES

1. van Bommel EF. Retroperitoneal fibrosis. Neth J Med 2002;60(6):231–42.
2. Marzano A, Trapani A, Leone N, et al. Treatment of idiopathic retroperitoneal fibrosis using cyclosporin. Ann Rheum Dis 2001;60(4):427–8.
3. Scavalli AS, Spadaro A, Riccieri V, et al. Long-term follow-up of low-dose methotrexate therapy in one case of idiopathic retroperitoneal fibrosis. Clin Rheumatol 1995;14(4):481–4.
4. Zen Y, Fujii T, Harada K, et al. Th2 and regulatory immune reactions are increased in immunoglobulin G4-related sclerosing pancreatitis and cholangitis. Hepatology 2007;45(6):1538–46.
5. Aalberse RC, Stapel SO, Schuurman J, et al. Immunoglobulin G4: an odd antibody. Clin Exp Allergy 2009;39(4):469–77.
6. Grotz W, von Zedtwitz I, Andre M, et al. Treatment of retroperitoneal fibrosis by mycophenolate mofetil and corticosteroids. Lancet 1998;352(9135):1195.
7. Catanoso MG, Spaggiari L, Magnani L, et al. Efficacy of infliximab in a patient with refractory idiopathic retroperitoneal fibrosis. Clin Exp Rheumatol 2012; 30(5):776–8.
8. Kamisawa T, Anjiki H, Egawa N, et al. Allergic manifestations in autoimmune pancreatitis. Eur J Gastroenterol Hepatol 2009;21(10):1136–9.
9. Vega J, Goecke H, Tapia H, et al. Treatment of idiopathic retroperitoneal fibrosis with colchicine and steroids: a case series. Am J Kidney Dis 2009;53(4): 628–37.
10. Spillane RM, Whitman GJ. Treatment of retroperitoneal fibrosis with tamoxifen. AJR Am J Roentgenol 1995;164(2):515–6.

11. Scheel PJ Jr, Feeley N. Retroperitoneal fibrosis: the clinical, laboratory, and radiographic presentation. Medicine (Baltimore) 2009;88(4):202–7.

12. Li KP, Zhu J, Zhang JL, et al. Idiopathic retroperitoneal fibrosis (RPF): clinical features of 61 cases and literature review. Clin Rheumatol 2011;30(5):601–5.

13. Gomez Garcia I, Sanchez Castano A, Romero Molina M, et al. Retroperitoneal fibrosis: single-centre experience from 1992 to 2010, current status of knowledge and review of the international literature. Scand J Urol 2012. [Epub ahead of print].

14. Scheel PJ Jr, Feeley N, Sozio SM. Combined prednisone and mycophenolate mofetil treatment for retroperitoneal fibrosis: a case series. Ann Intern Med 2011;154(1):31–6.

15. Uibu T, Oksa P, Auvinen A, et al. Asbestos exposure as a risk factor for retroperitoneal fibrosis. Lancet 2004;363(9419):1422–6.

16. Koep L, Zuidema GD. The clinical significance of retroperitoneal fibrosis. Surgery 1977;81(3):250–7.

17. Lepage-Savary D, Vallieres A. Ergotamine as a possible cause of retroperitoneal fibrosis. Clin Pharm 1982;1(2):179–80.

18. Ahmad S. Association of metoprolol and retroperitoneal fibrosis. Am Heart J 1996;131(1):202–3.

19. Doherty CC, McGeown MG, Donaldson RA. Retroperitoneal fibrosis after treatment with atenolol. Br Med J 1978;2(6154):1786.

20. Rimmer E, Richens A, Forster ME, et al. Retroperitoneal fibrosis associated with timolol. Lancet 1983;1(8319):300.

21. Lewis CT, Molland EA, Marshall VR, et al. Analgesic abuse, ureteric obstruction, and retroperitoneal fibrosis. Br Med J 1975;2(5962):76–8.

22. Ahmad S. Methyldopa and retroperitoneal fibrosis. Am Heart J 1983;105(6): 1037–8.

23. Waters VV. Hydralazine, hydrochlorothiazide and ampicillin associated with retroperitoneal fibrosis: case report. J Urol 1989;141(4):936–7.

24. Sauni R, Oksa P, Jarvenpaa R, et al. Asbestos exposure: a potential cause of retroperitoneal fibrosis. Am J Ind Med 1998;33(4):418–21.

25. Uibu T, Jarvenpaa R, Hakomaki J, et al. Asbestos-related pleural and lung fibrosis in patients with retroperitoneal fibrosis. Orphanet J Rare Dis 2008;3:29.

26. Rodemann HP, Bamberg M. Cellular basis of radiation-induced fibrosis. Radiother Oncol 1995;35(2):83–90.

27. Brandt AS, Kamper L, Kukuk S, et al. Associated findings and complications of retroperitoneal fibrosis in 204 patients: results of a urological registry. J Urol 2011;185(2):526–31.

28. Doolin EJ, Goldstein H, Kessler B, et al. Familial retroperitoneal fibrosis. J Pediatr Surg 1987;22(12):1092–4.

29. Phills JA, Geggie P, Hidvegi RI, et al. Retroperitoneal fibrosis in three siblings with the sickle cell trait. Can Med Assoc J 1973;108(8):1025–9.

30. Duffy PG, Johnston SR, Donaldson RA. Idiopathic retroperitoneal fibrosis in twins. J Urol 1984;131(4):746.

31. Martorana D, Vaglio A, Greco P, et al. Chronic periaortitis and HLA-DRB1*03: another clue to an autoimmune origin. Arthritis Rheum 2006;55(1):126–30.

32. Vivas I, Nicolas AI, Velazquez P, et al. Retroperitoneal fibrosis: typical and atypical manifestations. Br J Radiol 2000;73(866):214–22.

33. van Bommel EF, Jansen I, Hendriksz TR, et al. Idiopathic retroperitoneal fibrosis: prospective evaluation of incidence and clinicoradiologic presentation. Medicine (Baltimore) 2009;88(4):193–201.

34. Vaglio A, Palmisano A, Ferretti S, et al. Peripheral inflammatory arthritis in patients with chronic periaortitis: report of five cases and review of the literature. Rheumatology (Oxford) 2008;47(3):315–8.
35. Stone JH, Zen Y, Deshpande V. IgG4-related disease. N Engl J Med 2012;366(6): 539–51.
36. Vaglio A, Corradi D, Manenti L, et al. Evidence of autoimmunity in chronic periaortitis: a prospective study. Am J Med 2003;114(6):454–62.
37. Vaglio A, Greco P, Corradi D, et al. Autoimmune aspects of chronic periaortitis. Autoimmun Rev 2006;5(7):458–64.
38. Vaglio A, Salvarani C, Buzio C. Retroperitoneal fibrosis. Lancet 2006;367(9506): 241–51.
39. Mitchinson MJ. Retroperitoneal fibrosis revisited. Arch Pathol Lab Med 1986; 110(9):784–6.
40. Parums DV, Chadwick DR, Mitchinson MJ. The localisation of immunoglobulin in chronic periaortitis. Atherosclerosis 1986;61(2):117–23.
41. Parums DV, Brown DL, Mitchinson MJ. Serum antibodies to oxidized low-density lipoprotein and ceroid in chronic periaortitis. Arch Pathol Lab Med 1990;114(4):383–7.
42. Ormond JK. Idiopathic retroperitoneal fibrosis: a discussion of the etiology. J Urol 1965;94(4):385–90.
43. Mitchinson MJ. The pathology of idiopathic retroperitoneal fibrosis. J Clin Pathol 1970;23(8):681–9.
44. Moroni G, Del Papa N, Moronetti LM, et al. Increased levels of circulating endothelial cells in chronic periaortitis as a marker of active disease. Kidney Int 2005; 68(2):562–8.
45. Klein J, Sato A. The HLA System. N Engl J Med 2000;343(11):782–6.
46. Lichon FS, Sequeira W, Pilloff A, et al. Retroperitoneal fibrosis associated with systemic lupus erythematosus: a case report and brief review. J Rheumatol 1984;11(3):373–4.
47. LeBlanc CM, Inman RD, Dent P, et al. Retroperitoneal fibrosis: an extraarticular manifestation of ankylosing spondylitis. Arthritis Rheum 2002;47(2):210–4.
48. De la Iglesia Martinez F, Grana Gil J, Gomez Veiga F, et al. The association of idiopathic retroperitoneal fibrosis and ankylosing spondylitis. J Rheumatol 1992; 19(7):1147–9.
49. Plaza JA, Garrity JA, Dogan A, et al. Orbital inflammation with IgG4-positive plasma cells: manifestation of IgG4 systemic disease. Arch Ophthalmol 2011; 129(4):421–8.
50. Deshpande V, Gupta R, Sainani N, et al. Subclassification of autoimmune pancreatitis: a histologic classification with clinical significance. Am J Surg Pathol 2011; 35(1):26–35.
51. Geyer JT, Deshpande V. IgG4-associated sialadenitis. Curr Opin Rheumatol 2011;23(1):95–101.
52. Lindstrom KM, Cousar JB, Lopes MB. IgG4-related meningeal disease: clinicopathological features and proposal for diagnostic criteria. Acta Neuropathol 2010;120(6):765–76.
53. Leporati P, Landek-Salgado MA, Lupi I, et al. IgG4-related hypophysitis: a new addition to the hypophysitis spectrum. J Clin Endocrinol Metab 2011;96(7):1971–80.
54. Sato Y, Notohara K, Kojima M, et al. IgG4-related disease: historical overview and pathology of hematological disorders. Pathol Int 2010;60(4):247–58.
55. Dahlgren M, Khosroshahi A, Nielsen GP, et al. Riedel's thyroiditis and multifocal fibrosclerosis are part of the IgG4-related systemic disease spectrum. Arthritis Care Res (Hoboken) 2010;62(9):1312–8.

56. Inoue D, Zen Y, Abo H, et al. Immunoglobulin G4-related lung disease: CT findings with pathologic correlations. Radiology 2009;251(1):260–70.

57. Stone JR. Aortitis, periaortitis, and retroperitoneal fibrosis, as manifestations of IgG4-related systemic disease. Curr Opin Rheumatol 2011;23(1):88–94.

58. Sah RP, Chari ST, Pannala R, et al. Differences in clinical profile and relapse rate of type 1 versus type 2 autoimmune pancreatitis. Gastroenterology 2010;139(1): 140–8 [quiz: e12–3].

59. Saeki T, Nishi S, Imai N, et al. Clinicopathological characteristics of patients with IgG4-related tubulointerstitial nephritis. Kidney Int 2010;78(10):1016–23.

60. Finkelberg DL, Sahani D, Deshpande V, et al. Autoimmune pancreatitis. N Engl J Med 2006;355(25):2670–6.

61. Ghazale A, Chari ST, Zhang L, et al. Immunoglobulin G4-associated cholangitis: clinical profile and response to therapy. Gastroenterology 2008;134(3): 706–15.

62. Umemura T, Zen Y, Hamano H, et al. Clinical significance of immunoglobulin G4-associated autoimmune hepatitis. J Gastroenterol 2011;46(Suppl 1):48–55.

63. Miyoshi H, Uchida K, Taniguchi T, et al. Circulating naive and CD4+ CD25 high regulatory T cells in patients with autoimmune pancreatitis. Pancreas 2008;36(2): 133–40.

64. Zen Y, Onodera M, Inoue D, et al. Retroperitoneal fibrosis: a clinicopathologic study with respect to immunoglobulin G4. Am J Surg Pathol 2009;33(12): 1833–9.

65. Corradi D, Maestri R, Palmisano A, et al. Idiopathic retroperitoneal fibrosis: clinicopathologic features and differential diagnosis. Kidney Int 2007;72(6): 742–53.

66. Mirault T, Lambert M, Puech P, et al. Malignant retroperitoneal fibrosis: MRI characteristics in 50 patients. Medicine (Baltimore) 2012;91(5):242–50.

67. van Bommel EF, Siemes C, van der Veer SJ, et al. Clinical value of gallium-67 SPECT scintigraphy in the diagnostic and therapeutic evaluation of retroperitoneal fibrosis: a prospective study. J Intern Med 2007;262(2):224–34.

68. Vaglio A, Versari A, Fraternali A, et al. (18)F-fluorodeoxyglucose positron emission tomography in the diagnosis and followup of idiopathic retroperitoneal fibrosis. Arthritis Rheum 2005;53(1):122–5.

69. Vaglio A, Palmisano A, Alberici F, et al. Prednisone versus tamoxifen in patients with idiopathic retroperitoneal fibrosis: an open-label randomised controlled trial. Lancet 2011;378(9788):338–46.

70. van Bommel EF, Pelkmans LG, van Damme H, et al. Long-term safety and efficacy of a tamoxifen-based treatment strategy for idiopathic retroperitoneal fibrosis. Eur J Intern Med 2012. [Epub ahead of print].

71. Paz Z, Shoenfeld Y. Antifibrosis: to reverse the irreversible. Clin Rev Allergy Immunol 2010;38(2–3):276–86.

72. van Bommel EF, Hendriksz TR, Huiskes AW, et al. Brief communication: tamoxifen therapy for nonmalignant retroperitoneal fibrosis. Ann Intern Med 2006;144(2): 101–6.

73. Owens LV, Cance WG, Huth JF. Retroperitoneal fibrosis treated with tamoxifen. Am Surg 1995;61(9):842–4.

74. Tonietto G, Agresta F, Della Libera D, et al. Treatment of idiopathic retroperitoneal fibrosis by tamoxifen. Eur J Surg 1997;163(3):231–5.

75. Kramer S, Loof T, Martini S, et al. Mycophenolate mofetil slows progression in anti-thy1-induced chronic renal fibrosis but is not additive to a high dose of enalapril. Am J Physiol Renal Physiol 2005;289(2):F359–68.

76. Badid C, Vincent M, McGregor B, et al. Mycophenolate mofetil reduces myofibro-blast infiltration and collagen III deposition in rat remnant kidney. Kidney Int 2000; 58(1):51–61.
77. Ormond JK. Bilateral ureteral obstruction due to envelopment and compression by an inflammatory retroperitoneal process. J Urol 1948;59(6):1072–9.
78. Abbasi A, Wyre H, Ogan K. Use of full-length metallic stents in malignant ureteral obstruction. J Endourol 2012. [Epub ahead of print].

Hypertrophic Osteoarthropathy
What a Rheumatologist Should Know About this Uncommon Condition

Carlos Pineda, MD[a],*, Manuel Martínez-Lavín, MD[b]

KEYWORDS

- Clubbing • Hypertrophic osteoarthropathy • Pachydermoperiostosis • Periostosis
- Acropachy

KEY POINTS

- Hypertrophic osteoarthropathy (HOA) syndrome comprises the combined presence of digital clubbing, periostosis, and joint swelling.
- HOA is divided into primary and secondary forms. Primary HOA is also known as pachydermoperiostosis. The secondary form of HOA has been associated with a wide variety of medical conditions, including malignancies.
- Involvement of vascular endothelial growth factor, platelet-derived growth factor, platelets, and genetically determined increased prostaglandin E_2 levels has been postulated in its pathogenesis.
- If clubbing or periostosis become evident in a previously healthy individual, a thorough search for an underlying illness should be undertaken.
- The management of HOA is dependent on the correction of the underlying disease. Analgesics, nonsteroidal antiinflammatory drugs, and bisphosphonates may relieve bone pain.

DEFINITION

Hypertrophic osteoarthropathy (HOA) is a syndrome characterized by abnormal proliferation of the skin and osseous tissues at the distal parts of the extremities. Three features are typically present: a peculiar bulbous deformity of the tips of the digits conventionally described as clubbing, periostosis of the tubular bones, and synovial effusions.[1]

Funding Sources: None.
Conflict of Interest: None.
[a] Instituto Nacional de Rehabilitación, Calzada Mexico-Xochimilco 289, Col. Arenal de Guadalupe, Mexico City, 14389, Mexico; [b] Department of Rheumatology, Instituto Nacional de Cardiología Ignacio Chávez, Juan Badiano 1, Mexico City, 14080, Mexico
* Corresponding author.
E-mail address: carpineda@yahoo.com

HISTORICAL OVERVIEW

Digital clubbing is one of the oldest clinical signs in medicine. Its original recognition has been attributed to Hippocrates (circa 450 BC).[2] He described a patient with empyema and curved nails. Marie, in 1890,[3] and Bamberger, in 1891,[4] described the fully developed syndrome. Marie distinguished it from acromegaly and suggested the term pulmonary HOA. Paleopathologic studies have shown changes consistent with HOA in human skeletal remains from both pre-Hispanic Mesoamerica[5] and in a medieval skeleton from southwest Hungary.[6]

EPIDEMIOLOGY

There are no systematic studies on the prevalence of digital clubbing in the general population. A retrospective study of 1226 patients with lung cancer showed that 4.5% of these had findings suggestive of periostosis by bone scintigraphy and only 0.8% displayed clubbing and joint pain.[7] In another study,[8] clubbing was present in 1% of 1511 patients admitted over 1-year period to a general internal medicine department.

Clubbing is usually associated with a variety of internal illnesses. Thus, most clinicians, regardless of their specialty, may have encounters with patients who display this finger abnormality.

Veterinary literature contains reports of this illness in different species of mammals, including dogs, cats, horses, and cattle,[9] in which the syndrome appears in response to the same diseases, mainly neoplasms and chronic infections or inflammatory conditions, such as those reported for humans. HOA has been artificially produced in dogs by surgically induced right-to-left shunts of blood or by chemically induced lung cancer. However, a stable animal model of the syndrome, accessible for systematic studies, has not been developed.

NOMENCLATURE

The term acropachy is etymologically the most appropriate and has been used to describe either clubbing or the fully developed syndrome. Synonyms for clubbing include drumstick, pendulum, and Hippocratic fingers. Primary HOA is also known as pachydermoperiostosis.

There is evidence to sustain the belief that clubbing and HOA represent different stages of the same disease process.[10] In most cases, the finger deformity is the first manifestation and, as the syndrome progresses, periostosis becomes evident. The degree of association of clubbing with the diverse illnesses varies from its being a constant finding, as in cases with cyanotic heart diseases, to its being a rare manifestation, as in patients with lung cancer, cirrhosis of the liver, or Graves disease.

PATHOLOGY

An excessive soft tissue deposit of collagen fibers and interstitial edema are responsible for the bulbous deformity of the digits. Furthermore, small blood vessels are dilated and the number of arteriovenous anastomoses is increased. In addition, there is vascular hyperplasia and thickening of the vessel walls, with perivascular infiltration of lymphocytes.[11]

Electron microscopic studies have confirmed the structural vessel damage shown by the presence of Weibel-Palade bodies, the prominence of Golgi complexes,[12] activated endothelia, thickened, reduplicated capillary basal membranes, and perivascular infiltrate.[13]

The outer portion of the bones is laminated in appearance. At this level, excessive connective tissue elevates the periosteum and new osteoid matrix is deposited underneath.

Histologic studies of the joints have found minimal synovial cell proliferation but prominent arterial-wall thickening, with intravascular deposition of electron-dense material.[14]

CLASSIFICATION

As shown in **Table 1**, HOA is divided into primary and secondary forms. Primary HOA is also known as pachydermoperiostosis (MIM numbers 259100 and 167100), or Touraine-Solente-Golé syndrome. It is a rare hereditary condition with variable expressivity. According to several reports, from 33% up to 73% of patients with primary HOA have a close relative with the same illness.[15] The male/female ratio is 9:1. Primary cases are prone to displaying a more disseminated skin hypertrophy, hence the term pachydermoperiostosis.[11] Secondary HOA is most commonly associated with an intrathoracic malignancy, which may be carcinoma of the lung or the pulmonary metastases of other tumors. HOA is a constant finding in congenital cyanotic heart diseases and is less frequent in other conditions depicted in **Box 1**, such as cirrhosis of the liver, inflammatory bowel disease, gastrointestinal polyposis, thymoma, achalasia, and polyneuropathy, organomegaly, endocrinopathy, monoclonal proteins, and skin changes (POEMS) syndrome.[16] Forms of HOA localized to 1 or 2 limbs may be observed. Most of these occur as a result of a prominent endothelial injury of that particular limb, such as in cases of arterial aneurysms or endothelial infections. A growing number of cases with localized HOA secondary to the infection of an arterial graft have been reported.[17] These are characterized by painful swelling of the affected limb, associated with radiographic periostosis; clubbing has been reported in a few such cases.[17] Another form of localized HOA is patent ductus arteriosus complicated by pulmonary hypertension. In these instances, clubbing and sometimes periostosis are limited to the cyanotic limbs.[18] Cases of unilateral clubbing have been associated with hemiplegia.[19]

CAUSE AND PATHOGENESIS

Significant advances in the understanding of HOA have been made in recent decades.[18] Any valid theory attempting to unravel its pathogenesis must explain the peculiarities of the syndrome, namely, how such different diseases can induce so unique a deformity. It must also explain the reason for the acropachy: why the syndrome begins at the most distal parts of the extremities and evolves in a centripetal

Table 1 Classification of HOA		
HOA		
Primary HOA	**Secondary HOA**	
	Generalized	**Localized**
	Pulmonary	Aneurysms
	Cardiac	Infective arteritis
	Hepatic	Patent ductus arteriosus
	Intestinal	Hemiplegia
	Mediastinal	
	Miscellaneous	

Box 1 **Causes of secondary HOA**
Pulmonary diseases
Chronic infections
Arteriovenous fistula
Mesothelioma
Pulmonary fibrosis
Cystic fibrosis
Metastasis
Cancer
Cardiac diseases
Infective endocarditis
Congenital cyanotic diseases
Liver diseases
Cirrhosis
Carcinoma
Biliary atresia
Primary sclerosing cholangitis
Gastrointestinal diseases
Chronic infections
Laxative abuse
Gastrointestinal polyposis
Cancer
Crohn disease
Ulcerative colitis
Achalasia
Miscellaneous conditions
Thymoma, POEMS syndrome, thalassemia, persistent ductus arteriosus, myelofibrosis

fashion. It must also account for the pathologic features of edema, localized endothelial hyperplasia, and excessive collagen deposition. Several hypotheses that have been proposed to explain these peculiarities are now supported by experimental data.[20–22]

Most diseases associated with HOA have in common alteration of lung function. Such an alteration may be the result of the exclusion of this organ from part of the circulation, a phenomenon evident in cyanotic heart diseases but also present to a lesser degree in some cases of cancer of the lung, intestinal polyposis, cirrhosis of the liver, and hepatopulmonary syndrome. In hepatopulmonary syndrome, there is intrapulmonary shunting of blood.[23] A particularly strong argument in favor of the key role of lung bypass in the development of HOA is the existence of patients with patent ductus arteriosus complicated by pulmonary hypertension in whom the acropachy is limited to the cyanotic limbs.[18]

With a few exceptions,[24] the lack of inflammatory and autoimmune phenomena by conventional serology, in addition to the excessive collagen deposition evident in histologic studies, led to a proposal that a fibroblast growth factor could be at the epicenter of the syndrome.[10] This factor would normally be present in central venous circulation and removed in the lung. A platelet-derived growth factor (PDGF) was chosen from a mathematical model, suggesting that, under normal circumstances, large platelets are fragmented in pulmonary circulation. It was suggested that, in patients with right-to-left shunts of blood, large thrombocytes that escaped fragmentation in the lung would enter the systemic circulation and reach its most distal parts on axial streams, there releasing growth factors and inducing acropachy.[22]

Studies of patients with HOA associated with cyanotic heart diseases are consistent with these explanations. Patients with diverse types of cyanotic congenital heart diseases have a bizarre platelet population, which is characterized by the presence of macrothrombocytes with aberrant volume-distribution curves.[20] Such patients with cyanosis also display alterations in another distal part of the circulation: the renal glomeruli. Histologic studies have disclosed glomerular enlargement, with trapped megakaryocyte nuclei inside,[25] leading to the denomination of cyanotic nephropathy.[26] These features concur with the theory of platelet fragmentation in the lung. Furthermore, patients with cyanosis and patients with primary HOA have increased circulating concentrations of von Willebrand factor antigen, an abnormality that reflects activation of the platelet/endothelial cell.[27] There are theoretic grounds to suggest that similar mechanisms may be operative in other acropachy-associated diseases. Endothelial cell activation is a prominent feature of endarteritis and endocarditis of infective cause.

These data suggest that localized activation of the platelet/endothelial cells, with the subsequent release of growth factor(s), plays a key role in the development of HOA. Recent evidence suggests that vascular endothelial growth factor (VEGF) may play a key role in the pathogenesis of HOA. VEGF is one of the PDGFs released during platelet-endothelial cell activation. It is also produced by malignant tumors as a mechanism of cancer growth. Furthermore, VEGF is a hypoxia-induced agent. These peculiarities may explain how different hypoxic and malignant illnesses may induce VEGF overexpression. On the other hand, VEGF induces vascular hyperplasia, new bone formation, and edema, which are precisely histologic landmarks of HOA. These theoretic considerations are now supported by experimental data. Plasma and serum concentrations of VEGF are significantly greater in patients with primary HOA and with lung cancer–associated HOA compared with those in normal controls.[28] Histology has shown that VEGF is overexpressed in the stroma of clubbed digits.[29]

Recent genomic evidence proposes that prostaglandins may play a key role in the pathogenesis of HOA. Study of several families with primary HOA disclosed homozygous and compound heterozygous mutations in the 15-hydroxyprostaglandin-dehydrogenase encoding gene *HPGD,* the main enzyme of prostaglandin degradation, located at 4q33-q34. Affected individuals had chronically high prostaglandin E_2 levels and its metabolite PGE-M.[30–32] Furthermore, different mutations in the prostaglandin transporter encoding the *SLCO2A1* gene, which presumably result in reduced metabolic clearance by 15-hydroxyprostaglandin dehydrogenase caused by diminished cellular uptake of prostaglandin E_2 by mutant prostaglandin transporter, were associated with severe primary HOA phenotype and with isolated digital clubbing.[32]

However, it seems unlikely that prostaglandins could play a direct final role in the pathogenesis of HOA. There is no evidence that the skeletal syndrome regresses with the use of nonsteroidal antiinflammatory drugs (NSAIDs). These drugs are potent prostaglandin inhibitors. Rather, prostaglandin E_2 may act as facilitator for VEGF action on osteoblasts. The action of prostaglandins on bones is mediated precisely through VEGF expression.[22] It is clear that more research is needed to elucidate the nature of HOA pathogenesis.

SIGNS AND SYMPTOMS

In HOA, there is a continuum of signs and symptoms. At one end of the spectrum, patients may be asymptomatic and unaware of the deformity of their digits. On the other end, some patients, in particular those with lung malignancies, complain of a burning sensation of the fingertips and may also suffer from excruciating bone pain. Characteristically, this pain is deep seated, more prominent in the lower extremities, and aggravated by the dependency of the limbs.

Physical examination is of utmost importance in diagnosis, because the bulbous deformity of the fingertips is distinctive. The nail becomes progressively convex (watch-crystal nail), and the skin overlying its base becomes thin and shiny, with the disappearance of normal creases. The edema and increased soft tissue produce rocking of the nail bed on palpation, adopting a drumstick appearance. Toes are also affected, but early changes are more difficult to distinguish because of the splaying of the normal toe tip.

The Digital Index provides a practical method for quantifying this finger deformity. With the use of a nonelastic string, the perimeter of each finger is measured at the distal interphalangeal (DIP) joint and at the nail bed. If the sum of the 10 nail bed/distal interphalangeal ratios is greater than 10, clubbing is probably present. There is variation in the prominence of clubbing, and the Digital Index serves to assess the severity of the deformity or to compare groups of patients or treatment responsiveness (sensitivity to change).[20] The most advanced stages, with a Digital Index greater than 11, are observed mainly among patients with cyanotic heart diseases and in those with primary HOA.

In most cases, clubbing is the sole clinical manifestation of the syndrome. However, when the complete features of HOA are present, skin hypertrophy may be evident at additional levels, with facial feature coarsening or nonpitting, cylindrical soft tissue swelling of the legs (elephant legs as shown in **Fig. 1**). Thickening of the tubular bones may be evident in areas of the extremities not covered by muscles, such as the ankles and wrists.

Periostosis may be accompanied by tenderness on palpation of the involved anatomic area, but in some instances is asymptomatic. Effusions into the large joints are frequently observed, and are more easily detected in the knees and wrists. At the ankle, these effusions are more difficult to detect because of the surrounding soft tissue swelling. On palpation, there is no hypertrophy of the synovial membrane. The range of motion of the joints may be slightly decreased. Arthrocentesis usually yields a thick fluid with a tendency to spontaneous clotting. There is little inflammatory cell exudation; in consequence, the white blood cell count is usually less than $500/mm^3$ in the synovial fluid.[33] All of these features reflect the fact that HOA is neither an inflammatory joint disease nor a proliferative synovial disease. Joint effusions are most likely to represent a sympathetic reaction to nearby periostosis. Gout may coexist with HOA in patients with cyanotic heart diseases.[34] Palindromic rheumatism manifested by intermittent episodes of asymmetric, migratory oligoarthritis associated with primary HOA has been reported.[35]

There are additional clinical findings associated with particular types of HOA that echoes the dysfunction of an internal organ (**Table 2**). Cyanosis is prominent in congenital heart malformations associated with right-to-left shunts. These patients

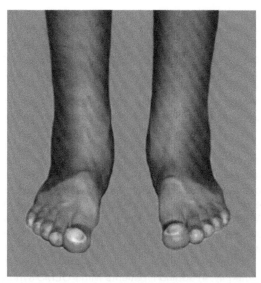

Fig. 1. A young male with primary hypertrophic osteoarthropathy displaying cylindrical swelling of the lower legs. Clubbed toes are also evident.

Table 2
Clinical features of HOA

Disease	Signs and Symptoms
Primary HOA	Digital clubbing
	Periostosis
	Joint effusion
	Soft tissue swelling of the ankles (elephant legs)
	Pachydermia with skin hypertrophy, coarsening facial features, and cutis verticis gyrata
	Hyperhidrosis, seborrhea, acne
	Hypertrophic gastropathy
Secondary HOA	Prominent cyanosis
Congenital cyanotic heart disease	Right-to-left shunts
	Lifelong digital clubbing
	Fully developed syndrome in 33%
Graves disease	Thyroid acropachy
	Clubbing
	Periosteal reaction in hand and feet
	Exophthalmos
	Pretibial myxedema
POEMS syndrome	Digital clubbing
	Skin hypertrophy
	Hyperhidrosis
Chronic pulmonary diseases	Mild digital clubbing
	Cyanosis
Lung cancer	Digital clubbing
	Burning sensation in fingertips
	Bone pain
Liver diseases	Jaundice
	Ascites
	Palmar erythema

are the prototype of HOA, because nearly all have a lifelong presence of clubbing, and more than 33% show the fully developed syndrome.[14] No other internal disease is so closely associated with HOA. A lesser degree of cyanosis is observed when the acropachy is associated with cystic fibrosis, pulmonary fibrosis, or chronic infections, and chronic obstructive pulmonary disease. Jaundice, ascites, and palmar erythema are common findings when the syndrome is secondary to chronic liver disease, as in liver cirrhosis, hepatopulmonary syndrome,[36] biliary atresia,[37] primary sclerosing cholangitis,[38] and rejected liver transplant.[39] Chronic diarrhea is a constant finding in intestinal HOA.

Thyroid acropachy is an extreme manifestation of autoimmune thyroid disease. It presents with digital clubbing, swelling of digits and toes, and exuberant periosteal proliferation, located mainly at the small tubular bones of the hands and feet. It is nearly always associated with exophthalmos and pretibial myxedema (thyroid dermopathy).[40] Myxedema bears a resemblance to the elephant legs described in other types of HOA.[41] Patients with the POEMS syndrome display a multisystem disorder associated with plasma cell dyscrasia. A high serum level, a strong promoter of both neovascularization and vasopermeability (VEGF), is considered to be responsible for characteristic POEMS features such as angiomata, pleural effusion/ascites, edema, and organomegaly. In addition, patients with POEMS syndrome often display features of HOA, such as digital clubbing, skin thickening, and hyperhidrosis.[16]

In primary HOA, or pachydermoperiostosis, disseminated skin hypertrophy is noticeable. This overgrowth roughens the facial features and can reach the extreme of cutis verticis gyrata, the most advanced stage of cutaneous hypertrophy. In such cases, the scalp takes on a cerebroid appearance. Another cutaneous alteration more frequently observed in idiopathic cases is glandular dysfunction, manifested as hyperhidrosis, seborrhea, or acne, or combinations thereof. A variety of associated abnormalities have been described in primary HOA: in early childhood, delayed closure of cranial sutures and fontanels, males with female escutcheon, and hypertrophic gastropathy may occur.[42,43] In primary HOA, disease activity is usually limited to the growth period, with adults becoming asymptomatic. There are cases of primary HOA that show an enigmatic clinical palindrome. Such cases show, as late manifestation, diseases that under other circumstances are known causes of HOA. In this palindrome, persistent ductus arteriosus, Crohn disease, or myelofibrosis can be the cause or the effect of HOA.[44]

WORKUP
Laboratory Studies

There are no useful serologic tests for HOA. However, an array of biochemical abnormalities may be found, reflecting the pathophysiologic process of underlying disease. Isolated reports have shown increased bone-formation marker levels, such as total alkaline phosphatase, bone alkaline phosphatase, the amino terminal propeptide of type I procollagen, and osteocalcin. Also, bone resorption markers including the serum carboxy terminal telopeptide of type I collagen, and the urinary amino terminal telopeptide of type I collagen have been found in some patients. These reports suggest that measuring these markers could be useful in the clinical monitoring of disease activity in individuals with either primary or secondary HOA.[45,46] In addition, increased serum levels of interleukin 6 and the receptor activator of nuclear factor κB ligand have been related with bone resorption in acute phases of patients with primary HOA, suggesting a possible role of these cytokines in the regulation of bone turnover in this process.[47] Further investigations are needed to establish whether bone turnover markers are useful for monitoring HOA disease activity.

Serum and urinary levels of prostaglandin E_2, a recently implicated mediator in this disorder, have been reported to be increased in isolated cases.[45] The role of this cytokine in the pathogenesis of this syndrome, and its value as a diagnostic tool in patients with the primary form of HOA, remains to be elucidated.

Imaging Evaluation

Of utmost importance for correct assessment of HOA are plain radiographs of the extremities, which may detect both soft tissue and bony abnormalities, even in asymptomatic patients.[11]

Radiographically, digital clubbing is recognized by the presence of various degrees of bulbous deformity of the soft tissues located at the distal end of the fingers. Abnormal curvature of the nails also is evident on plain radiographs, as a loss of the radiolucent line normally present between the nail and skin. Long-standing clubbing is characterized by a bone remodeling process, which usually takes the form of acro-osteolysis and, more rarely, tuftal overgrowth. Characteristically, the bone changes of clubbing are observed first at the toes; the fingers are affected in more advanced cases **(Fig. 2)**.[48,49]

Additional soft tissue abnormalities include a cylindrical leg deformity called elephant leg, and the hypertrophy of the scalp skin present in some cases of primary HOA, known as cutis verticis gyrata, which in extreme cases results in a cerebroid appearance of the scalp and forehead of the affected individual. Both abnormalities are well depicted by plain radiography.[50]

Periostosis is an orderly, evolutionary process that depends on the chronicity of the disease and the intensity of the underlying stimuli. It progresses in 3 dimensions: in the number of affected bones; at the site of involvement of a given bone; and in the shape of the periosteal apposition. In mild cases, few bones are affected (usually tibias and fibulas); periostosis is limited to the diaphysis and it has a monolayer configuration, increasing the circumference of the affected bones without otherwise altering its shape **(Fig. 3)**. With disease progression, periosteal new bone formation becomes more prominent, extends into the epiphyses, and is laminated or multilayered in appearance. In advanced cases, all tubular bones are affected: in addition to the diaphysis, the metaphysis and epiphysis are also involved and the periostosis acquires an irregular configuration **(Fig. 4)**.[51]

Periostosis has a symmetric distribution and evolves in centripetal fashion. It is independent of the underlying disease; primary and secondary cases feature similar

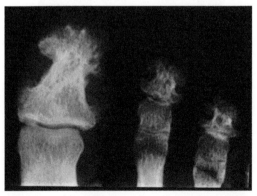

Fig. 2. Anteroposterior radiograph of the distal foot in a patient with primary hypertrophic osteoarthropathy. There is both tuftal overgrowth and acroosteolysis.

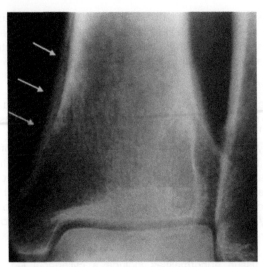

Fig. 3. Early radiographic changes in a patient with hypertrophic osteoarthropathy associated with congenital cyanotic heart disease. Monolayer periosteal reaction of the distal tibia (*arrows*) is evident.

changes.[48] Joint involvement in HOA is radiographically characterized by the presence of synovial effusion, preservation of joint spaces, and the absence of erosions or para-articular osteopenia, thus reflecting its noninflammatory nature. Chest radiographs may reveal the underlying cause of secondary HOA.

Radionuclide bone scanning is a sensitive method for showing periosteal involvement. Nuclear medicine studies reveal early evidence of disease. There is increased

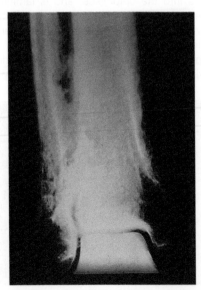

Fig. 4. Anteroposterior radiograph of a patient with primary hypertrophic osteoarthropathy. There is thickening of the tibia and fibula with florid periosteal proliferation.

uptake of the bone-seeking tracer at the periosteum, often appearing as symmetric and linear uptake in the cortical margins of the diaphysis and metaphysis of the tubular long bones.[52] Using this imaging technique, the diagnosis of HOA is sometimes performed serendipitously in patients with known malignant disease who develop bone pain, with the study requested in the evaluation of metastatic cancer. Clubbed digits may also show increased uptake in early passage flow studies.

Although isotope bone scanning is a highly sensitive means of assessing HOA, its findings are nonspecific, and similar results can occur in other forms of periosteal proliferation. Recently, it has been suggested that single-photon emission computed tomography/computed tomography (CT) is able to improve the specificity of the planar scintigraphic findings by confirming tracer uptake localized to the periosteum, as expected for HOA, thereby excluding the presence of skeletal metastases.[53]

[18]F-Fluorodeoxyglucose positron emission tomography in combination with CT may show increased symmetric metabolic activity along the contours of the long tubular bones compatible with periostitis, as well as tracer accumulation in internal organs, indicating the possible origin of secondary HOA.[54]

CT scanning is useful in elucidating the cause of HOA in cases of intrathoracic or abdominal disease. In addition, it may aid in detecting nonneoplastic causes of HOA, such as infected vascular grafts. Regarding magnetic resonance imaging (MRI), the experience is insufficient for assessing its reliability in the diagnosis of skeletal manifestations of HOA. Apparently, in a reported case, the soft tissue component of the disease was better depicted in MRI than in other imaging techniques.[55]

DIFFERENTIAL DIAGNOSIS

When HOA is fully expressed, the drumstick fingers are unique to such a degree that its recognition poses no dilemma. However, there are borderline cases in which neither careful examination nor the Digital Index clarify the situation.[20] The most appropriate approach for such cases is to assume the presence of clubbing and to search for an underlying disease.[11]

Diagnostic criteria for HOA include the combined presence of clubbing and radiographic evidence of periostosis of the tubular bones. Synovial effusion is not essential for the diagnosis.[1] However; in some patients, particularly in those with malignant lung tumors, painful arthropathy may be the presenting manifestation of the syndrome, before clubbing. Such cases could be misdiagnosed as suffering from an inflammatory type of arthritis.[56] Important clinical features in the differential diagnosis comprise the site of the pain (in HOA, not only the joint but also the adjacent bone are involved) plus the fact that the rheumatoid factor is usually absent and synovial fluid is noninflammatory. Furthermore, with the advent of modern imaging techniques, it is now possible to detect cases of early HOA with the presentation of only periostitis and limb pain, without clubbing.[55]

Both clubbing and pseudoclubbing present as a bulbous deformity of the soft tissue in the fingertips; in pseudoclubbing, distinctive clinical features are the preservation of the angle between nail bed and proximal nail fold or Lovibond angle (normal 160° angle), and asymmetric finger involvement.[57] This condition is usually caused by an underlying process of acro-osteolysis, with the resulting collapse of the soft tissues, as in the case of hyperparathyroidism, scleroderma, chromosomal deletion, and subungueal hemangioma.[58,59]

Some patients with HOA show exuberant skin hypertrophy, which may resemble acromegaly. The presence of clubbing and periostosis, plus the absence of prognathism, enlarged sella turcica, or abnormal circulating concentrations of growth hormone, should lead to the correct diagnosis. A patient should be classified as having the primary form of the syndrome only after careful scrutiny fails to reveal an underlying disease.

Several cases of painful multifocal nodular periostitis in recipients of transplants taking voriconazole have recently been described. Voriconazole is a new fluoride-containing antifungal medication used to treat serious, invasive fungal infections, which are generally observed in immunocompromised patients. Fluorosis seems to be the underlying pathogenesis. Symptoms subsided after medication withdrawal.[60,61]

The importance of recognizing HOA cannot be overstated. If, in a previously healthy individual, any of the manifestations of the syndrome become evident, a thorough search for an underlying disease should be undertaken. Special attention must be directed to the chest, because at present the most frequent cause of acute onset of HOA in adults is malignant lung tumor, either primary or metastatic.[62] Conversely, if a patient previously diagnosed with any of the chronic diseases listed in **Box 1** develops clubbing, this alone is an unfavorable prognostic sign, indicating that the disease has reached an advanced stage.

In some clinical situations, the presence of acropachy signals a serious but treatable complication. If clubbing appears in a patient with known rheumatic heart disease, infective endocarditis should be strongly suspected. A similar consideration applies to patients with a previous history of prosthetic vascular surgery who develop periostosis of a limb.

Because periostosis is the radiographic hallmark of HOA, the presence of periosteal new bone formation of multiple bones, especially in the long tubular bones of the lower limbs, should alert the clinician to the underlying presence of HOA. **Box 2** presents a list of conditions associated with polyostotic periosteal reaction.

| Box 2 |
Periostosis of multiple bones: differential diagnosis
HOA
Thyroid acropachy
Hypervitaminosis A
Venous stasis
Fluorosis
Leukemia
Trauma
Multifocal osteomyelitis
Eosinophilic granuloma
Polyostotic bone tumors
Psoriatic arthritis
Infantile cortical hyperostosis
Child abuse
Juvenile idiopathic arthritis
Scurvy
Drug-induced
Sickle cell dactylitis

Table 3
Rheumatic conditions associated with HOA

Rheumatic Disease	Reference
Antiphospholipid syndrome	63
Behçet disease	64,65
Takayasu arteritis	66,67
Polyarteritis nodosa	68–70
Systemic lupus erythematosus	71,72
Rheumatoid arthritis	73,74
Spondyloarthropathies	75–77
Palindromic rheumatism	35
Gout	34
Pseudogout	78

RHEUMATIC DISEASES ASSOCIATED WITH HOA

As shown in **Table 3**, a variety of the more common rheumatic diseases have been associated with or coexist either with clubbing, periostosis or, less frequently, with the fully developed HOA syndrome.

TREATMENT

Aside from its unsightliness, clubbing is usually asymptomatic and does not require treatment. For patients with painful osteoarthropathy, pharmacologic treatment with analgesics and NSAIDs is effective in relieving pain in most patients. There are isolated case reports from different parts of the world stating that intravenous infusions of bisphosphonates are effective in cases of HOA with refractory bone pain.[79,80] Bisphosphonates are not only osteoclastic bone resorption antagonists but also VEGF inhibitors. Octreotide relieved pain associated with cyanotic congenital heart disease and lung cancer-related HOA. The pain- relieving efficacy of octreotide for HOA may partly be attributed to its inhibitory effects on the production of VEGF and endothelial proliferation.[81] Botulinum toxin type A is a simple procedure that may be of value in temporarily improving the cosmetic appearance of pachydermia in patients with pachydermoperiostosis.[82] A patient with the primary form of HOA, who had refractory bone pain and arthritis and who responded partially to infliximab treatment, was recently described.[83] Hyperhidrosis could be eased with the use of glycopyrrolate, clonidine, botulinum toxin injections, or regional sympathectomy.[84] Gefetinib, a selective epidermal growth factor receptor tyrosine kinase inhibitor, induced the disappearance of periostitis in a case of HOA with advanced lung adenocarcinoma.[85]

Management of HOA is dependent on the underlying disease. Removal of a lung tumor, chemotherapy,[86] correction of a heart malformation, or successful treatment of infective endocarditis is followed by a dramatic regression of all features of the syndrome. In addition, lung transplantation has been reported to improve HOA in cystic fibrosis.[87]

REFERENCES

1. Martínez-Lavín M, Matucci-Cerinic M, Jajic I, et al. Hypertrophic osteoarthropathy, consensus on its definition, classification, assessment and diagnostic criteria. J Rheumatol 1993;20:1386–7.

2. Lyons AS, Petrucelli RJ. Medicine: an illustrated history. New York: Abrams; 1978. p. 216.
3. Marie P. De l'ostéo-arthrophie hypertrophiante pneumique. Rev Med 1890;10: 1–36 [in French].
4. Bamberger E. Uber Knochenveränderugen bei chronishen Lungen und Herz-krankheiten. Z Klin Med 1891;18:193–217 [in German].
5. Martínez-Lavín M, Mansilla J, Pineda C, et al. Evidence of hypertrophic osteo-arthropathy in human skeletal remains from proHispanic Mesoamerica. Ann Intern Med 1994;12:238–41.
6. Christensen T, Martínez-Lavín M, Pineda C. Periostitis and osteolysis in a medieval skeleton from South-West Hungary: (leprosy, treponematosis, tuberculosis or hypertrophic osteoarthropathy): a diagnostic challenge! Int J Osteoarchaeol 2013;23:69–82.
7. Izumi M, Takayama K, Yabuuchi H, et al. Incidence of hypertrophic pulmonary osteo-arthropathy associated with primary lung cancer. Respirology 2010;15(5):809–12.
8. Vandemergel X, Renneboog B. Prevalence, aetiologies and significance of club-bing in a department of general internal medicine. Eur J Intern Med 2008;19(5): 325–9.
9. Guyot H, Sandersen C, Rollin F. A case of hypertrophic osteoarthropathy in a Belgian blue cow. Can Vet J 2011;52(12):1308–11.
10. Martínez-Lavín M. Digital clubbing and hypertrophic osteoarthropathy: a unifying hypothesis. J Rheumatol 1987;14:6–8.
11. Martínez-Lavín M, Pineda C. Digital clubbing and hypertrophic osteoarthropathy. In: Hochberg M, Silman AJ, Smolen JS, et al, editors. Rheumatology. 5th edition. Philadelphia: Mosby Elsevier; 2011. p. 1701–5.
12. Padula S, Broketa G, Sampieri A, et al. Increased collagen synthesis in skin fibro-blasts from patients with primary hypertrophic osteoarthropathy. Arthritis Rheum 1994;37:1386–94.
13. Fara EF, Baughman RP. A study of capillary morphology in the digits of patients with acquired clubbing. Am Rev Respir Dis 1989;140:1063–6.
14. Martínez-Lavín M, Bobadilla M, Casanova J, et al. Hypertrophic osteoarthropathy in cyanotic congenital heart disease. Arthritis Rheum 1982;25:1186–93.
15. Jajic Z, Jajic I, Nemcic T. Primary hypertrophic osteoarthropathy: clinical, radio-logic, and scintigraphic characteristics. Arch Med Res 2001;32:136–42.
16. Martínez-Lavín M, Vargas AS, Cabré J, et al. Features of hypertrophic osteoarthr-opathy in patients with POEMS syndrome: a meta-analysis. J Rheumatol 1997;24: 2268–9.
17. Ahrenstorf G, Rihl M, Pichlmaier MA, et al. Unilateral hypertrophic osteoarthrop-athy in a patient with a vascular graft infection. J Clin Rheumatol 2012;18(6): 307–9.
18. Martínez-Lavín M. Elucidation of digital clubbing may help in understanding the pathogenesis of pulmonary hypertension associated with congenital heart defects. Cardiol Young 1994;4:228–31.
19. Velur P, Kalamangalam GP. Teaching neuroimages: unilateral clubbing in hemi-plegia [abstract]. Neurology 2012;78(19):e122.
20. Vázquez-Abad D, Pineda C, Martínez-Lavín M. Digital clubbing: a numerical assessment of the deformity. J Rheumatol 1989;16:518–20.
21. Martínez-Lavín M. Exploring the cause of the most ancient clinical sign of medi-cine: digital clubbing. Semin Arthritis Rheum 2007;36:380–5.
22. Dickinson CJ, Martin JF. Megakaryocytes and platelet clumps as the cause of finger clubbing. Lancet 1987;2:1434–5.

23. Stoller J, Moodie D, Schiavone W, et al. Reduction of intrapulmonary shunt and resolution of digital clubbing associated with primary biliary cirrhosis after liver transplantation. Hepatology 1990;11:54–8.
24. Cruz C, Rocha M, Andrade D, et al. Hypertrophic pulmonary osteoarthropathy with positive antinuclear antibodies: case report. Case Rep Oncol 2012;5:308–12.
25. Perloff JK, Latta H, Barsotti P. Pathogenesis of the glomerular abnormality in cyanotic congenital heart disease. Am J Cardiol 2000;86:1198–204.
26. Inatomi J, Matsuoka K, Fujimaru R, et al. Mechanisms of development and progression of cyanotic nephropathy. Pediatr Nephrol 2006;21(10):1440–5.
27. Matucci-Cerinic M, Martínez-Lavín M, Rojo F, et al. Von Willebrand factor antigen in hypertrophic osteoarthropathy. J Rheumatol 1992;19:765–7.
28. Silveira LH, Martínez-Lavín M, Pineda C, et al. Vascular endothelial growth factor and hypertrophic osteoarthropathy. Clin Exp Rheumatol 2000;18:57–62.
29. Atkinson S, Fox SB. Vascular endothelial growth factor (VEGF)-A and platelet-derived growth factor (PDGF) play a central role in the pathogenesis of clubbing. J Pathol 2004;203:721–8.
30. Uppal S, Diggle CP, Carr IM, et al. Mutations in 15-hydroxyprostaglandin-dehydrogenase cause primary hypertrophic osteoarthropathy. Nat Genet 2008;40:789–93.
31. Diggle CP, Parry DA, Logan CV, et al. Prostaglandin transporter mutations cause pachydermoperiostosis with myelofibrosis. Hum Mutat 2012;33(8):1175–81.
32. Seifert W, Kühnisch J, Tüysüz B, et al. Mutations in the prostaglandin transporter encoding gene SLCO2A1 cause primary hypertrophic osteoarthropathy and isolated digital clubbing. Hum Mutat 2012;33(4):660–4.
33. Schumacher R. Articular manifestations of hypertrophic pulmonary osteoarthropathy in bronchogenic carcinoma. Arthritis Rheum 1976;19:629–35.
34. Martínez-Lavín M, Amigo MC, Castillejos G, et al. Coexistent gout and hypertrophic osteoarthropathy in patients with cyanotic heart disease. J Rheumatol 1984;11(6):832–4.
35. Shinjo SK, Levy-Neto M, Borba EF. Palindromic rheumatism associated with primary hypertrophic osteoarthropathy. Clinics (Sao Paulo) 2006;61(6):581–3.
36. Ede K, McCurdy D, García-Lloret M. Hypertrophic osteoarthropathy in the hepatopulmonary syndrome. J Clin Rheumatol 2008;14(4):230–3.
37. Kuloğlu Z, Kansu A, Ekici F, et al. Hypertrophic osteoarthropathy in a child with biliary atresia. Scand J Gastroenterol 2001;39(7):698–701.
38. Reginato AJ, Petrokubi R, Jasper CA. Juvenile hypertrophic osteoarthropathy associated with primary sclerosing cholangitis. Arthritis Rheum 1980;23(12):1391–5.
39. Wolfe SM, Aelion JA, Gupta RC. Hypertrophic osteoarthropathy associated with a rejected liver transplant. J Rheumatol 1987;14(1):147–51.
40. Fatourechi V, Ahmed DD, Schwartz KM. Thyroid acropachy: report of 40 patients treated at a single institution in a 26-year period. J Clin Endocrinol Metab 2002;87(12):5435–41.
41. Martínez-Lavín M, Pineda C, Valdez T, et al. Primary hypertrophic osteoarthropathy. Semin Arthritis Rheum 1988;17:156–62.
42. Martínez-Lavín M. Pachydermoperiostosis. Best Pract Res Clin Rheumatol 2011;25:727–34.
43. Seifert W, Beninde J, Hoffmann K, et al. HPGD mutations cause cranioosteoarthropathy but not autosomal dominant digital clubbing. Eur J Hum Genet 2009;17:1570–6.
44. Martínez-Lavín M, Vargas A, Rivera-Viñas M. Hypertrophic osteoarthropathy: a palindrome with a pathogenic connotation. Curr Opin Rheumatol 2008;20:88–91.

45. Martínez Ferrer A, Peris P, Alós LI, et al. Prostaglandin E2 and bone turnover markers in the evaluation of primary hypertrophic osteoarthropathy (pachydermoperiostosis): a case report. Clin Rheumatol 2009;28:1229–33.

46. Jojima H, Kinoshita K, Naito M. A case of pachydermoperiostosis treated by oral administration of a bisphosphonate and arthroscopic synovectomy. Mod Rheumatol 2007;17:330–2.

47. Rendina D, De Filippo G, Viceconti R, et al. Interleukin (IL)-6 and receptor activator of nuclear factor (NF)-κB ligand (RANKL) are increased in the serum of a patient with primary pachydermoperiostosis. Scand J Rheumatol 2008;37: 225–9.

48. Pineda C, Fonseca C, Martínez-Lavín M. The spectrum of soft tissue and skeletal abnormalities of hypertrophic osteoarthropathy. J Rheumatol 1990;17:626–32.

49. Pineda CJ, Guerra J Jr, Weisman MH, et al. The skeletal manifestations of clubbing: a study in patients with cyanotic congenital hearth disease and hypertrophic osteoarthropathy. Semin Arthritis Rheum 1985;14(4):263–73.

50. Pineda C. Diagnostic imaging in hypertrophic osteoarthropathy. Clin Exp Rheumatol 1992;10(Suppl 7):27–33.

51. Pineda CJ, Martínez-Lavín M, Goobar JE, et al. Periostitis in hypertrophic osteoarthropathy: relationship to disease duration. AJR Am J Roentgenol 1987;148(4): 773–8.

52. Mudalsha R, Jacob MJ, Jora C, et al. Tc-99m MDP bone scintigraphy in a case of Touraino Solente-Gole syndrome. Indian J Nucl Med 2011;26:46–8.

53. Russo RR, Lee A, Mansberg R, et al. Hypertrophic pulmonary osteoarthropathy demonstrated on SPECT/CT. Clin Nucl Med 2009;34(9):628–31.

54. Manger B, Wacker J, Schmidt D, et al. Clinical images: hippocrates confirmed by positron emission tomography [abstract]. Arthritis Rheum 2011;63(4):1150.

55. Sainani NI, Lawande MA, Parikh VP, et al. MRI diagnosis of hypertrophic osteoarthropathy from a remote childhood malignancy. Skeletal Radiol 2007;36(Suppl 1): S63–6.

56. Segal A, Mackenzie A. Hypertrophic osteoarthropathy: a 10-year retrospective analysis. Semin Arthritis Rheum 1982;12:220–32.

57. Lovibond JL. Diagnosis of clubbed fingers. Lancet 1938;1:363–4.

58. Farzaneh-Far A. Images in clinical medicine. Pseudoclubbing [abstract]. N Engl J Med 2006;354(15):e14.

59. Santiago MB, Lima I, Feitosa AC, et al. Pseudoclubbing: is it different from clubbing? Semin Arthritis Rheum 2009;38(6):452–7.

60. Lustenberger DP, Granata JD, Scharschmidt TJ. Periostitis secondary to prolonged voriconazole therapy in a lung transplant recipient. Orthopedics 2011; 34:e793–6.

61. Rossier C, Dunet V, Tissot F, et al. Voriconazole-induced periostitis. Eur J Nucl Med Mol Imaging 2012;39(2):375–6.

62. Yao Q, Altman RD, Brahn E. Periostitis and hypertrophic pulmonary osteoarthropathy: report of 2 cases and review of the literature. Semin Arthritis Rheum 2009; 38(6):458–66.

63. Harris AW, Harding TA, Gaitonde MD, et al. Is clubbing a feature of the antiphospholipid antibody syndrome? Postgrad Med J 1993;69(815):748–50.

64. de Lastours V, Lidove O, Lieberherr D, et al. Lower limb hypertrophic osteoarthropathy can reveal aortic graft infection in Behcet syndrome. Rheumatology (Oxford) 2006;45(1):117–8.

65. Benekli M, Güllü IH. Hippocratic fingers in Behçet's disease. Postgrad Med J 1997;73(863):575–6.

66. Kim JE, Kolh EM, Kim DK. Takayasu's arteritis presenting with focal periostitis affecting two limbs. Int J Cardiol 1998;67(3):267–70.

67. Matucci-Cerinic M. Takayasu's arteritis and hypertrophic osteoarthropathy: a real association? Clin Exp Rheumatol 1988;6(3):329–30.

68. Astudillo LM, Rigal F, Couret B, et al. Localized polyarteritis nodosa with periostitis. J Rheumatol 2001;28(12):2758–9.

69. Meijers KA, Pare DM, Loose H, et al. Periarteritis nodosa and subperiosteal new bone formation. J Bone Joint Surg Br 1982;64(5):592–6.

70. Vedrine L, Rault A, Debourdeau P, et al. Polyarteritis nodosa manifesting as tibial periostitis. Ann Med Interne (Paris) 2001;152(3):213–4.

71. Burson JS, Grana J, Varela J, et al. Laminar periostitis and multiple osteonecrosis in systemic lupus erythematosus. Clin Rheumatol 1990;9(4):535–8.

72. Di Cataldo A, Villari L, Milone P, et al. Thymic carcinoma, systemic lupus erythematosus, and hypertrophic pulmonary osteoarthropathy in an 11-year-old boy: a novel association. Pediatr Hematol Oncol 2000;17(8):701–6.

73. Diamond S, Momeni M. Primary hypertrophic osteoarthropathy in a patient with rheumatoid arthritis. J Clin Rheumatol 2007;13(4):242–3.

74. Schechter SL, Bole GG. Hypertrophic osteoarthropathy and rheumatoid arthritis: simultaneous occurrence in association with diffuse interstitial fibrosis. Arthritis Rheum 1976;19(3):639–43.

75. Shinjo SK, Borba EF, Goncalves CR, et al. Ankylosing spondylitis in a patient with primary hypertrophic osteoarthropathy [abstract]. J Clin Rheumatol 2007; 13(3):175.

76. Jalan KN, Prescott RJ, Walker RJ, et al. Arthropathy, ankylosing spondylitis, and clubbing of fingers in ulcerative colitis. Gut 1970;11(9):748–54.

77. Ramonda R, Zucchetta P, Contessa C, et al. The psoriatic great toe or the psoriatic onycho-pachydermo-periostitis of great toe (OP3gt). Reumatismo 2004;56(4):282–5.

78. Zyskowski LP, Silverfield JC, O'Duffy JD. Pseudogout masking other arthritides. J Rheumatol 1983;10(3):449–53.

79. Jayakar BA, Abelson AG, Yao Q. Treatment of hypertrophic osteoarthropathy with zoledronic acid: case report and review of the literature. Semin Arthritis Rheum 2011;41:291–6.

80. Ammital H, Applbaum YH, Vasiliey L, et al. Hypertrophic pulmonary osteoarthropathy: control of pain and symptoms with pamidronate. Clin Rheumatol 2004;23(4): 330–2.

81. Angel-Moreno Maroto A, Martínez-Quintana E, Suárez-Castellano L, et al. Painful hypertrophic osteoarthropathy successfully treated with octreotide. The pathogenetic role of vascular endothelial growth factor (VEGF). Rheumatology (Oxford) 2005;44(10):1326–7.

82. Ghosn S, Uthman I, Dahdah M, et al. Treatment of pachydermoperiostosis pachydermia with botulinum toxin type A. J Am Acad Dermatol 2010;63(6):1036–41.

83. da Costa FV, de Magalhães Souza Fialho SC, Zimmermann AF, et al. Infliximab treatment in pachydermoperiostosis: a rare disease without an effective therapeutic option. J Clin Rheumatol 2010;16(4):183–4.

84. Walling HW, Swick BL. Treatment options for hyperhidrosis. Am J Clin Dermatol 2011;12:285–95.

85. Hayashi M, Sekikawa A, Saijo A, et al. Successful treatment of hypertrophic osteoarthropathy by gefitinib in a case with lung adenocarcinoma. Anticancer Res 2005;25(3c):2435–8.

86. Ulusakarya A, Gumus Y, Brahmi N, et al. Symptoms in cancer patients and an unusual tumor: case 1. Regression of hypertrophic pulmonary osteoarthropathy

following chemotherapy for lung metastases of a nasopharyngeal carcinoma. J Clin Oncol 2005;23(36):9422–3.

87. Augarten A, Goldman R, Laufer J, et al. Reversal of digital clubbing after lung transplantation in cystic fibrosis patients: a clue to the pathogenesis of clubbing. Pediatr Pulmonol 2002;34(5):378–80.

SAPHO Syndrome

Sueli Carneiro, MD, PhD[a,b], Percival D. Sampaio-Barros, MD, PhD[c],*

KEYWORDS

- SAPHO • Acne conglobata • Pustulosis palmoplantaris • Hyperostosis
- Chronic recurrent multifocal osteomyelitis • Therapy

KEY POINTS

- SAPHO syndrome is a disorder characterized by Synovitis, Acne, Pustulosis, Hyperostosis, and Osteitis.
- As the osteoarticular and skin manifestations often do not occur simultaneously and there are no validated diagnostic criteria, the diagnosis can be difficult.
- Clinical and imaging investigation is necessary to establish the many differential diagnoses of SAPHO syndrome.
- The etiopathogenesis involves infectious (probably *Propionibacterium acnes*), immunologic, and genetic factors.
- Treatment is based on information gathered from case reports and small series, and is related to specific skin or articular symptoms.

INTRODUCTION

In 1987 a group of French researchers, after conducting a national investigation, proposed the acronym SAPHO syndrome to encompass a group of clinical and radiographic entities constituted by specific skin, bone, and joint manifestations.[1] The meaning of this acronym was initially Syndrome Acne Pustulosis Hyperostosis Osteitis, and the "S" was changed to Synovitis in the following year.[2] Twenty-five years after its inception, the complete syndrome described by the acronym is not common; moreover, the dermatologic manifestations are not frequently concomitant with the

Funding Sources: S. Carneiro: None; P.D. Sampaio-Barros: Federico Foundation.
Conflict of Interest: S. Carneiro: Consultant for MSD; P.D. Sampaio-Barros: Consultant for Abbott, Janssen, MSD, and Pfizer.
[a] State University of Rio de Janeiro - Rua Farme de Amoedo 140/601, Ipanema, Rio de Janeiro 22420-020, Brazil; [b] Federal University of Rio de Janeiro - Hospital Universitario Clementino Fraga Filho, Rua Prof. Rodolpho Paulo Rocco, 250 - Cidade Universitária, Ilha do Fundão, Rio de Janeiro 22590-213, Brazil; [c] Division of Rheumatology, Faculdade de Medicina, Universidade de São Paulo, School of Medicine, Av. Dr Arnaldo, 455 – 3° Andar, Cerqueira César, São Paulo 01246-903, Brazil
* Corresponding author.
E-mail address: pdsampaiobarros@uol.com.br

Rheum Dis Clin N Am 39 (2013) 401–418
http://dx.doi.org/10.1016/j.rdc.2013.02.009
0889-857X/13/$ – see front matter © 2013 Elsevier Inc. All rights reserved.
rheumatic.theclinics.com

joint symptoms, with its distinct clinical and radiographic manifestations occurring in isolation in a significant number of patients. In the twenty-first century, with the development of new perspectives on treatment, interest in the SAPHO syndrome has increased significantly.

EPIDEMIOLOGY

SAPHO is a rare disorder that affects predominantly children and adults. It is not common in individuals older than 60 years. The high variability in the clinical and imaging presentation depends on the stage of the lesions and the imaging method.[3–6]

There is no predilection for gender, except for the male predominance in patients with severe acne. The estimated prevalence is 1 in 10,000 and the largest series are European.[5,7,8] There are also descriptions from China[9] and Australia.[10] It is not frequent in United States, Canada, and Latin America. SAPHO is most severe in African Americans with hidradenitis suppurativa, and presents with heterogeneous musculoskeletal and cutaneous manifestations, including erosive polyarthritis or oligoarthritis with nonspecific mild inflammatory fluid.[11]

In a French study analyzing 120 patients with SAPHO syndrome, of whom 102 were followed up prospectively, 9 patients had the diagnosis of inflammatory bowel disease, and no severe or disabling complications were noted. Except for a significant association of palmoplantar pustulosis or psoriasis vulgaris with axial osteitis ($P = .07$), the dermatologic presentation had no significant influence on rheumatic symptoms.[7]

An Italian study analyzed 71 patients with SAPHO syndrome who had a minimum follow-up of 2 years. Six patients were diagnosed as having Crohn disease and 14 had never had cutaneous involvement. After a median disease duration of 10 years, 13% presented a limited (<6 months) disease course, 35% had a relapsing-remitting course, and 52% had an acute painful phase and a chronic course.[5]

A retrospective study in a single center in Spain reported 52 patients with SAPHO syndrome between 1984 and 2007 (26 men, mean age at diagnosis 42 ± 12 years), with articular involvement preceding cutaneous involvement in 59.6% of patients. Anterior chest wall pain was the most frequent manifestation (73%), followed by peripheral arthritis (32%) and pain in the sacroiliac joints (26.9%); skin manifestations were referred by 63.5% and human leukocyte antigen (HLA) B27 was positive in 8% of the patients.[8]

CLINICAL PICTURE

It is important for the rheumatologist, dermatologist, and clinician to understand the distinct signs and symptoms that constitute the core manifestations of the SAPHO syndrome, as they are predominantly nonspecific and overlap with many other diseases.

Osteoarticular Manifestations

The most common musculoskeletal manifestations of SAPHO syndrome include erosive or nonerosive oligoarthritis affecting knees, ankles, metacarpal phalangeal and metatarsal phalangeal joints; enthesitis; sclerosis of the sacroiliac joints; and osteitis of the anterior chest wall (sternum, clavicle, ribs), axial skeleton, and pelvis. The affected bones are painful; the painful swelling of the anterior chest wall is caused by hyperostosis and osteitis.[11]

The characteristic synovitis affecting peripheral joints is referred by around one-third of patients.[8,12] The peripheral arthritis is frequently insidious at onset, associated with morning stiffness. The joints are swollen and painful, and it is suggested that the articular involvement is an extension of the adjacent osteitis, especially when affecting sternocostal, sternoclavicular, sacroiliac, and hip joints. Enthesitis can represent an initial symptom of SAPHO syndrome in some patients.[13] Inflammatory enthesopathies can cause ossification, contributing to the formation of bone bridges.[6] The mandible is affected in approximately 10% of cases.[14] The lesions are radiolucent and well defined with evidence of osteitis and sclerosis, causing edema and pain without suppuration and/or joint limitation.[15] Chronic recurrent multifocal osteomyelitis (CRMO) usually manifests as recurrent flares of bone pain and inflammation without fever. Kahn and Khan[3] consider that the presence of CRMO, even in the absence of cutaneous manifestations, is sufficient to establish the diagnosis of SAPHO. Nowadays, CRMO is considered the pediatric equivalent of SAPHO syndrome, and recent data suggest its inclusion as an autoinflammatory disease.[16,17] The articular involvement is frequently intermittent, with exacerbations and remissions, and there is no correlation with cutaneous activity of the disease.[7] In the follow-up of at least 2 years of 71 patients with SAPHO syndrome, the presence of peripheral synovitis was associated with a chronic disease course ($P = .0036$).[5]

Skin Manifestations

The characteristic skin manifestations are severe acne (conglobata or fulminans) (**Fig. 1**) and pustulosis palmoplantaris (PPP) (**Fig. 2**). Severe acne can affect around one-fourth of patients, and PPP 50% to 75% of patients. The largest cohorts of SAPHO syndrome have shown that the skin involvement preceded musculoskeletal symptoms in 40% to 68%, occurred simultaneously in 30%, and was a late manifestation in 32% to 60% of patients.[5,7,8] At least 15% of adults and more than 70% of children may never experience skin manifestations.[6]

Other Manifestations

Rare and uncommon manifestations of SAPHO syndrome are muscular weakness and generalized seizures due to central nervous system involvement[18]; venous thrombosis[19,20]; and bilateral optic canal involvement with retrobulbar pain, decreased vision, and a protruding appearance of the left eye.[21] SAPHO has also been described as a widespread bony metastatic disease of unknown origin.[22]

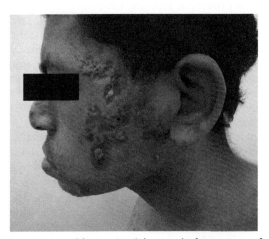

Fig. 1. Severe acne in a 22-year-old man. Partial control of symptoms after long-term antibiotic treatment, with successive flares.

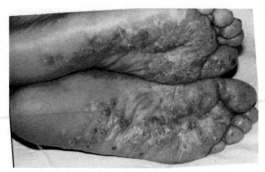

Fig. 2. Pustulosis palmoplantaris.

Is SAPHO a Spondyloarthritis?

Although SAPHO syndrome can share clinical and radiologic features with spondyloarthritis (SpA), including sacroiliitis, enthesitis, paravertebral ossifications, and ankylosis, and many times is associated with psoriasis and inflammatory bowel disease, its consideration as a variant of the SpA is controversial and not definitely established.[6] A genetic study analyzing the HLA profile in 25 patients with SAPHO syndrome in a comparison with 50 patients with psoriasis vulgaris, 150 with psoriatic arthritis, and 170 healthy blood donors, found a different genetic background in the patients with SAPHO syndrome compared with the group with psoriasis and psoriatic arthritis.[23]

IMAGING

There is a great variability in imaging, which depends on the stage of the lesion and the imaging method. Special attention should be given to examination of the spine, which can facilitate an early diagnosis and prevent inadequate biopsies and unnecessary surgery.[15,24–26]

Radiography

Two important osteoarticular manifestations are hyperostosis and osteitis, which are chronic inflammatory reactions involving the cortical and medullary bone. Radiographs of the affected areas are frequently normal at the initial stages of the disease. Early lesions are often purely osteolytic, with or without a sclerotic margin. With disease progression these lesions become lytic/sclerotic or entirely sclerotic. Chronic lesions are predominantly sclerotic.[6,16] The anterior chest wall can involve any component of the sternoclavicular region; adjacent joints may develop arthritis or ankylosis. In contrast to adults, only the clavicle is involved in children.[6,15,26] Mandibular lesions are characterized by diffuse sclerosis of the affected area, often associated with pronounced periosteal reaction.[14]

Spinal involvement has a variety of forms, including vertebral hyperostosis; osteolytic lesions with vertebral collapse; spondylitis with or without discitis; paravertebral ossifications and further syndesmophytes; and sacroiliitis.[15,26]

Ultrasonography

Ultrasonography can be indicated to investigate the presence and the characteristics of enthesitic manifestations. Queiro and colleagues[27] analyzed the ultrasonographic findings in 210 entheses of SAPHO patients and 420 entheses in a control group, and found significant statistical prevalence of ultrasonographic alterations in the

SAPHO group (15%) compared with controls (4.8%: $P<.01$); the most frequently affected entheses were patellar and Achilles tendon, and no control patient presented signs of enthesitis or perienthesitis on power Doppler.

Bone Scintigraphy

Bone scintigraphy can be useful because it not only shows increased uptake in the affected joints, but also frequently reveals clinically silent lesions. The sternoclavicular joint can present the characteristic "bullhead sign," with the manubrium sterni representing the upper skull and the inflamed sternoclavicular joint with the adjacent claviculae forming the horns.[28]

Computed Tomography

Computed tomography (CT) is important for the investigation of the sternoclavicular region, which is frequently difficult to be visualized by conventional radiography because of the superimposition of ribs, spine, and mediastinum. CT examination can show cortical bone erosions, joint-space narrowing, ligament ossification, subchondral sclerosis, and periosteal bone formation.[8,29] ^{18}F-Fluorodeoxyglucose positron emission tomography (PET)/CT can help differentiate SAPHO syndrome from suspected metastatic bone disease in patients who present several sites of bone involvement but no primary malignancy.[30]

Magnetic Resonance Imaging

Nowadays, magnetic resonance imaging (MRI) is the most sensitive technique in the evaluation of soft-tissue swelling, intra-articular effusion, and synovial reaction in SAPHO syndrome.[8,29] MRI can also show vertebral corner erosion lesions early in the diagnosis of SAPHO syndrome in patients with spinal symptoms.[31]

When bone tumors are considered in the differential diagnosis of SAPHO syndrome, a bone biopsy guided by CT or MRI can be performed to confirm the diagnosis.

DIAGNOSIS

The frequent atypical or incomplete presentation, and the clinical mimicry with other diseases such as osteomyelitis, can delay the diagnosis of SAPHO syndrome. Unfortunately, there are no validated criteria for the diagnosis of SAPHO syndrome, and most patients do not fulfill the diagnosis of complete SAPHO. In 1988, Benhamou and colleagues[2] proposed a group of inclusion and exclusion criteria (**Box 1**) that are still used by many physicians. In 2003, Khan proposed new classification criteria for SAPHO syndrome at the ACR 67th Annual Scientific Meeting (cited in Ref.[14] but not published) (**Box 2**).

DIFFERENTIAL DIAGNOSIS

The differential diagnosis among these different syndromes will help to avoid inappropriate diagnostic procedures and treatment.[3] Briefly discussed here are the main syndromes that are considered important in the differential diagnosis of SAPHO syndrome (**Box 3**).

Synovitis. The peripheral involvement in the patients with the diagnosis of SAPHO syndrome and related diseases is completely nonspecific.

Acne. The association of the characteristic acne conglobata or acne fulminans with arthritis has appeared in the literature since 1961.[49] In fact, there are many different acne-associated syndromes, revised by Chen and colleagues.[32] SAPHO syndrome and 2 other diseases (PAPA and PASH) highlight the attributes of

Box 1
Inclusion and exclusion criteria for SAPHO syndrome

Inclusion Criteria[a]

- Osteoarticular manifestations of acne conglobata, acne fulminans, or hidradenitis suppurativa
- Osteoarticular manifestations of PPP
- Hyperostosis (of the anterior chest wall, limbs, or spine) with or without dermatosis
- CRMO involving the axial or peripheral skeleton with or without dermatosis

Sometimes Reported

- Possible association with psoriasis vulgaris
- Possible association with inflammatory enterocolopathy
- Features of ankylosing spondylitis
- Presence of low-virulence bacterial infections

Exclusion Criteria

- Septic osteomyelitis
- Infectious chest wall arthritis
- Infectious PPP
- Palmoplantar keratoderma
- Diffuse idiopathic skeletal hyperostosis, except for fortuitous association
- Osteoarticular manifestations of retinoid therapy

[a] The presence of 1 of the 4 inclusion features is sufficient for a diagnosis of SAPHO syndrome.
Data from Benhamou CL, Chamot AM, Kahn MF. Synovitis-acne-pustulosis-hyperostosis-osteomyelitis syndrome (SAPHO): a new syndrome among the spondyloarthropathies? Clin Exp Rheumatol 1988;6(2):109–12.

Box 2
Proposed classification criteria for SAPHO syndrome

Inclusion

Bone ± joint involvement associated with PPP and psoriasis vulgaris

Bone ± joint involvement associated with severe acne

Isolated[a] sterile hyperostosis/osteitis (adults)

Chronic recurrent multifocal osteomyelitis (children)

Bone ± joint involvement associated with chronic bowel diseases

Exclusion

Infectious osteitis

Tumoral conditions of the bone

Noninflammatory condensing lesions of the bone

[a] Exception: growth of *Propionibacterium acnes*.

Box 3
Differential diagnosis of SAPHO syndrome

- Acne-associated syndrome[32]
- PAPA (Pyogenic sterile Arthritis, Pyoderma gangrenosum, and Acne) syndrome[33]
- PASH (Pyoderma gangrenosum, Acne, and Suppurative Hidradenitis) syndrome[34]
- Arthritis associated with hidradenitis suppurativa (also called acne inversa)[35]
- Follicular occlusion triad, in particular with acne conglobata[36]
- Behçet disease[37]
- Minocycline-induced autoimmume syndromes[38]
- Isotretinoin side effect[39]
- Pustular psoriasis[6]
- Sneddon-Wilkinson disease[40]
- Pustulotic arthro-osteitis[41]
- Acquired hyperostosis syndrome (AHS)[42]
- Chronic recurrent multifocal osteomyelitis (CRMO)[43]
- Diffuse sclerosing osteomyelitis of the mandible (DSOM)[44]
- Majeed syndrome[45]
- Nonbacterial osteitis (NBO)[46]
- Tuberculous spondylitis[47]
- Secondary syphilis[48]
- Primary bone tumors[30]
- Metastatic tumors[30]

inflammation for the formation of acne. PAPA (*Pyogenic sterile Arthritis, Pyoderma gangrenosum, and Acne*)[33] syndrome is an autosomal dominant disease that shares several features with SAPHO syndrome. Recently, the PASH (*Pyoderma gangrenosum, Acne, and Suppurative Hidradenitis*)[34] syndrome has been proposed, which is similar to PAPA with acute and recurrent acne conglobata, but without aseptic abscesses. Although uncommon, there are descriptions of arthritis associated with hidradenitis suppurativa (also called acne inversa) (**Fig. 3**); these patients have predominantly peripheral arthritis, with rare and frequently asymptomatic axial involvement.[35] When acne conglobata is associated with hidradenitis suppurativa and dissecting cellulitis, it is called the follicular occlusion triad.[36] Acneiform skin lesions, more frequently papulopustular, can be observed in patients with Behçet disease with arthritis.[37] A concern related to acne conglobata is the side effects of minocycline, a drug frequently used for the treatment of acne. There are specific minocycline-induced autoimmume syndromes, characterized by serum sickness, drug-induced lupus, autoimmune hepatitis, and vasculitis.[38] Another drug used in the treatment of acne, isotretinoin, also can cause musculoskeletal or mucocutaneous symptoms in 2% to 5% of treated patients.[39]

Pustulosis. The characteristic PPP is a common cutaneous manifestation of SAPHO syndrome, affecting around 65% of patients.[8,12,50] PPP cannot be distinguished from pustular psoriasis in many cases. Although psoriasis vulgaris can affect one-third of patients with SAPHO syndrome, its presence is almost always associated with PPP

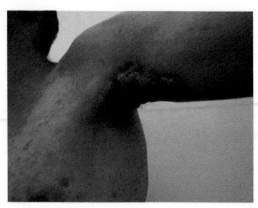

Fig. 3. Hidradenitis suppurativa.

or severe acne, which is the reason why it is not considered as a skin manifestation of SAPHO syndrome.[6] Subcorneal pustular dermatosis (Sneddon-Wilkinson syndrome) is considered a variant of pustular psoriasis.[40] Pustulotic arthro-osteitis is a disorder characterized by PPP and osteoarticular inflammation, affecting predominantly the anterior chest wall, spine, pelvis, sacroiliac joint, and long bones.[41]

Hyperostosis. Hyperostosis is a chronic inflammatory reaction involving the cortical and medullary bones. It affects more frequently the axial skeleton, particularly the anterior chest wall and sternoclavicular joints. The chronic hyperostosis of the spine may result in bony bridges that can evolve to ankylosis.[5] AHS is a chronic inflammatory hyperostosis that affects the sternoclavicular joint in 80% of cases, also presenting skin manifestations (PPP, pustular psoriasis, or severe acne) in 20% to 60% of patients.[42]

Osteitis. In 1972, CRMO was described as a chronic inflammatory process in children and young adults.[43] DSOM was initially considered a disease restricted to temporomandibular joints, but many researchers have observed that many patients also presented with PPP, cutaneous psoriasis, and/or osteitis in various different locations.[44,51] Majeed syndrome is characterized by CRMO of early onset and lifelong course, associated with congenital dyserythropoietic anemia that presents with hypochromic microcytic anemia during the first year of life and ranges to transfusion-dependent, with transient inflammatory dermatosis often manifest as Sweet syndrome (neutrophilic skin infiltration).[45] NBO is characterized by sterile bone lesions with nonspecific histopathologic features of inflammation; only when it is chronic and recurrent can it be considered CRMO.[46] Sterile bone inflammation in children demands various differential diagnoses, including genetic mutations and autoinflammatory diseases.[52] Tuberculous spondylitis,[47] secondary syphilis,[48] primary bone tumors, and metastatic tumors[30] also represent differentials of SAPHO syndrome. An example of osteitis observed on MRI is shown in **Fig. 4**.

Etiopathogenesis

Although the pathogenesis of SAPHO syndrome is not yet completely understood, one may consider that infectious, immunologic, and genetic factors are involved in this multifactorial process. One important hypothesis for SAPHO syndrome considers it to result from an autoimmune response caused by microorganisms in a genetically predisposed individual, leading to a "reactive arthritis."[53]

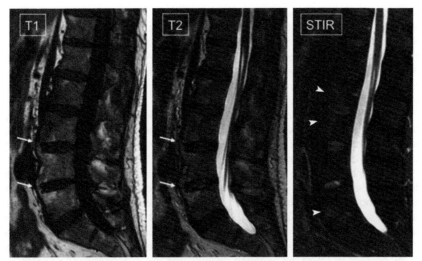

Fig. 4. MRI of lumbar spine (T1, T2, STIR, sagital imaging): Anterior syndesmophytes from L3 to L5 (*arrows*), with bone marrow edema in the anterior segments of L2, L3, and L5 (*arrow heads*), corresponding to the classical osteitis of SAPHO syndrome. (*Courtesy of* Dr Marcelo Bordalo, Head of the MRI Section, Institute of Orthopedics and Traumatology, University of São Paulo, Brazil).

Infection

The infectious or postinfectious theory considers that SAPHO syndrome can be the result of an autoimmune process generated by the long-term persistence of low-virulence pathogens.[54] The corynebacterium *Propionibacterium acnes* is a gram-positive bacterium that constitutes part of the normal flora of the skin, oral cavity, conjunctiva, and external ear canal. Although primarily recognized for its role in acne, *P acnes* is an opportunistic pathogen, causing a range of postoperative and device-related infections in bones and joints, mouth, eye, and brain. It may play a role in SAPHO syndrome, PPP, pyoderma gangrenosum, and other clinical conditions.[55] *P acnes* has been identified in bone biopsies of the affected chest anterior wall, and in spinal and peripheral lesions.[54–57] Clinical improvement after long-term antibiotics, mainly tetracycline or azithromycin, for the treatment of bone erosions caused by intra-articular injections of inactivated *P acnes* supports the infectious hypothesis.[53,58,59] The immune response elicited by *P acnes* can be partially explained by a dysfunction of the toll-like receptors.[60] Nevertheless, in many cases the tests for *P acnes* are negative, and the response to antibiotics is not completely satisfactory.[61]

Immunologic Factors

SAPHO syndrome is associated with high serum levels of proinflammatory cytokines, such as interleukin (IL)-8, IL-18, and tumor necrosis factor (TNF)-α, and these cytokines can be responsible for the maintenance of the clinical manifestations.[62] SAPHO syndrome was also described after immunotherapy with bacillus Calmette-Guérin (BCG) for bladder cancer. It is known that IL-8 level is a good predictive factor for successful outcome after BCG immunotherapy following bladder transurethral resection.[63] TNF overexpression in mandible osteitis has been documented, and some reports have shown a good clinical response to TNF-α inhibitors.[6,64–66]

Colina and colleagues[67] measured IL-1β secretion in the presence of stimulators or blockers of the P2X$_7$ receptor, a major activator of the inflammasome complex, and therefore of IL-1β processing and release, and found that the level of expression of the P2X$_7$ receptor was about 1.75-fold higher in SAPHO than in healthy control leukocytes, suggesting a possible dysregulation of the IL-1β processing machinery. P acnes also induces the production of proinflammatory cytokines such as IL-1, IL-8, and TNF-α.[61]

Patients with SAPHO syndrome can present with leukocytosis, elevated erythrocyte sedimentation rate, and elevated C-reactive protein. The analysis of the most frequent autoantibodies in a group of 90 patients with SAPHO syndrome found antinuclear antibodies (ANA) in 15.5%, antithyroid peroxidase in 3.3%, antigastric parietal cells in 3.3%, anti–smooth-muscle antibodies in 4.4%, and anti-Ro in 2.3% of the tested patients; other common autoantibodies (anti–cyclic citrullinated peptide, anti–double-stranded DNA, antimitochondria) were negative in all the tested patients.[12] In a cross-sectional study analyzing 252 patients with acne vulgaris, there was no difference in the positivity of ANA in patients exposed (14%) and not exposed (11%) to minocycline; however, the positivity of anti-neutrophil cytoplasmic antibody (ANCA), present in 7% of the exposed patients and 0% in nonexposed patients, was statistically significantly associated with the development of an autoimmune disease.[68]

Genetic Factors

Genetic susceptibility and familial clustering have been reported in pairs of monozygotic twins and in siblings.[69–71] HLA-B27 haplotypes are less frequent in SAPHO syndrome than in other forms of SpA.[8] HLA-B51, B52, and A26 were reported in Japanese patients with SAPHO syndrome with mucosal lesions.[72]

The mouse model derived from a BALB/c.DBA/2 strain spontaneously develops aseptic multifocal osteomyelitis similar to those lesions observed in SAPHO syndrome, has a susceptibility gene localized in chromosome 18 (locus cmo), and transmits the disease in a recessive way.[73] Analysis of the locus cmo suggests that a mutation on gene pstpip2 (proline-serine-threonine phosphatase-interacting protein2) may be the genetic explanation for the autoinflammatory phenotype seen in the cmo mouse.[74] PSTPIP2, the human equivalent of the murine pstpip2, is involved in the regulation of the immune response mediated by T cells and apoptosis, and has been implicated in some chronic inflammatory diseases such as psoriasis.[62,75] The study of 27 patients with chronic recurrent multifocal osteitis and their parents has shown a susceptibility gene inherited in dominant way with variable penetrance, also localized on chromosome 18q near the D18S60 marker.[76]

A study of genetic polymorphisms among patients with psoriasis and psoriatic arthritis detected no differences in allele or genotype frequencies of the p53-gene single-nucleotide polymorphism (SNP) G72C and Mdm2-gene SNP T309G. However, in patients with SAPHO, the frequencies of the Mdm2 SNP 309G allele and the genotype SNP 309GG were significantly increased compared with the controls. In addition, the frequencies of the p53 SNP 72C allele and the genotype SNP 72CC were also increased in the SAPHO cohort, suggesting that SAPHO syndrome may be linked to an imbalance between Mdm2 and p53 regulation, with a "weak" p53 response associated with the Mdm2 SNP 309G allele.[77] PAPA syndrome is an autosomal dominant disease that shares several features with SAPHO syndrome, but its susceptibility locus has been mapped in the long arm of chromosome 15.[78,79] The gene NOD2/CARD15, frequently present in Crohn disease, encodes the intracellular receptor for a bacterial wall component, muramyl dipeptide, involved in the activation of nuclear factor (NF)-κB and in the caspase pathway, and the altered recognition of *P acnes* by this gene can lead to an overactivation of NF-κB with exacerbated inflammatory response.[80,81]

TREATMENT

As SAPHO syndrome is a rare disease, there are no placebo-controlled randomized trials analyzing its treatment. All the published experience regarding the treatment of SAPHO syndrome derives from case reports and a few series of patients. Among the drugs that can be used in the treatment of SAPHO syndrome are nonsteroidal anti-inflammatory drugs (NSAIDs), analgesics, oral and intra-articular corticosteroids, antibiotics, bisphosphonates, and biologics (**Box 4**).[6,82]

As the initial osteoarticular symptom in SAPHO syndrome is pain, NSAIDs and analgesics are commonly the first drugs prescribed, but they are effective in just a few patients.[2,5,7]

Intra-articular instillations of corticosteroids were performed in the sternoclavicular joints in 10 patients with SAPHO syndrome; despite good initial clinical improvement in some patients, there were no observed improvements in the MRI scores after 12 weeks of follow-up.[83]

Although the use of antibiotics (doxycycline, azithromycin, or clindamycin) can be indicated, their efficacy is observed only in some cases, suggesting that the disease process can be an inflammatory and immunologic reaction.[44,84] A study analyzing 27 patients with SAPHO syndrome using antibiotics (25 using azithromycin, 500 mg twice a week) showed significant improvement in the MRI score of osteitis after 16 weeks of treatment, but this improvement did not persist at week 28, 12 weeks after stopping antibiotic treatment.[84]

Isotretinoin, frequently indicated for the treatment of acne, is also described in the treatment of flares of SAPHO syndrome.[4]

Conventional DMARDs used in the treatment of chronic inflammatory arthritis were prescribed in patients with SAPHO syndrome. Methotrexate, 20 mg weekly, stabilized disease flares in a patient with SAPHO syndrome who presented with flares after the use of corticosteroids and isotretinoin.[85] There are also reports of the use of sulfasalazine[82] and leflunomide.[86]

Refractory cases of arthritis, osteitis, and enthesitis associated with acne conglobata or fulminans, and hidrosadenitis, other cutaneous manifestations, or isolated CRMO were treated with anti–TNF-α agents (infliximab, etanercept, or adalimumab).

Box 4
Therapeutic options for SAPHO syndrome

- Analgesics
- NSAIDs
- Corticosteroids: intralesional/oral
- Oral antibiotics (doxycycline, azithromycin, clindamycin)
- Isotretinoin
- Conventional disease-modifying antirheumatic drugs (DMARDs): methotrexate, sulfasalazine, leflunomide
- Biologics: anti–TNF-α, anti–IL-1
- Bisphosphonates: alendronate, risedronate, pamidronate, zoledronate

A good and fast initial clinical response is frequently obtained, but there are no descriptions of series of long-term use of these drugs.[64,66,87–91] Some relapses and cases with silent asymptomatic activity were also described.[6,87] Anakinra, a recombinant human IL-1 receptor antagonist, is also indicated for the treatment of refractory cases of SAPHO syndrome.[92,93]

As bisphosphonates can exert an anti-inflammatory effect modulating the proinflammatory cytokines, they have been used for the treatment of SAPHO syndrome. Case reports have shown good clinical response with oral bisphosphonates, such as alendronate[94] and ibandronate.[95] The use of intravenous pamidronate can produce partial or complete remission in a significant number of patients.[96–99] A study analyzing 14 patients with SAPHO syndrome who had a predominantly relapsing-remitting course and were prescribed intravenous pamidronate, 60 mg daily for 3 consecutive days, showed a good response in 12 patients and sustained remission in 8 patients.[100] The association of pamidronate with isotretinoin has also produced good results.[101] Pamidronate was associated with marked improvement in function and well-being in 7 children with SAPHO, producing a reduction in pain and in the concomitant use of other medications, with no significant side effects.[102] A case of the association of SAPHO syndrome with ulcerative colitis showed a good response to pamidronate.[103] Successful treatment with zoledronic acid has also been reported in a patient with refractory disease.[104] Mandible osteomyelitis has been reported to show a satisfactory response to the use of bisphosphonates.[105] In a series of 13 patients with SAPHO syndrome treated with intravenous pamidronate, increased serum crosslaps (sCTx) represented a good prognostic factor in the small group of 6 patients considered good responders after 3 months.[106]

Radical surgery is rarely indicated, because decortication and partial resection was ineffective in most patients. In a rare case of SAPHO syndrome with unilateral hyperostosis of the mandible and massive painful swelling of the surrounding soft tissues, leading to facial disfiguration, resection of the affected bone followed by immediate reconstruction with microvascular iliac crest flap was effective.[44] Reconstructive surgery can also be indicated in rapidly progressive cases affecting thoracic spine that leads to severe destruction and kyphotic deformity followed by paralysis.[107]

SUMMARY

SAPHO syndrome is a chronic disease of unknown origin characterized by bone, joint, and skin manifestations, which probably represents a chronic "reactive" osteitis that develops according to a sequence involving an initial infectious phase with P acnes, followed by an immunologic and autoimmune phase with strong humoral and cellular proinflammatory responses under the influence of genetic factors, although P acnes is not often found in bone lesions. It may be underrecognized, as skin manifestations are frequently mild or absent. Although SAPHO syndrome is an entity that shares features that fit into a variety of established disease categories and bridges multiple medical specialties, it has a clinical and radiologic pattern that is officially recognized as an independent entity. The evaluation of the anterior chest wall in patients with different rheumatic disorders represents a difficult diagnostic problem, because of the anatomic complexity of the region and the variability of the radiographic findings. To avoid misdiagnosis the integrated use of radiography, CT, MRI, and nuclear medicine is suggested. Although optimal therapy for these patients remains unclear, it is important to make the diagnosis of SAPHO so as to avoid unnecessary investigations and treatment, and a bone biopsy may represent a useful procedure for corroborating the diagnosis or for excluding other diseases only in specific cases. Bisphosphonates represent an interesting therapeutic option, and TNF-α blockers should be considered in the therapeutic strategy of refractory cases of SAPHO syndrome, despite their effect seeming to be less impressive than in other spondyloarthritic conditions.

REFERENCES

1. Chamot AM, Benhamou CL, Khan MF, et al. Le syndrome acné pustulose hyperostose ostéite. Résultats d'une enquête nationale; 85 observations. Rev Rhum Mal Osteoartic 1987;54:187–96 [in French].
2. Benhamou CL, Chamot AM, Kahn MF. Synovitis-acne-pustulosis-hyperostosis-osteomyelitis syndrome (SAPHO) A new syndrome among the spondyloarthropathies? Clin Exp Rheumatol 1988;6(2):109–12.
3. Kahn MF, Khan MA. The SAPHO syndrome. Baillieres Clin Rheumatol 1994;8(2):333–62.
4. Beretta-Picolli BC, Sauvin MJ, Gal I, et al. Synovitis, acne, pustulosis, hyperostosis, osteitis (SAPHO) syndrome: a report of ten cases and review of the literature. Eur J Pediatr 2000;159(8):594–601.
5. Colina M, Govoni M, Orzincolo C, et al. Clinical and radiologic evolution of synovitis, acne, pustulosis, hyperostosis, and osteitis syndrome: a single center study of a cohort of 71 patients. Arthritis Rheum 2009;61(6):813–21.
6. Nguyen MT, Borchers A, Selmi C, et al. The SAPHO syndrome. Semin Arthritis Rheum 2012;42(3):254–65.
7. Hayem G, Bouchaud-Chabot A, Benali K, et al. SAPHO syndrome: a long-term follow-up study of 120 cases. Semin Arthritis Rheum 1999;29(3):159–71.
8. Sallés M, Olivé A, Perez-Andres R, et al. The SAPHO syndrome: a clinical and imaging study. Clin Rheumatol 2011;30(2):245–9.
9. Zhao Z, Li Y, Li Y, et al. Synovitis, acne, pustulosis, hyperostosis and osteitis (SAPHO) syndrome with review of the relevant published work. J Dermatol 2011;38(2):155–9.
10. Van Doornum S, Baraclough D, McColl G, et al. SAPHO: rare or just not recognized? Semin Arthritis Rheum 2000;30(1):70–7.
11. Steinhoff JP, Cilursu A, Falasca GF, et al. A study of musculoskeletal manifestations in 12 patients with SAPHO syndrome. J Clin Rheumatol 2002;8(1):13–22.
12. Grosjean C, Hurtado-Nedelec M, Nicaise-Roland P, et al. Prevalence of autoantibodies in SAPHO syndrome: a single-center study of 90 patients. J Rheumatol 2010;37(3):639–43.
13. Maugars Y, Berthelot JM, Ducloux JM, et al. SAPHO syndrome: a followup study of 19 cases with special emphasis on enthesis involvement. J Rheumatol 1995;22(11):2135–41.
14. McPhillips A, Wolford LM, Rodrigues DB. SAPHO syndrome with TMJ involvement: review of the literature and case presentation. Int J Oral Maxillofac Surg 2010;39(12):1160–7.
15. Earwaker JW, Cotten A. SAPHO: syndrome or concept? Imaging findings. Skeletal Radiol 2003;32(6):311–27.
16. Tlougan BE, Podjasek JO, O'Haver J, et al. Chronic recurrent multifocal osteomyelitis (CRMO) and synovitis, acne, pustulosis, hyperostosis, and osteitis (SAPHO) syndrome with associated neutrophilic dermatoses: a report of seven cases and review of the literature. Pediatr Dermatol 2009;26(5):497–505.
17. Wipff J, Adamsbaum C, Kahan A, et al. Chronic recurrent multifocal osteomyelitis. Joint Bone Spine 2011;78(6):555–60.

18. Abul-Kasim K, Nilsson T, Turesson C. Intracranial manifestations in SAPHO syndrome: the first case report in literature. Rheumatol Int 2012;32(6):1797–9.
19. Legoupil N, Révelon G, Allain J, et al. Iliac vein thrombosis complicating SAPHO syndrome: MRI and histologic features of soft tissue lesions. Joint Bone Spine 2001;68(1):79–83.
20. Kawabata T, Morita Y, Nakatsuka A, et al. Multiple venous thrombosis in SAPHO syndrome. Ann Rheum Dis 2005;64(3):505–6.
21. Smith M, Buller A, Radford R, et al. Ocular presentation of the SAPHO syndrome. Br J Ophthalmol 2005;89(8):1069–70.
22. Mann B, Shaerf DA, Sheeraz A, et al. SAPHO syndrome presenting as widespread bony metastatic disease of unknown origin. Rheumatol Int 2012;32(2):505–7.
23. Queiro R, Moreno P, Sarasqueta C, et al. Synovitis-acne-pustulosis-hyperostosis-osteitis syndrome and psoriatic arthritis exhibit a different immunogenetic profile. Clin Exp Rheumatol 2008;26(1):125–8.
24. Akisue T, Yamamoto T, Marui T, et al. Lumbar spondylodiscitis in SAPHO syndrome: multimodality imaging findings. J Rheumatol 2002;29(5):1100–1.
25. Tohme-Noun C, Feydy A, Belmatoug N, et al. Cervical involvement in SAPHO syndrome: imaging findings with a 10-year follow-up. Skeletal Radiol 2003;32(2):103–6.
26. Depasquale R, Kumar N, Lalam RK, et al. SAPHO: what radiologists should know. Clin Radiol 2012;67(3):195–206.
27. Queiro R, Alonso S, Alperi M, et al. Entheseal ultrasound abnormalities in patients with SAPHO syndrome. Clin Rheumatol 2012;31(6):913–9.
28. Freyschmidt J, Sternberg A. The bullhead sign: scintigraphic pattern of sternocostoclavicular hyperostosis and pustulotic arthroosteitis. Eur Radiol 1998;8:807–12.
29. Guglielmi G, Cascavilla A, Scalzo G, et al. Imaging of sternocostoclavicular joint in spondyloarthropathies and other rheumatic conditions. Clin Exp Rheumatol 2009;27(3):402–8.
30. Patel CN, Smith JT, Rankine JJ, et al. F18 FDG PET/CT can help differentiate SAPHO syndrome from suspected metastatic bone disease. Clin Nucl Med 2009;34(4):254–7.
31. Laredo JV, Vuillemin-Bodaghi V, Butry N, et al. SAPHO syndrome: MR appearance of vertebral involvement. Radiology 2007;242(3):825–31.
32. Chen W, Obermayer-Pietsch B, Hong JB, et al. Acne-associated syndromes: models for better understanding of acne pathogenesis. J Eur Acad Dermatol Venereol 2011;25(6):637–46.
33. Lindor NM, Arsenault TM, Solomon H, et al. A new autosomal dominant disorder of pyogenic sterile arthritis, pyoderma gangrenosum, and acne: PAPA syndrome. Mayo Clin Proc 1997;72(7):611–5.
34. Braun-Falco M, Kovnerystyy O, Lohse P, et al. Pyoderma gangrenosum, acne, and suppurative hidradenitis (PASH)—a new autoinflammatory syndrome distinct from PAPA syndrome. J Am Acad Dermatol 2012;66(3):409–15.
35. Bhalla R, Sequeira W. Arthritis associated with hidradenitis suppurativa. Ann Rheum Dis 1994;53(1):64–6.
36. Olafsson F, Khan MA. Musculoskeletal features of acne, hidradenitis suppurativa, and dissecting cellulitis of the scalp. Rheum Dis Clin North Am 1992;18(1):215–24.
37. Diri E, Mat C, Hamuryudan V, et al. Papulopustular skin lesions are seen more frequently in patients with Behçet's syndrome who have arthritis: a controlled and masked study. Ann Rheum Dis 2001;60(11):1074–6.

38. Elkayam O, Yaron M, Caspi D. Minocycline-induced autoimmune syndromes: an overview. Semin Arthritis Rheum 1999;28(6):392–7.

39. Goulden V, Layton AM, Cunliffe WJ. Long-term safety of isotretinoin as a treatment for acne vulgaris. Br J Dermatol 1994;131(3):360–3.

40. Scarpa R, Lubrano E, Cozzi R, et al. Subcorneal pustular dermatosis (Sneddon-Wilkinson syndrome): another cutaneous manifestation of SAPHO syndrome? Br J Rheumatol 1997;36(5):602–3.

41. Hyodoh K, Sugimoto H. Pustulotic arthro-osteitis: defining the radiologic spectrum of the disease. Semin Musculoskelet Radiol 2001;5(2):89–93.

42. Dihlmann W, Schnabel A, Gross WL. The acquired hyperostosis syndrome: a little known skeletal disorder with distinctive radiological and clinical features. Clin Investig 1993;72(1):4–11.

43. Giedion A, Holthusen W, Masel LF, et al. Subacute and chronic "symmetrical" osteomyelitis. Ann Radiol (Paris) 1972;15(3):329–42 [in Multiple languages].

44. Zemann W, Pau M, Feichtinger M, et al. SAPHO syndrome with affection of the mandible: diagnosis, treatment, and review of literature. Oral Surg Oral Med Oral Pathol Oral Radiol Endod 2011;111(2):190–5.

45. Ferguson PJ, Chen S, Tayeh MK, et al. Homozygous mutations in LPIN2 are responsible for the syndrome of chronic recurrent multifocal osteomyelitis and congenital dyserythropoietic anaemia (Majeed syndrome). J Med Genet 2005; 42(7):551–7.

46. Gikas PD, Islam L, Aston W, et al. Nonbacterial osteitis: a clinical, histopathological, and imaging study with a proposal for protocol-based management of patients with this diagnosis. J Orthop Sci 2009;14(5):505–16.

47. Nakamura J, Yamada K, Mitsugi N, et al. A case of SAPHO syndrome with destructive spondylodiscitis suspicious of tuberculous spondylitis. Mod Rheumatol 2010;20(1):93–7.

48. Arnson Y, Rubinow A, Amital H. Secondary syphilis presenting as SAPHO syndrome features. Clin Exp Rheumatol 2008;26(6):1119–21.

49. Windom RE, Sanford JP, Ziff M. Acne conglobata and arthritis. Arthritis Rheum 1961;4:632–5.

50. Hurtado-Nedelec M, Chollet-Martin S, Chapeton D, et al. Genetic susceptibility factors in a cohort of 38 patients with SAPHO syndrome: a study of PSTPIP2, NOD2, and LPIN2 genes. J Rheumatol 2010;37(2):401–9.

51. Suei Y, Taguchi A, Tanimoto K. Diagnostic points and possible origin of osteomyelitis in synovitis, acne, pustulosis, hyperostosis and osteitis (SAPHO) syndrome: a radiographic study of 77 mandibular osteomyelitis cases. Rheumatology (Oxford) 2003;42:1398–403.

52. Twilt M, Laxer RM. Clinical care of children with sterile bone inflammation. Curr Opin Rheumatol 2011;23(5):424–31.

53. Assmann G, Simon P. The SAPHO syndrome—are microbes involved. Best Pract Res Clin Rheumatol 2011;25(3):423–34.

54. Govoni M, Colina M, Massara A, et al. SAPHO syndrome and infections. Autoimmun Rev 2009;8(3):256–9.

55. Perry A, Lambert P. *Propionibacterium acnes*: infection beyond the skin. Expert Rev Anti Infect Ther 2011;9(12):1149–56.

56. Kotilainen P, Merilahti-Palo R, Lehtonen OP, et al. *Propionibacterium acnes* isolated from sternal osteitis in a patient with SAPHO syndrome. J Rheumatol 1996; 23(7):1302–4.

57. Magrey M, Khan MA. New insights into synovitis, acne, pustulosis, hyperostosis, and osteitis (SAPHO) syndrome. Curr Rheumatol Rep 2009;11(5):329–33.

58. Trimble BS, Evers CJ, Ballaron AS, et al. Intraarticular injection of *Propionibacterium acnes* causes an erosive arthritis in rats. Agents Actions 1987;21(3–4): 281–3.
59. Kirchhoff T, Merkesdal S, Rosenthal H, et al. Diagnostic management of patients with SAPHO syndrome: use of MRI imaging to guide bone biopsy at CT for microbiological and histological work-up. Eur Radiol 2003;13:2304–8.
60. Kallis C, Gumenscheimer M, Freudenberg N, et al. Requirement for TLR9 in the immunomodulatory activity of *Propionibacterium acnes*. J Immunol 2005;174(7): 4295–300.
61. Hayem G. Valuable lessons from SAPHO syndrome [editorial]. Joint Bone Spine 2007;74(2):123–6.
62. Hurtado-Nedelec M, Chollet-Martin S, Nicaise-Roland P, et al. Characterization of the immune response in the Synovitis, Acne, Pustulosis, Hyperostosis, Osteitis (SAPHO) syndrome. Rheumatology (Oxford) 2008;47:1160–7.
63. Matsumaru K, Nagai K, Murakami T, et al. SAPHO syndrome with bacillus Calmette-Guerin (BCG) immunotherapy for bladder cancer. BMJ Case Rep 2010;2010:2591.
64. Ben Abdelghani K, Dran DG, Gottenberg JE, et al. Tumor necrosis factor-alpha blockers in SAPHO syndrome. J Rheumatol 2010;37(8):1699–704.
65. Burgemeister LT, Baeten DL, Tas SW. Biologics for rare inflammatory diseases: TNF blockade in the SAPHO syndrome. Neth J Med 2012;70(10):444–9.
66. Garcovich S, Amelia R, Magarelli N, et al. Long-term treatment of severe SAPHO syndrome with adalimumab: case report and a review of the literature. Am J Clin Dermatol 2012;13(1):55–9.
67. Colina M, Pizzirani C, Khodeir M, et al. Dysregulation of P2X7 receptor-inflammasome axis in SAPHO syndrome: successful treatment with anakinra. Rheumatology (Oxford) 2010;49(7):1416–8.
68. Marzo-Ortega H, Baxter K, Strauss RM, et al. Is minocycline therapy in acne associated with antineutrophil cytoplasmic antibody positivity? A cross-sectional study. Br J Dermatol 2007;156(5):1005–9.
69. Darley CR, Currey HL, Baker H. Acne fulminans with arthritis in identical twins treated with isotretinoin. J R Soc Med 1984;77:328–30.
70. Dumolard A, Gaudin P, Juvin R, et al. SAPHO syndrome or psoriatic arthritis? A familial case study. Rheumatology (Oxford) 1999;38(5):463–7.
71. Gonzalez T, Gantes M, Bustabad S, et al. Acne fulminans associated with arthritis in monozygotic twins. J Rheumatol 1985;12(2):389–91.
72. Yabe H, Ohshima H, Takano Y, et al. Mucosal lesions may be a minor complication of SAPHO syndrome: a study of 11 Japanese patients with SAPHO syndrome. Rheumatol Int 2010;30(10):1277–83.
73. Byrd L, Grossmann M, Potter M, et al. Chronic multifocal osteomyelitis, a new recessive mutation on chromosome 18 of the mouse. Genomics 1991;11(4): 794–8.
74. Ferguson PJ, Bing X, Vasef MA, et al. A missense mutation in pstpip2 is associated with the murine autoinflammatory disorder chronic multifocal osteomyelitis. Bone 2006;38(1):41–7.
75. Baum W, Kirkin V, Fernandez SB, et al. Binding of the intracellular Fas ligand (FasL) domain to the adaptor protein PSTPIP results in a cytoplasmic localization of FasL. J Biol Chem 2005;280(48):40012–24.
76. Golla A, Jansson A, Ramser J, et al. Chronic recurrent multifocal osteomyelitis (CRMO): evidence for a susceptibility gene located on chromosome 18q21.3-18q22. Eur J Hum Genet 2002;10(3):217–21.

77. Assmann G, Wagner AD, Monika M, et al. Single-nucleotide polymorphisms p53 G72C and Mdm2 T309G in patients with psoriasis, psoriatic arthritis, and SAPHO syndrome. Rheumatol Int 2010;30(10):1273–6.
78. Yeon HB, Lindor NM, Seidman JG, et al. Pyogenic arthritis, pyoderma gangrenosum, and acne syndrome maps to chromosome 15q. Am J Hum Genet 2000; 66(4):1443–8.
79. Wise C, Gillum J, Seidman C, et al. Mutations in CD2BP1 disrupt binding to PTP PEST and are responsible for PAPA syndrome, an autoinflammatory disorder. Hum Mol Genet 2002;11(8):961–9.
80. Hampe J, Grebe J, Nikolaus S, et al. Association of NOD2 (CARD 15) genotype with clinical course of Crohn's disease: a cohort study. Lancet 2002;359: 1661–5.
81. Giardin SE, Boneca IG, Viala J, et al. Nod2 is a general sensor of peptidoglycan through muramyl dipeptide (MDP) detection. J Biol Chem 2003;278(11): 8869–72.
82. Olivieri I, Padula A, Palazzi C. Pharmacological management of SAPHO syndrome. Expert Opin Investig Drugs 2006;15(10):1229–33.
83. Jung J, Molinger M, Kohn D, et al. Intra-articular glucocorticosteroid injection into sternocostoclavicular joints in patients with SAPHO syndrome. Semin Arthritis Rheum 2012;42(3):266–70.
84. Assmann G, Kueck O, Kirchhoff T, et al. Efficacy of antibiotic therapy for SAPHO syndrome is lost after its discontinuation: an interventional study. Arthritis Res Ther 2009;11(5):R140.
85. Azevedo VF, Dal Pizzol VI, Lopes H, et al. Methotrexate to treat SAPHO syndrome with keloidal scars. Acta Reumatol Port 2011;36(2):167–70 [in Portuguese].
86. Scarpato S, Tirri E. Successful treatment of SAPHO syndrome with leflunomide. Report of two cases. Clin Exp Rheumatol 2005;23(5):731.
87. Eleftheriou D, Gerschman T, Sebire N, et al. Biologic therapy in refractory chronic non-bacterial osteomyelitis of childhood. Rheumatology (Oxford) 2010;49(8): 1505–12.
88. De Souza A, Solomon GE, Strober BE. SAPHO syndrome associated with hidradenitis suppurativa successfully treated with infliximab and methotrexate. Bull NYU Hosp Jt Dis 2011;69(2):185–7.
89. Vilar-Alejo J, Dehesa L, de la Rosa-del Rey P, et al. SAPHO syndrome with unusual cutaneous manifestations treated successfully with etanercept. Acta Derm Venereol 2010;90(5):531–2.
90. Arias-Santiago S, Sanchez-Cano D, Callejas-Rubio JL, et al. Adalimumab treatment for SAPHO syndrome. Acta Derm Venereol 2010;90(3):301–2.
91. Castelví I, Bonet M, Narváez JA, et al. Successful treatment of SAPHO syndrome with adalimumab: a case report. Clin Rheumatol 2010;29(10):1205–7.
92. Pazyar N, Feily A, Yaghoobi R. An overview of interleukin-1 receptor antagonist, anakinra, in the treatment of cutaneous diseases. Curr Clin Pharmacol 2012; 7(4):271–5.
93. Wendling D, Prati C, Aubin F. Anakinra treatment of SAPHO syndrome: short-term results of an open study. Ann Rheum Dis 2012;71(6):1098–100.
94. Fioravanti A, Cantarini L, Burroni L, et al. Efficacy of alendronate in the treatment of the SAPHO syndrome. J Clin Rheumatol 2008;14(3):183–4.
95. Soyfoo MS, Gangji V, Margaux J. Successful treatment of SAPHO syndrome with ibandronate. J Clin Rheumatol 2010;16(5):253.
96. Courtney PA, Hosking DJ, Fairbairn KJ, et al. Treatment of SAPHO with pamidronate. Rheumatology (Oxford) 2002;41(10):1196–8.

97. Marshall H, Bromilow J, Thomas AL, et al. Pamidronate: a novel treatment for the SAPHO syndrome? Rheumatology (Oxford) 2002;41(2):231–3.

98. Guignard S, Job-Deslandre C, Sayag-Boukris V, et al. Pamidronate treatment in SAPHO syndrome. Joint Bone Spine 2002;69(4):392–6.

99. Amital H, Applbaum YH, Aamar S, et al. SAPHO syndrome treated with pamidronate: an open-label study of 10 patients. Rheumatology (Oxford) 2004;43(5): 658–61.

100. Colina M, La Corte R, Trotta F. Sustained remission of SAPHO syndrome with pamidronate: a follow-up of fourteen cases and a review of the literature. Clin Exp Rheumatol 2009;27(1):112–5.

101. Galadari H, Bishop AG, Venna SS, et al. Synovitis, acne, pustulosis, hyperostosis, and osteitis syndrome treated with a combination of isotretinoin and pamidronate. J Am Acad Dermatol 2009;61(1):123–5.

102. Kerrison C, Davidson JE, Cleary AG, et al. Pamidronate in the treatment of childhood SAPHO syndrome. Rheumatology (Oxford) 2004;43(10):1246–51.

103. Siau K, Laversuch C. SAPHO syndrome in an adult with ulcerative colitis responsive to intravenous pamidronate: a case report and review of the literature. Joint Bone Spine 2010;30(8):1085–8.

104. Kopterides P, Pikazis D, Koufos C. Successful treatment of SAPHO syndrome with zoledronic acid. Arthritis Rheum 2004;50(9):2970–3.

105. Hatano H, Shigeishi H, Higashikawa K, et al. A case of SAPHO syndrome with diffuse sclerosing osteomyelitis of the mandible treated successfully with prednisolone and bisphosphonate. J Oral Maxillofac Surg 2012;70(3): 626–31.

106. Solau-Gervais E, Soubrier M, Gerot I, et al. The usefulness of bone remodeling markers in predicting the efficacy of pamidronate treatment of SAPHO syndrome. Rheumatology (Oxford) 2006;45(3):339–42.

107. Takigawa T, Tanaka M, Nakahara S, et al. SAPHO syndrome with rapidly progressing destructive spondylitis: two cases treated surgically. Eur Spine J 2008;17(Suppl 2):S331–7.

Joint Hypermobility Syndrome

Asma Fikree, BM BCh, MA, MRCP[a], Qasim Aziz, PhD, FRCP[a],
Rodney Grahame, CBE, MD, FRCP[b],*

KEYWORDS

- Hypermobility • Hypermobility syndrome • Ehlers-Danlos syndrome • Dysautonomia
- Functional gastrointestinal disorder

KEY POINTS

- Joint hypermobility syndrome is a common, heritable disorder of connective tissue that is frequently overlooked.
- It is almost certainly identical to the Ehlers-Danlos Syndrome, hypermobility type.
- It is not a trivial articular problem occurring in healthy individuals; it is now recognized as a multisystemic disorder and a major source of chronic widespread pain, dysautonomias, and gastrointestinal dysmotility. It is a neglected area within rheumatology.

INTRODUCTION

Most rheumatologists have a basic appreciation of joint hypermobility (JH). They know that the term refers to the increased passive or active movement of a joint beyond its normal range. They are familiar with the 9-point Beighton score[1] and many see this as the gold standard for recognizing JH. On an all-or-none basis, it signals the flexibility of 5 body areas (spine/hips and paired elbows, fifth metacarpophalangeals, thumb/wrists, and knees) as shown in **Table 1**, but takes no account of the rest. The maximum score is 9 out of 9. Higher scores do not represent greater degrees of JH, merely the number of joints affected out of a limited selection. A score of 4 or more out of 9 is arbitrarily considered to show the presence of generalized JH. However, it was introduced as an instrument for epidemiologic research; it was never intended to become a tool for clinical diagnosis. It is with the interpretation of hypermobility that most rheumatologists have difficulties. The wherewithal to establish a definitive

Disclosure of relationships with commercial companies: None.
[a] Wingate Institute of Neurogastroenterology, Centre for Gastroenterology, Blizard Institute, Barts and The London School of Medicine and Dentistry, Queen Mary University of London, 26 Ashfield Street, London E1 2AJ, UK; [b] Centre for Rheumatology, University College London Hospitals, 3rd Floor Central, 250 Euston Road, London NW1 2PQ, UK
* Corresponding author.
E-mail address: r.grahame@ucl.ac.uk

Rheum Dis Clin N Am 39 (2013) 419–430
http://dx.doi.org/10.1016/j.rdc.2013.03.003
0889-857X/13/$ – see front matter © 2013 Elsevier Inc. All rights reserved.

Table 1 Nine-point Beighton hypermobility score		
The Ability to:	Right	Left
(1) Passively dorsiflex the fifth metacarpophalangeal joint to ≥90°	1	1
(2) Oppose the thumb to the volar aspect of the ipsilateral forearm	1	1
(3) Hyperextend the elbow to ≥10°	1	1
(4) Hyperextend the knee to ≥10°	1	1
(5) Place hands flat on the floor without bending the knees	1	
TOTAL	9	

One point may be gained for each side for maneuvers 1 to 4 so that the hypermobility score has a maximum of 9 points if all are positive.

differential diagnosis and thereby to develop an appropriate management plan is often lacking. This article is intended to assist colleagues in this critical task.

RECOGNIZING HYPERMOBILITY
The 5-Point Questionnaire

JH can also be identified reliably with the use of the 5-point questionnaire, which is a simple statistically validated questionnaire that accurately predicts the presence of hypermobility according to the individual's response to 5 questions. It has an 84% sensitivity and an 80% specificity when 2 or more questions are answered in the affirmative (**Box 1**).[2] This questionnaire is particularly useful as a screening tool when the person is not present or available for examination. It is easy and quick to complete, and therefore a useful research tool. It has been successfully used to estimate the heritability of hypermobility in a twin study.[3]

Hypermobility Syndrome

Hypermobility syndrome (HMS; later termed joint hypermobility syndrome [JHS]) is a poorly understood clinical entity, the nature of which has changed almost beyond recognition since it was first described by Kirk and colleagues[4] in 1967. It was originally conceived as the occurrence of musculoskeletal symptoms in the presence of generalized joint hypermobility. These early workers in the field (being eminent rheumatologists) thought of it as a purely rheumatologic disorder that occurred in healthy individuals who happened (by chance) to be at the upper end of the spectrum of

Box 1 Validated 5-point questionnaire for generalized JH
1. Can you now (or could you ever) place your hands flat on the floor without bending your knees?
2. Can you now (or could you ever) bend your thumb to touch your forearm?
3. As a child, did you amuse your friends by contorting your body into strange shapes or could you do the splits?
4. As a child or teenager, did your kneecap or shoulder dislocate on more than 1 occasion?
5. Do you consider yourself 'double-jointed'?
Data from Hakim AJ, Grahame R. A simple questionnaire to detect hypermobility: an adjunct to the assessment of patients with diffuse musculoskeletal pain. Int J Clin Pract 2003;57(3):163–6.

normal joint mobility. Although in their discussion they considered the alternative interpretation, namely that these individuals might have a heritable disorder of connective tissue (HDCT) akin to Ehlers-Danlos syndrome (EDS) or Marfan syndrome (MFS), they rejected it outright, without stating their reasons for doing so, carrying with them most of the rheumatologic community worldwide. It has taken nearly half a century to set the record straight. This realization arose from the steady acquisition by a handful of interested investigators of new knowledge that gradually accrued during the second half of the twentieth century. It started in the 1980s, with the observation that patients with JHS showed phenotypic overlap with patients with other HDCTs, notably with skin and skeletal manifestations,[5] so that JHS began to seem more and more like EDS type III than a seemingly trivial rheumatologic disorder occurring in healthy people, as it was widely perceived. This change was swiftly followed by the revelation that gynecologic abnormalities arising from pelvic floor weakness, such as uterine prolapse, were frequently found among women with JHS.[6] In the 1990s, the focus moved to the further revelations that chronic pain and dysautonomia were also becoming recognized as complications associated with JHS.[7–10] It is only in the last decade that interest has focused on the gastrointestinal (GI) tract with the discovery of a strong association between JHS and functional disorders of the GI tract (functional GI disorders [FGID]).[11]

Recognizing Hypermobility Syndrome: the Brighton Criteria for JHS

The Beighton score identifies JH but not the symptoms that may have arisen as a result of it. It could, therefore, never be used to diagnose JHS. Thus, before 2000, there was no reliable way of identifying the syndrome other than by using the 1967 definition, which was too inclusive to be of use for this purpose, and therefore research was hampered by the lack of any means of defining the phenotype or classifying the syndrome. The Brighton criteria were conceived in the 1990s and published in 2000 for the purpose of addressing this need.[12] Like its predecessors, the Ghent criteria for MFS[13] and the Villefranche criteria for EDS,[14] the Brighton criteria comprise major and minor criteria and incorporated the Beighton score and, in addition, included the principal symptoms, notably joint/spinal pain, dislocations, soft tissue lesions, as well as overlap features of connective tissue disorder such as hernias, uterine/rectal prolapse, marfanoid features, and skin changes. The full criteria are shown in **Box 2**. The diagnosis of JHS should always be considered against the background of the other HDCTs, and the clinician must be alert to the wider differential diagnosis, so that a working knowledge of the clinical features including prognosis and availability, or otherwise, of genetic testing of the other major HDCTs, such as MFS, EDS (other than type III), and osteogenesis imperfecta (OI) is important (**Fig. 1**). There is currently no genetic test or other biological marker for EDS III or JHS. A recent guide to the diagnosis of HDCTs written from a rheumatologist's perspective may assist readers in this task.[15]

Epidemiology of JH and JHS

The epidemiology of JH and JHS are in their infancy. There are many published surveys of JH in different parts of the world among peoples of different ethnic origin, and it has long been recognized that the prevalence is highest among those of Asian origin, followed by those of African and then European origin. Strict comparisons have been hampered by the differing use of criteria and methodology.

It is now more than a decade since the Brighton criteria for JHS were introduced, but there have been no large epidemiology studies conducted to determine the prevalence of JHS using this (or any other) instrument.

Box 2
The 1998 Brighton criteria for the classification of benign JHS

Major criteria

1. A Beighton score of 4/9 or greater (either currently or historically)
2. Arthralgia for longer than 3 months in 4 or more joints

Minor criteria

1. A Beighton score of 1, 2, or 3/9 (0, 1, 2, or 3 if aged 50 years or older)
2. Arthralgia in 1 to 3 joints or back pain or spondylosis, spondylolysis/spondylolisthesis
3. Dislocation in more than 1 joint, or in 1 joint on more than 1 occasion
4. Three or more soft tissue lesions (eg, epicondylitis, tenosynovitis, bursitis)
5. Marfanoid habitus (tall, slim, span > height, upper segment/lower segment ratio less than 0.89, arachnodactyly)
6. Skin striae, hyperextensibility, thin skin, or abnormal scarring
7. Eye signs: drooping eyelids or myopia or antimongoloid slant
8. Varicose veins or hernia or uterine/rectal prolapse

JHS is diagnosed in the presence 2 major criteria, or 1 major and 2 minor criteria, or 4 minor criteria. Two minor criteria suffice if there is an unequivocally affected first-degree relative. JHS is excluded by presence of MFS or EDS (other than the EDS hypermobility type, formerly EDS III) as defined by the De Paepe 1996[13] and Beighton 1998[14] criteria respectively.

Data from Grahame R, Bird HA, Child A, et al. The revised (Brighton 1998) criteria for the diagnosis of benign joint hypermobility syndrome (BJHS). J Rheumatol 2000;27(7):1777–9.

In one district hospital–based study, it was observed that 45% of all attenders to a rheumatology clinic satisfied the Brighton criteria for JHS.[16] This percentage was unexpectedly high, but similarly high prevalences have also have been shown in a clinic with an interest in heritable disorders of connective tissue in Santiago, Chile,[17] and in a population of 365 French undergraduate students (39.5%).[18]

Systemic Complications of JHS

Many rheumatologists still harbor an outdated view that symptoms in JHS are confined to the musculoskeletal system and that noninflammatory joint, spinal, and soft tissue pain are a mechanical consequence of increased joint laxity, devoid of any systemic elements. This idea was the original concept in the 1960s when it was first described and in the decades that followed. However, despite mounting evidence to the contrary, showing that JHS is a systemic disorder, the concept proved difficult to shake, which explains why there is such confusion surrounding JHS today.[19]

The multisystemic disorder incorporates 3 principal components: (1) chronic pain, (2) autonomic dysfunction, and (3) pan-GI dysmotility. These three aspects, either singly or in unison, emerge to become part of the natural history of the condition usually in the third decade,[20] although it is increasingly recognized today in adolescents or even in younger children (Ninis N and Grahame R, unpublished data, 2013).

Chronic pain can either present as a significant intensification of preexisting joint and/or spinal pain or as a superadded layer of whole-body (or hemibody) pain that adds to the preexisting pain. Its advent may be triggered by unaccustomed physical exercise (like running a marathon), a road traffic accident or other traumatic event, or it may develop for no obvious reason. The distribution is nonanatomic. The pain is

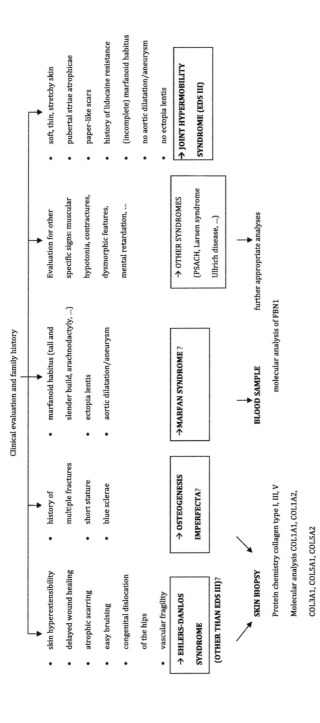

Fig. 1. Differential diagnosis of a patient presenting with JH. (*Data from* Malfait F, Hakim AJ, De PA, et al. The genetic basis of the joint hypermobility syndromes. Rheumatology (Oxford) 2006;45(5):502–7; and *Reproduced from* Oxford University Press, with permission.)

usually resistant even to the most potent analgesics, including opiates. For this reason, pain management using cognitive behavior therapy (CBT) has become the treatment of choice.[21] Chronic pain in JHS is often labeled fibromyalgia. Unless they are specifically sought, the features of JHS are overlooked and the true diagnosis missed.[22,23]

Autonomic dysfunction is a frequently occurring feature of JHS. In one series it was identified (by the Brighton criteria) in 78% of patients with JHS compared with 21% of controls.[7] The most common type of dysautonomia seen in JHS is postural tachycardia syndrome (PoTS), defined as an increase in heart rate of greater than or equal to 30 beats per minute on 60° head-up tilt table[10] or on rising from the lying to the erect posture. Symptoms include palpitations, orthostatic intolerance (dizziness, presyncope, or syncope on standing), headache, impaired concentration, forgetfulness, irritability, fatigue, and heat intolerance.

GI Manifestations

The existence of JHS-related GI manifestations as distinct clinical entities is a recent discovery. The ramifications in terms of symptoms, altered physiology and morbidity, and treatment are currently being studied for the first time. As a consequence, few clinicians are yet aware of its occurrence or of the impact it can have on an affected patient's quality of life. Because few readers are likely to have encountered this complication in their clinical practice, the remainder of this article concentrates on this aspect.

Hypermobility and Abnormal GI Anatomy

Hypermobility is associated with several anatomic abnormalities in both the upper and lower GI tract. In a study of 100 patients attending an endoscopy unit, the prevalence of JH in patients with hiatus hernias (22%) was significantly increased compared with age-matched and sex-matched controls without hernias (6%, $P<.001$).[24]

In patients with constipation and symptoms of rectal evacuatory dysfunction, those with JH had an increased prevalence of rectal morphologic anomalies compared with those without JH,[25] most commonly large functional rectoceles (24%) and external compression of the anterior rectal wall (11%). Lower GI symptoms in JHS frequently overlap with urinary symptoms, and a urologic study of patients with lower urinary tract dysfunction similarly showed that patients with JHS were significantly more likely to have symptoms of rectal evacuatory dysfunction and evidence of rectal morphologic anomalies (eg, rectal prolapses) compared with those without JHS.[26]

Case reports of patients with JHS describe further anatomic abnormalities in small numbers of patients, including diverticular disease[27] and visceroptosis of the bowel.[28] The latter is rare and refers to the downward displacement of abdominal organs below their natural position. It can cause kinking of blood vessels and nerves and thereby cause symptoms that can be severe. In one case, the patient presented with a 4-year history of abdominal distension and bloating that interfered with her eating and activities of daily living.

Hypermobility and Abnormal GI Physiology

There is a physiologic association between JH and constipation.[26,29] In young boys, a higher prevalence of JH was shown in those with slow transit constipation compared with those without.[29] Adults seem to have a different pattern of constipation and, in a study of patients referred for investigation of severe constipation, those with JH had a higher prevalence of rectal evacuatory dysfunction but not slow transit constipation, with more severe constipation, greater abdominal pain, increased laxative use, and need for manual evacuation.[25]

Association Between JHS and GI Symptoms

The association between JHS and GI symptoms was first described 8 years ago by Hakim and Grahame (**Fig. 2**).[30] Patients with JHS attending a hypermobility clinic had significantly more GI symptoms compared with age-matched and sex-matched controls (37% vs 11%). The most common GI symptoms were nausea, abdominal pain, constipation, and diarrhea. It was thought that dysautonomia was one mechanism by which this may occur,[7,30] and since then it has been shown that PoTS is associated with GI symptoms such as nausea, reflux, bloating, constipation, and diarrhea.[11] Thus it seems that JHS, autonomic symptoms, and GI symptoms are linked, although the exact mechanism for the association is unknown.

Since that landmark study, other studies worldwide in specialist hospital settings have confirmed that GI symptoms are common in patients with an existing diagnosis of JHS. In a study of 21 patients with JHS attending a genetics clinic in Italy, 87% of patients had GI symptoms, most commonly dyspepsia (67%), gastroesophageal reflux (57%), recurrent abdominal pain (62%), alternating constipation and diarrhea (33%), and abdominal hernias (5%).[31] Furthermore, the incidence of GI symptoms increased with age, and older patients with JHS were more likely to have GI symptoms than their younger counterparts.[20]

Another study showed not only that GI symptoms such as constipation, diarrhea, bloating, and swallowing problems were associated with JHS but that these GI symptoms were also associated with clusters of other extra-articular symptoms, particularly cognitive problems, insomnia, postural dizziness, and syncope,[31] which supported previous findings.[29] Furthermore, there was large heterogeneity in presentation and with cluster analysis it was shown that 2 main clusters of symptoms, and therefore patients, were present. Musculoskeletal symptoms were prominent in both clusters but GI symptoms were particularly prominent in the group that also had high levels

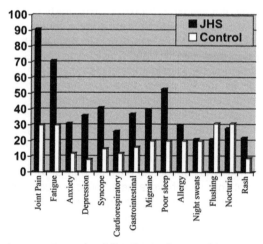

Fig. 2. Extra-articular symptoms in JHS. (*Data from* Hakim AJ, Grahame R. Non-musculoskeletal symptoms in joint hypermobility syndrome. Indirect evidence for autonomic dysfunction? Rheumatology (Oxford) 2004;43(9):1194–5; and *Reproduced from* Oxford University Press, with permission.)

of fatigue, cutaneous changes, and orthostatic, immune, urogynecologic, visual, and respiratory problems.[32]

Thus the association between GI symptoms and JHS in specialist hospital settings seems to be consistent. Furthermore, there seems to be clustering of JHS and GI symptoms with several other symptoms, including musculoskeletal pain, fatigue, autonomic symptoms, and urologic symptoms, to varying degrees.

From a gastroenterology point of view, GI symptoms can be caused by organic disorders or FGID, the latter referring to disorders whereby symptoms arise in the absence of demonstrable changes on conventional testing (eg, irritable bowel syndrome [IBS]). There is literature, albeit limited, that associates JHS with both types of disorder.

JHS and Organic GI Disorders

Only 2 published studies exist that show a possible association between hypermobility and organic disorders. The first compared 69 patients with IBD with 67 age-matched and sex-matched controls. A significantly higher prevalence of JH was found in patients with Crohn's disease (70%) compared with controls (25%) and with patients with ulcerative colitis (36%),[33] suggesting a possible association between JH and Crohn's disease, although this has not yet been replicated. In addition, only JH was assessed, so it is questionable whether the findings can be generalized to JHS.

The other study assessed 31 patients with JHS for celiac disease. Five (16%) had a confirmed diagnosis based on both serologic and histologic testing,[34] which was significantly higher than the estimated population prevalence (1%). However, the patients were a highly selected group, attending specialist genetics clinics, and so may not represent most patients with JHS, most of whom remain undiagnosed and do not present to clinics.

Hypermobility and FGID

The only direct evidence for an association between FGID and hypermobility comes from a single retrospective observational study in the tertiary gastroenterology setting.[11] In this study, the validated 5-point hypermobility questionnaire was used to screen for JH in 129 consecutive patients attending a neurogastroenterology clinic. The prevalence of JH in these patients was 49%, 3 times higher than the prevalence in healthy controls (17%). Those with JH were more likely to have GI symptoms without a known underlying structural, biochemical, metabolic, or autoimmune cause compared with those without JH (ie, the symptoms were more likely to be unexplained). A subgroup of these patients were assessed further by a rheumatologist and found to have JHS. These patients with JHS tended to have motility problems in their gut on physiologic testing, such as small bowel dysmotility, delayed gastric emptying, and delayed colonic transit. This study confirmed that, in a tertiary neurogastroenterology setting, JH was strongly associated with unexplained GI symptoms or FGID. It also showed that GI dysmotility is common in patients with GI symptoms and JHS, suggesting that these patients may have a neuromuscular basis for their symptoms. The cause of the dysmotility and the GI symptoms is as yet unknown but research is ongoing to determine whether this is a direct consequence of abnormal connective tissue in the gut, or of associated dysautonomia.

Although no large observational studies have been published that confirm an association between JHS and FGID, smaller studies have shown not only that IBS symptoms are common in JHS[30,31,35] but that patients with JHS with GI symptoms often have a preexisting diagnosis of IBS.[26,31]

Further support for the association between JHS and FGID comes from both disorders sharing several features, in particular an association with several medically unexplained disorders, also known as functional somatic syndromes (**Table 2**). There is speculation that the same underlying process, involving a combination of somatic hypersensitivity, chronic pain, and dysautonomia, underlies all the functional somatic syndromes and that JHS is the common link (**Fig. 3**).[36]

Management of JHS

A full consideration of the treatment of JHS and related conditions is outside the scope of this article and can be found elsewhere.[37,38] Physical therapies (in particular physiotherapy) has traditionally played the leading role in the rehabilitation of patients with JHS, although many patients question its benefit, whereas others attest to its counterproductive effects when inappropriately applied. It is only within the last couple of decades that pioneers in physiotherapy have studiously adapted the principles of physiotherapy to the needs of patients with lax and fragile tissues to good effect.[39] The important discovery that joint proprioception is significantly impaired in JHS, and that its correction by physiotherapeutic means is beneficial in terms that go beyond the locomotor system, has laid the foundations of an evidence-based approach to management.[40] As mentioned previously, the application of cognitive behavioral techniques to pain management plays an important role

Table 2
Similarities between JHS and FGID

	JHS	FGID
Demographics		
Population prevalence (%)	5–17	2.5–13
Gender	More common in women	More common in women
Age	Incidence decreases with age	Incidence decreases with age
Symptoms		
Chronic pain	Yes	Yes
Hypersensitivity	Somatic	Visceral
Diagnosis		
Validated biomarker	Yes	Yes
Criteria based diagnosis	Yes	Yes
Disease Associations		
Fibromyalgia[a]	Yes	Yes
Chronic fatigue syndrome[a]	Yes	Yes
Anxiety	Yes	Yes
Depression	Yes	Yes
Migraine[a]	Yes	Yes
Temporomandibular joint disorder[a]	Yes	Yes
Pelvic/bladder pain[a]	Yes	Yes
Insomnia	Yes	Yes
Allergies/atopy	Yes	Yes
Autonomic dysfunction	Yes	Yes

[a] Functional somatic syndromes.

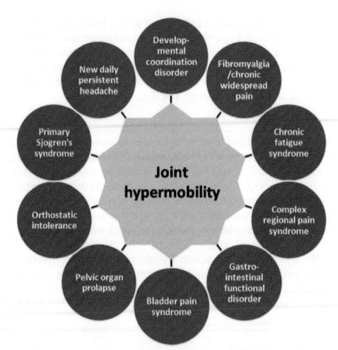

Fig. 3. Functional somatic syndromes. (*Reproduced from* Castori M, Celletti C, Camerota F. Ehlers-Danlos syndrome hypermobility type: a possible unifying concept for various functional somatic syndromes. Rheumatol Int 2013;33(3):819–21; with permission of Springer Science and Business Media.)

in enabling patients with secondary chronic pain to achieve an improved quality of life.[21]

REFERENCES

1. Beighton P, Solomon L, Soskolne CL. Articular mobility in an African population. Ann Rheum Dis 1973;32(5):413–8.
2. Hakim AJ, Grahame R. A simple questionnaire to detect hypermobility: an adjunct to the assessment of patients with diffuse musculoskeletal pain. Int J Clin Pract 2003;57(3):163–6.
3. Hakim AJ, Cherkas LF, Grahame R, et al. The genetic epidemiology of joint hypermobility: a population study of female twins. Arthritis Rheum 2004;50(8):2640–4.
4. Kirk JA, Ansell BM, Bywaters EG. The hypermobility syndrome. Musculoskeletal complaints associated with generalized joint hypermobility. Ann Rheum Dis 1967; 26(5):419–25.
5. Grahame R, Edwards JC, Pitcher D, et al. A clinical and echocardiographic study of patients with the hypermobility syndrome. Ann Rheum Dis 1981;40(6):541–6.
6. Al-Rawi ZS, Al-Rawi ZT. Joint hypermobility in women with genital prolapse. Lancet 1982;1(8287):1439–41.
7. Gazit Y, Nahir AM, Grahame R, et al. Dysautonomia in the joint hypermobility syndrome. Am J Med 2003;115(1):33–40.
8. Sacheti A, Szemere J, Bernstein B, et al. Chronic pain is a manifestation of the Ehlers-Danlos syndrome. J Pain Symptom Manage 1997;14(2):88–93.

9. Grahame R. Pain, distress and joint hyperlaxity. Joint Bone Spine 2000;67(3): 157–63.

10. Mathias CJ, Lowe DA, Iodice V, et al. Postural tachycardia syndrome–current experience and concepts. Nat Rev Neurol 2011;8(1):22–34.

11. Zarate N, Farmer AD, Grahame R, et al. Unexplained gastrointestinal symptoms and joint hypermobility: is connective tissue the missing link? Neurogastroenterol Motil 2010;22:252.e78.

12. Grahame R, Bird HA, Child A, et al. The revised (Brighton 1998) criteria for the diagnosis of benign joint hypermobility syndrome (BJHS). J Rheumatol 2000; 27(7):1777–9.

13. De Paepe A, Devereux RB, Dietz HC, et al. Revised diagnostic criteria for the Marfan syndrome. Am J Med Genet 1996;62(4):417–26.

14. Beighton P, De Paepe A, Steinmann B, et al. Ehlers-Danlos syndromes: revised nosology, Villefranche, 1997. Ehlers-Danlos National Foundation (USA) and Ehlers-Danlos Support Group (UK). Am J Med Genet 1998;77(1):31–7.

15. Grahame R, Hakim AJ. Arachnodactyly - a key to diagnosing heritable disorders of connective tissue. Nat Rev Rheumatol 2013. [Epub ahead of print].

16. Grahame R, Hakim AJ. Joint hypermobility syndrome is highly prevalent in general rheumatology clinics, its occurrence and clinical presentation being gender, age and race-related [abstract]. Ann Rheum Dis 2006;65(Suppl 2):263.

17. Bravo JF, Wolff C. Clinical study of hereditary disorders of connective tissues in a Chilean population: joint hypermobility syndrome and vascular Ehlers-Danlos syndrome. Arthritis Rheum 2006;54(2):515–23.

18. Baeza-Velasco C, Gely-Nargeot MC, Vilarrasa AB, et al. Association between psychopathological factors and joint hypermobility syndrome in a group of undergraduates from a French university. Int J Psychiatry Med 2011;41(2):187–201.

19. Grahame R. Hypermobility: an important but often neglected area within rheumatology. Nat Clin Pract Rheumatol 2008;4(10):522–4.

20. Castori M, Sperduti I, Celletti C, et al. Symptom and joint mobility progression in the joint hypermobility syndrome (Ehlers-Danlos syndrome, hypermobility type). Clin Exp Rheumatol 2011;29(6):998–1005.

21. Daniel HC. Pain management and cognitive behavioural therapy. In: Hakim AJ, Keer R, Grahame R, editors. Hypermobility, fibromyalgia and chronic pain. Oxford (England): Elsevier; 2010. p. 125–42.

22. Ross J, Grahame R. Joint hypermobility syndrome. BMJ 2011;342:c7167.

23. Grahame R. Joint hypermobility syndrome pain. Curr Pain Headache Rep 2009; 13(6):427–33.

24. Al-Rawi ZS, Al-Dubaikel KY, Al-Sikafi H. Joint mobility in people with hiatus hernia. Rheumatology (Oxford) 2004;43(5):574–6.

25. Mohammed PJ, Lunniss N, Zarate N. Joint hypermobility and rectal evacuatory dysfunction: an etiological link in abnormal connective tissue? Neurogastroenterol Motil 2010;22(10):1085.e283.

26. Manning J, Korda A, Benness C, et al. The association of obstructive defecation, lower urinary tract dysfunction and the benign joint hypermobility syndrome: a case-control study. Int Urogynecol J Pelvic Floor Dysfunct 2003; 14(2):128–32.

27. Lindor NM, Bristow J. Tenascin-X deficiency in autosomal recessive Ehlers-Danlos syndrome. Am J Med Genet A 2005;135(1):75–80.

28. Reinstein E, Pimentel M, Pariani M, et al. Visceroptosis of the bowel in the hypermobility type of Ehlers-Danlos Syndrome: presentation of a rare manifestation and review of the literature. Eur J Med Genet 2012;55:548–51.

29. Reilly DJ, Chase JW, Hutson JM, et al. Connective tissue disorder–a new sub-group of boys with slow transit constipation? J Pediatr Surg 2008;43(6):1111–4.

30. Hakim AJ, Grahame R. Non-musculoskeletal symptoms in joint hypermobility syndrome. Indirect evidence for autonomic dysfunction? Rheumatology (Oxford) 2004;43(9):1194–5.

31. Castori M, Camerota F, Celletti C, et al. Natural history and manifestations of the hypermobility type Ehlers-Danlos syndrome: a pilot study on 21 patients. Am J Med Genet A 2010;152A(3):556–64.

32. De Wandele I, Rombaut L, Malfait F, et al. Clinical heterogeneity in patients with the hypermobility type of Ehlers-Danlos Syndrome. Res Dev Disabil 2013;34(3): 873–81.

33. Vounotrypidis P, Efremidou E, Zezos P, et al. Prevalence of joint hypermobility and patterns of articular manifestations in patients with inflammatory bowel disease. Gastroenterol Res Pract 2009;2009:924138.

34. Danese C, Castori M, Celletti C, et al. Screening for celiac disease in the joint hypermobility syndrome/Ehlers-Danlos syndrome hypermobility type. Am J Med Genet A 2011;155A(9):2314–6.

35. Rombaut L, Malfait F, De Wandele I, et al. Medication, surgery, and physiotherapy among patients with the hypermobility type of Ehlers-Danlos syndrome. Arch Phys Med Rehabil 2011;92(7):1106–12.

36. Castori M, Celletti C, Camerota F. Ehlers-Danlos syndrome hypermobility type: a possible unifying concept for various functional somatic syndromes. Rheumatol Int 2013;33(3):819–21.

37. Keer R, Grahame R. Hypermobility syndrome: recognition and management for physiotherapists. 1st edition. Edinburgh, London, New York, Oxford (United Kingdom), Philadelphia, St Louis (MO), Sydney (Australia), Toronto: Butterworth Heinemann; 2003.

38. Hakim A, Keer R, Grahame R. Hypermobility, fibromyalgia and chronic pain. 1st edition. Edinburgh, London, New York, Philadelphia, St Louis (MO), Sydney (Australia), Toronto: Churchill Livingstone Elsevier; 2010.

39. Keer R, Simmonds J. Joint protection and physical rehabilitation of the adult with hypermobility syndrome. Curr Opin Rheumatol 2010;23(2):131–6.

40. Ferrell WR, Tennant N, Sturrock RD, et al. Amelioration of symptoms by enhancement of proprioception in patients with joint hypermobility syndrome. Arthritis Rheum 2004;50(10):3323–8.

Mucopolysaccharidoses and Other Lysosomal Storage Diseases

Christina Lampe, MD[a],*, Cinzia Maria Bellettato, PhD[b],
Nesrin Karabul, MD[a], Maurizio Scarpa, MD, PhD[b]

KEYWORDS

- Lysosomal storage diseases • Mucopolysaccharidosis • Joint stiffness
- Joint contractures • Dysostosis multiplex • Carpal tunnel syndrome • Hip dysplasia

KEY POINTS

- Lysosomal storage diseases (LSDs) are rare multisystemic and progressive genetic metabolic diseases, which present a wide heterogeneity and a clinical spectrum from severe to very attenuated.
- Typical musculoskeletal signs and symptoms of LSDs are bone abnormalities, osteopenia, osteonecrosis, secondary osteoarthritis, hip dysplasia, carpal tunnel in childhood, bone pain, and neuropathic pain.
- Key features, particularly in mucopolysaccharidosis (MPS), include joint pain, stiffness, and contractures in absence of inflammation.
- Therapies that address the causes of several LSDs (eg, Fabry disease, Gaucher disease, Pompe disease, and several forms of MPS) and slow disease progression are under clinical investigation or are commercially available.
- Diagnosis in attenuated affected LSD patients is often delayed. Timely diagnosis and early treatment lead to improve patient quality of life.

RARE DISEASES

In the United States, disorders with a prevalence of less than 200,000 persons are considered rare. It is estimated that in the United States, the rare disorders list comprises more than 6800 distinct rare diseases—commonly life-threatening or

Funding Sources: None.
Conflict of Interest: C. Lampe and N. Karabul received unrestricted research grants from Biomarin, Shire, and Genzyme. M. Scarpa received unrestricted research grants from Biomarin, Shire, Genzyme, and Actelion. C.M. Bellettato has no conflicts of interest.
[a] Department of Pediatric and Adolescent Medicine, Villa Metabolica, University Medical Center of the Johannes Gutenberg, University of Mainz, Langenbeckstrasse 2, Mainz 55131, Germany;
[b] Department of Pediatrics, Brains for Brain Foundation, University of Padua, Via Giustiniani 3, Padua 35128, Italy
* Corresponding author.
E-mail address: christina.lampe@unimedizin-mainz.de

chronically debilitating conditions—mostly inherited and affecting more than approximately 6% to 8% of the population.[1] These disorders affect 1 in 5000 children worldwide, 30% of whom die before the age of 5 years. Due to lack of knowledge and awareness of these diseases, diagnosis and treatment access are often delayed, when available.[2]

Although each single rare or orphan disease has little impact on society, in their sum they represent a burden not only for patients but also for their families, friends, caregivers, and society as a whole.

Many physicians think of LSDs as patients looking like gargoyles, dimly remembering long forgotten lessons in pediatrics and monochrome pictures in pediatric textbooks. This is far from truth. Given that the attenuated forms of LSDs have been recently recognized, it seems reasonable to presume that the clinical manifestations of these diseases represent a continuum from the most severely affected patients to individuals with nearly normal appearance and subclinical disease course not seeking medical advice. One focus of research should be the identification of the attenuated patients, thereby preventing medical odysseys and initiating appropriate therapy, even if only supportive.

LYSOSOMAL STORAGE DISEASES

LSDs are a heterogeneous group of more than 50 inherited metabolic disorders characterized by the absence or deficiency of one or more functional lysosomal enzymes responsible for the degradation and recycling of macromolecules.[3] As a consequence, undegraded or partially degraded macromolecules (proteins, polysaccharides, lipids, and so forth) accumulate progressively in the lysosomes of various tissues, activating a variety of pathogenetic cascades that lead to a systemic dysfunction of cells, tissues, and organs.[4] The lysosome is a complex and actively interacting intracellular organelle involved in phagocytosis, autophagy, exocytosis, receptor recycling and regulation, intracellular signaling, immunity, pigmentation, and bone biology. Accumulation of lysosomal storage material not only alters its functionality but also has an impact on the whole cell function.[5] The resulting dysfunction causes a multisystemic progressive physical and/or neurologic deterioration and, if not promptly diagnosed and treated, even death.[6–9] Generally, LSDs present a variable phenotypic expression, depending on the specific accumulated macromolecule, the site of production and degradation of the specific metabolites, the residual enzymatic expression, and the general genetic background of a patient.[10] All LSDs show a wide spectrum of heterogeneity, without a clear correlation between phenotype and genotype or course of the disease and the residual enzyme activity, when present.

The severity is correlated with the onset of the disease: the later the onset of symptoms, the more attenuated the phenotype of the disease. In general, 3 phenotypes are recognized: severe (mostly infantile), intermediate, and attenuated (mostly juvenile or adult). Such classification is sometimes useful, although such imposed distinctions are artificial, because often the early-onset and late-onset forms overlap. Early diagnosis has implications for patient quality of life; therapies for some of these disorders exist today and, if promptly used, these treatments can slow disease progression and increase life expectancy.

Some therapies also influence the pathologic process of neurodegeneration (hematopoietic stem cell transplantation [HSCT]). It is of paramount importance to diagnose these conditions as soon as possible. Unfortunately, some patients suffering from LSDs, in particular those with milder forms, have not been diagnosed in childhood and often seek rheumatologists without diagnosis.

COMMON FEATURES OF LYSOSOMAL STORAGE DISEASES

Although LSDs are characterized typically by a progressive and deteriorating course of neurodegenerative symptoms, there are various LDSs or disease subtypes without involvement of the central nervous system (CNS).

Somatic symptoms are hepatosplenomegaly, coarse facial features, and involvement of the skin, heart, eye, lung, and musculoskeletal system.[11] Musculoskeletal manifestations are, in early stages, commonly the reason why patients seek a physician's attention. For this reason, rheumatologists play an important role in timely diagnosis of LSDs: this group of diseases should be considered in the presence of bone abnormalities, osteopenia, osteonecrosis, secondary osteoarthritis or hip dysplasia, unexplained joint stiffness or contractures, bone pain, or burning neuropathic pain. These symptoms should alert a LSD to a rheumatologist, in particular when occurring in clusters or when suggesting a multisystemic nature. Unfortunately, these symptoms are not specific, and clinical presentation of LSDs can mimic rheumatologic conditions, such as rheumatoid arthritis or juvenile idiopathic arthritis, rheumatic fever, fibromyalgia/chronic fatigue syndrome, Raynaud disease, lupus erythematosus, and growth pain.

A rheumatologist's suspicion and diagnosis of LSDs is important, in particular with regard to LSDs, such as Gaucher disease, Fabry disease, Pompe disease, and MPSs, that are now treatable with, for example, enzyme replacement therapy (ERT) or HSCT.[12]

This review aims to illustrate the most recent signs and symptoms of LSDs manifestation, focusing on musculoskeletal involvement, that may lead to its clinical suspicion and an early diagnosis.

MUCOPOLYSACCHARIDOSES

MPSs are a heterogeneous group of LSDs, with a global incidence of 1:25,000,[13] caused by a deficit of lysosomal enzymes necessary to catalyze the stepwise degradation of mucopolysaccharides. The mucopolysaccharides, commonly called glycosaminoglycans (GAGs), are composed of long disaccharide chains. When linked to proteins, GAGs are called proteoglycans and are the essential part of the extracellular matrix. So far, 11 enzyme deficiencies, comprising 7 types of MPSs, have been identified (I, II, III, IV, VI, VII, and IX). Although the precise underlying pathophysiologic mechanisms are not completely understood yet,[14] recent data emphasize the concept that primary GAG storage alters cellular, tissue, and organ homeostasis, with consequent modification of complex cellular pathways, which induce secondary effects that play an important role as effectors of disease symptoms and progression.[15]

Except for MPS II (Hunter syndrome), which is an X-linked disease and in general affects boys and men (but some affected girls and women are described), all MPSs follow an autosomal recessive inheritance. In any type of MPS, the affected gene is clearly defined, but mutations leading to loss of function are multiple.

Common features of MPS in its most typical expression are dwarfism, short neck, coarse face, hepatosplenomegaly, corneal clouding, macroglossia, recurrent infections of ears and upper airways, hernias, cardiac and pulmonary involvement, thoracolumbar kyphoscoliosis, claw hands, joint stiffness and contractures, dysostosis multiplex, and, in some types, neurocognitive impairment, but symptoms depend on the specific type of stored GAGs.

Special symptoms of some types of MPS include the following: in MPS III patients, rapidly progressive dementia, sleep disturbance, and hyperactivity; MPS IV patients exhibit hypermobility of all joints but, in the authors' experience, mild stiffness of both shoulders; and corneal clouding occurs mainly in MPS I and MPS VI and more rarely in other MPS subtypes.

As discussed previously, disease severity in each MPS type varies from a grade of very severe phenotype, with fast progressive clinical course and multisystemic organ involvement, to a more attenuated grade, mainly affecting the musculoskeletal apparatus, with characteristic problems consisting of joint stiffness and joint pain (**Box 1, Table 1**).

PATHOGENETIC MECHANISMS RESPONSIBLE FOR MUSCULOSKELETAL SYMPTOMS IN MUCOPOLYSACCHARIDOSES

As discussed previously, primary GAG storages gives rise to a series of related secondary and complex pathogenetic cascades.[2,14,16,17]

Regarding the wide range of differences in severity of symptomatology and progression concerning joint mobility and functionality, the underlying pathologic mechanism is similar among the different types of MPSs and involves (1) the articular cartilage, (2) the surrounding connective tissue, and (3) the primary bone development.[15,18]

Typically, the joint involvement is characterized by absence of evident clinical signs of inflammation,[19] but animal model studies in MPSs I, II, VI, and VII have shown that there is local, intracellular inflammation caused by dermatan sulfate storage. Due to its structural similarity to lipopolysaccharide, dermatan sulfate is also activating the Toll-like receptor 4 signaling pathway. Dermatan sulfate storage results in stimulation of intracellular inflammation and alteration of growth of connective tissue and other cells.[20] Furthermore, this activation of inflammation causes production and release of several inflammatory cytokines, chemokines, proteases (such as tumor necrosis factor α, interleukin 1b, and macrophage inflammatory protein 1a), and nitric oxide that induce production of the proapoptotic lipid ceramide and, consequently, cartilage apoptosis, synovial hyperplasia, recruitment of macrophages, poorly organized and abnormal connective tissue matrices, and, finally, inflammatory joint destruction.[21] Thus, although not clinically evident, inflammation plays a pivotal role, particularly in MPSs I, II, III, VI, and VII,[15] which present progressive and diffuse joint stiffness and joint contractures and eventually destructive joint disease.[22]

Studies of growth plate and bone tissues from various MPS animal models showed that chondrocyte maturation, mineralization, and osteoblast differentiation were altered with consequent disordered bone architecture. In particular, it was shown that GAG storage inhibits the collagenolytic activity of cathepsin K with consequent impairment of the cartilage/bone resorption and chondrocyte apoptosis, leading to a high turnover and abnormal matrix homeostasis.[23] Summarizing, Toll-like receptor 4 signal pathways, together with inflammation and altered collagenase activity of cathepsin K, play a crucial role in the pathogenesis of the musculoskeletal symptoms of the MPSs.

MUSCULOSKELETAL SYMPTOMS OF MUCOPOLYSACCHARIDOSES

Because bone and joint manifestations and skeletal abnormalities are early and prominent features of MPSs, even in attenuated and mild affected patients, rheumatologists or orthopedists play a key role in disease recognition and timely diagnosis.[24,25] Severe forms of the disease commonly manifest with early and impressive symptoms affecting several organ systems at once and often also with significant cognitive impairment. In contrast, in an attenuated course of disease, patients do not present specific symptoms but more general manifestations, such as pain, stiffness, and contractures of joints, as well as hip and back pain, which overlap with other conditions, leading to misdiagnosis and remain undiagnosed for years.[26,27] The progressive joint disease in the absence of inflammation is a key element for detecting attenuated or slowly progressing forms of MPSs.[19] Furthermore, there is a significantly strong

Box 1
Mucopolysaccharidoses

- Heterogeneous group of genetically inherited diseases known as LSDs
- Eleven known lysosomal enzyme deficiencies embrace 7 different clinical MPS subtypes
- Highly variable clinical manifestations
- Rare (collective MPS incidence is 1/25,000 live births)

Pathogenesis

Accumulation of undegraded GAGs in lysosomes

Signs and symptoms

1. Appearance
   a. (Disproportioned) dwarfism
   b. Coarse facial features (eg, hypertelorism and flat nose)
   c. Short neck
   d. Hirsutism
2. Respiratory
   a. Upper airway obstruction
   b. Obstructive sleep apnea
   c. Restrictive lung disease
   d. Frequent airway infections
   e. Tracheal stenosis or tracheomalacia
3. Musculoskeletal
   a. Dysostosis multiplex
   b. Degenerative bilateral hip dysplasia
   c. Thoracolumbar kyphosis or kyphoscoliosis (gibbus)
   d. Joint contractures and stiffness
   e. Coxa and genua valga deformities
   f. Claw hands
   g. Hypermobility of joints (MPS IV)
4. Cardiac
   a. Cardiomyopathy
   b. Stenosis or insufficiency of heart valves
   c. Coronary artery disease
5. Gastrointestinal
   a. Hepatosplenomegaly
   b. Umbilical and inguinal hernia
   c. Swallowing problems
   d. Diarrhea, drooling
6. Peripheral nervous system
   a. Peripheral nerve entrapment (eg, carpal tunnel syndrome [CTS])

7. CNS
   a. Hydrocephalus
   b. Atlantoaxial instability
   c. Cervical cord compression
   d. Myelopathy
   e. Seizures
   f. Behavior problems (hyperactivity)
   g. Sleep disturbance
   h. Progressive mental retardation (MPS I Hurler, MPS II severe, MPS III, and MPS VII)

8. Eyes
   a. Visual impairment
   b. Glaucoma
   c. Retinal dystrophy
   d. Corneal clouding (except MPS II)

9. Ears, nose, and throat
   a. Macroglossia
   b. Hearing loss
   c. Recurrent otitis media

10. Dental
    a. Dental enamel defects
    b. Caries
    c. Dental abscess

correlation between severity of the dysostosis and the phenotypic expression of the disease.[28] The characteristic musculoskeletal alterations are summarized in **Box 2**.

The main features helpful for identifying patients with MPS are discussed.

Dysostosis Multiplex

As a clinical hallmark, the term, *dysostosis multiplex*, refers to the radiographic bone changes manifesting through short stature and progressive skeletal deformation, which are seen in some storage disorders (eg, mucolipidosis [ML]) and almost all different types of MPS with the exception of MPS III.[29]

Because some inflammatory and or primary degenerative joint diseases may mimic some of these findings, it is important to verify the origins of the radiographic findings and take into consideration the commonly symmetric and diffuse changes that are typical of MPS patients.[30] Moreover, the probability that a patient is affected by an MPS disorder correlates with the number of skeletal alterations; therefore, in presence of suspicious radiologic symptoms, it is important to perform more clinical investigations and send patients to a metabolic disease specialist.[28]

Typically, bony changes involve the skull, ribs and thorax, pelvis, hips, hands, long bones, vertebrae, and spine and lead to defects in bone formation and turnover (see **Box 2, Fig. 1**).[30,31]

Table 1
Enzyme defects and excretion products of mucopolysaccharidoses

Disorder	Eponym	Enzyme Deficiency	GAGs Excreted	CNS Involvement
MPS I	Hurler/Scheie	α-L-Iduronidase	DS/HS	Hurler + Hurler-Scheie ± Scheie −
MPS II	Hunter	Iduronate 2-sulfatase	DS/HS	Severe form + Attenuated form −
MPS III A	Sanfilippo A	Heparan N-sulfatase	HS	+
MPS III B	Sanfilippo B	N-acetyl-α-D-glucosaminidase	HS	+
MPS III C	Sanfilippo C	Acetyl-CoA: α-glucosaminide N-acetyltransferase	HS	+
MPS III D	Sanfilippo D	N-acetylglucosamine-6-sulfatase	HS	+
MPS IV A	Morquio A	Galactosamine-6-sulfatase	KS/CS	−
MPS IV B	Morquio B	β-Galactosidase	KS	−
MPS VI	Maroteaux-Lamy	Arylsulfatase B	DS	−
MPS VII	Sly	β-Glucuronidase	DS/HS/C6S	+
MPS IX	Hyaluronidase deficiency	Hyaluronidase	None	± (2 Families described)

Abbreviations: C6S, chondroitin sulfate; DS, dermatan sulfate; HS, heparan sulfate; KS, keratan sulfate.

The presence of any of the following red flag symptoms should warrant further investigation:

- Dysostosis multiplex in the skull: thickened diploic space and anomalous J-shaped sella turcica, which is a distinctive but not diagnostic feature of MPS disorders[28]
- Dysostosis multiplex in the thorax: paddle-shaped (oar-shaped) ribs, which are anteriorly enlarged and posteriorly narrowed; furthermore, the presence of shortened, often thickened, clavicles[28]
- Dysostosis multiplex in the spine: multiple superiorly notched (inferiorly beaked) vertebrae, often posterior scalloping at the thoracolumbar level. Typically, in MPS IV (Morquio syndrome), vertebral bodies at the thoracolumbar junction are more middle-beaked.[28]
- Dysostosis multiplex in the pelvis and hips: rounded iliac wings and inferiorly tapered ilia that inferiorly slope down to embrace the acetabular roof region and merge into it; furthermore, a double wall in the lower lateral portion of the ilium[28]
- Dysostosis multiplex in the long bones: mildly hypoplastic epiphyses but hypoplastic, dysplastic, or fragmented capital femoral heads or long and narrow femoral necks that can be eroded on both the lateral and the medial sides, proximal humeral notching, hypoplastic distal ulnae, and thickened short diaphyses[28]
- Dysostosis multiplex in the distal extremities (hands, knee, and feet): thick and short metacarpals and metatarsals, which can be proximally pointed

Hypoplastic carpal and/or tarsal bones of irregular shape are very common.

Box 2
Musculoskeletal manifestations of mucopolysaccharidoses

- Spine
  - Physiologic kyphosis of the spine
  - Platyspondyly (flattened vertebral bodies)
  - Thoracolumbar kyphosis
  - Hypoplastic odontoid process
  - Cervical myelopathy
  - Lumbar radiculopathy
  - Late degenerative arthritis
- Upper limbs
  - Stiffness of shoulder, elbow, and wrist
  - Claw hands
  - Shortness of phalanges
  - Contractures of fingers (in particular, distal parts)
  - Trigger finger deformity
  - CTS
  - Ulnar deviation of the hand
- Lower limbs
  - Flared pelvis
  - Hip dysplasia
  - Valgus knee and ankle (coxa valga)
  - Flat foot
  - Late degenerative arthritis

Growth Abnormalities

Patients with MPS are born with normal body length and weight but during growth fall below the 50th percentile up to less than the 3rd percentile. Attenuated patients, although they can still be characterized by lower stature, may also reach normal height.

Skeletal abnormalities in MPS patients (eg, kyphoscoliosis and genua valga) were initially proposed as the responsible factor in limiting growth and adult height, but it is now known that short stature features in MPS patients can be found even in the absence of severe abnormal spine curvatures or genu valgum.

Growth abnormalities might be related to GAG deposition in the growth plate consequent to disturbed endochondrial ossification that leads to a disproportional short stature. Short stature, however, can also be a secondary consequence of a permutation of structural, metabolic, and, in some cases, endocrine abnormalities.[32] Typically in the MPS forms, the axial growth is more affected than the appendicular growth and, as a consequence, generally, MPS patients are characterized by shortening of the trunk with a mild shortening of the limbs.[12] In the attenuated MPS subtypes (eg, MPS I [Scheie syndrome]), short stature is not necessarily a prominent feature, although the linear growth is usually below the target height.[33]

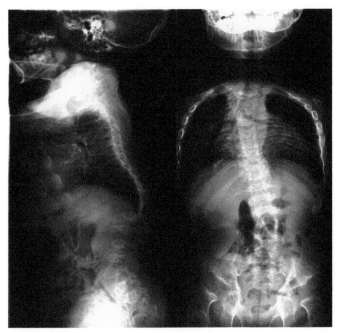

Fig. 1. Dysostosis multiplex in a 12-year-old patient with MPS IV (Morquio syndrome).

Many factors can have an impact on children's growth, such as poor nutrition, insufficient growth or thyroid hormones, abnormal bone metabolism, chronic disease, and social isolation, but growth abnormalities may also represent clinical signs of MPS and, therefore, MPS should be considered for differential diagnosis in children evaluated for short stature.[32]

Joint Stiffness and Contractures

Joint stiffness is a hallmark of almost all the MPS forms (only MPS IV and MPS IX do not present this manifestation),[12] probably due to storage of GAGs in the ligaments, tendons, and joint capsules and other soft tissues that along with epiphyseal and metaphyseal deformities give rise to defective skeletal remodeling.[34] Unfortunately, the majority of the people affected by the attenuated forms presenting stiffness or contractures of the joints are not promptly diagnosed because of the nonspecific and initially mild nature of these symptoms that physicians commonly attribute to more common diseases, such as juvenile idiopathic arthritis or rheumatoid arthritis (**Fig. 2**).[12,26] A main differential feature is the absence of typical signs of inflammation, such as redness, warmth, and tenderness, associated with joint stiffness. Moreover, systemic signs of inflammation, such as fever and/or elevated laboratory markers of inflammation (erythrocyte sedimentation rate, C-reactive protein, and white blood cell count), are not present, and autoimmune markers (rheumatoid factor and antinuclear antibodies) are not suggestive of a rheumatic disease, although their diagnostic utility is limited.[19] Another difference is that, compared with what happens in the case of inflammatory arthritis, in cases of MPSs, stiffness typically is not greater in the morning or intensified after a long period of rest and is not relieved by heat, gentle exercise, or assumption of steroids or anti-inflammatory drugs. Restricted joint mobility, although diffuse, preferentially involves the shoulders and distal interphalangeal joints

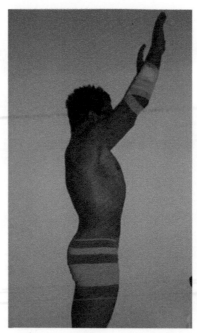

Fig. 2. Restricted shoulder mobility in a 30-year-old patient with MPS VI (Maroteaux-Lamy syndrome).

of the hands, giving rise to the characteristic claw hand deformities and impaired hand function. Joint swelling may occur along with joint stiffness and characteristically it is not due to synovial effusion but is consequent to the bony enlargement.[12]

Carpal Tunnel Syndrome

CTS is one of the most reported compressive neuropathy of the upper extremity of adults but it is rarely seen in children, and its clinical presentation in childhood is not the same as in adulthood. When present in children, it is strongly suggestive of LSDs (MPS and ML), which sometimes is the first sign of the disease.[35] CTS has been detected in the 58% of MPS-affected children.[36]

CTS is a common hallmark of the different MPSs group,[25] in which the compression of the nerve is consequent to the thickening of the flexor retinaculum and the tissues around the nerve sheaths.[37] It is essential to quickly recognize CTS in these children to prevent irreversible median nerve damage.[38] Unfortunately, in these cases, diagnosis is not a simple matter, considering patients' verbal and cognitive limitations; numbness and pain are often not referred symptoms[39] and can be masked by other features of the disease, such as joint stiffness and contractures. It is, therefore, difficult to perform and interpret appropriate neurophysiologic investigations.[40] Some clue manifestations are thenar hypotrophy and lack of thumb opposition and abduction, together with increased difficulties with fine motor skills and manual clumsiness (**Fig. 3**).[41]

Trigger finger, also known as stenosing tenosynovitis, together with CTS, is the entity more frequently found in MPS patients. Generally, this complication is caused by GAG deposits in the capsular tissues of joints or flexor tendons but can also be related to difficulties in fine motor abilities.[42]

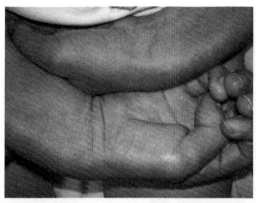

Fig. 3. Thenar atrophy in a 12-year-old patient with MPS II (Hunter syndrome).

Arm/hand and Leg/foot Abnormalities

Patients affected by MPSs share the common feature of presenting hand and foot deformities. These can be the consequence of the conditions discussed previously and result in GAG deposition, causing a typical thickening of the phalanges, which generally are proximally pointed and in some cases associated with oblique deformity of the distal terminal ends of the radius and ulna. Claw hand and the presence of thickened subcutaneous tissues on the hands, responsible for impaired ability of the fingers and CTS, are frequent findings. Hands are often short and broad with stubby fingers, especially in MPS I and MPS VI patients (**Fig. 4**).[43]

Coxa valga and genua valga deformities are further typical and frequent manifestations, which lead to immobility and pain (**Fig. 5**).[44]

Joint Hypermobility in Mucopolysaccharidoses IV

Joint hypermobility consists of the capacity to move limbs into unusual positions that are commonly impossible for the majority of people. It is the hallmark of the joint involvement in patients with MPS IV.[45] Hypermobility is a consequence of degradation of connective tissues around the joint, bones hypoplasia, and metaphyseal deformities. It is mainly characterized by distal joint hypermobility (eg, hand, wrist, knee, and ankle) in contrast to proximal joints stiffness.[46] As a consequence, patients manifest a very weak grip and progressive difficulties because these symptoms have an impact on their ability to conduct normal daily tasks, such as dressing, cooking, showering, and so forth (**Fig. 6**).

DIAGNOSIS

Clinical identification of MPS patients is not an easy task, and this is particularly true for patients with more attenuated forms of MPS. It was demonstrated that, for example, that the attenuated form of MPS I was recognized in less than 20% of cases.[19] As a consequence, patients commonly experience significant diagnostic delays. Because appropriate treatments for many of these conditions now exist, there is an imperative need to diagnose and recognize affected patients as soon as possible to stop the disease progression and prevent the occurrence of irreversible damages.[47]

A diagnostic algorithm for rheumatologic evaluation of joint and bone involvement has recently been proposed.[47] The algorithm underlines the importance of considering MPS diagnosis if the development of stiffness or contractures of joints is not followed

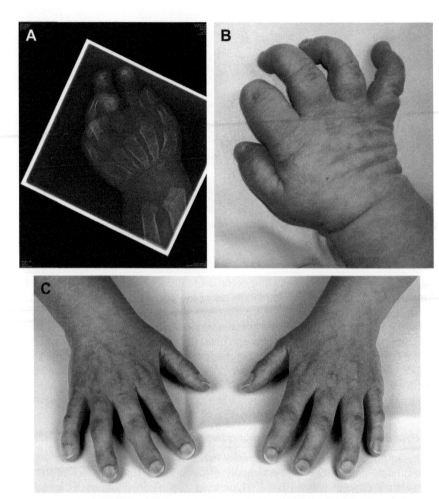

Fig. 4. Typical claw hands in an 18 year old with MPS VI (Maroteaux-Lamy syndrome); (*A*) Radiograph; (*B*) photograph; (*C*) hands of a mildly affected 36-year-old patient with MPS VI (Maroteaux-Lamy syndrome).

by concomitant signs of inflammation. Other red flag symptoms that could increase awareness of the necessity of consulting a geneticist or metabolic specialist are corneal clouding, frequent respiratory infections and gastrointestinal complaints, heart murmur, short stature, abnormal gait, hip dysplasia, and history of hernia repair.[47]

In general, the first step in diagnosis is the assessment of urinary GAG excretion, collected over 24 hours.[48] MPS patients show typically much higher urinary GAG levels compared with age-matched healthy subjects, but GAG excretion is age dependent (decrease by age) and can be of normal value in attenuated affected and adult MPS patients.

The gold standard of diagnosis is the demonstration of decreased enzyme activity in plasma, leukocytes, or fibroblasts. Although dried blood spot tests also provide clues for an MPS diagnosis, they are not available for all types of MPS and it is essential to confirm diagnosis by second enzyme measurement.[49] Genetic testing has a limited impact, however, on screening because of the wide genetic heterogeneity in all types

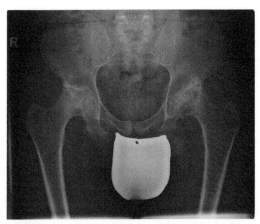

Fig. 5. Bilateral hip dysplasia/arthrosis in a 34 year old patient with MPS VI (Maroteaux-Lamy syndrome).

of MPSs; it should be performed not only in patients but also their parents to use for genetic counseling and prenatal diagnostics.[47]

Unfortunately, there is a lack of strict correlation between residual enzyme activity, genotype, and clinical phenotype, making the care of presymptomatic individuals more complicated.[50] Newborn screening also plays a role in reliable and prompt identification and classification of MPSs; however, technology requires some time before a routine application.[51,52]

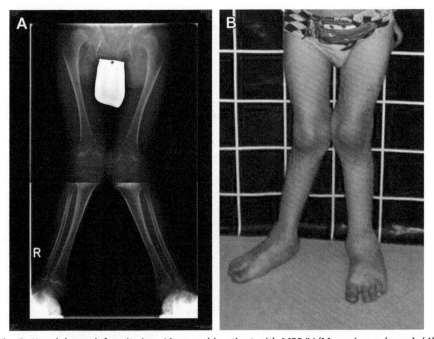

Fig. 6. Knock-knee deformity in a 10-year-old patient with MPS IV (Morquio syndrome). (*A*) Radiograph; (*B*) photograph.

Finally, diseases that present musculoskeletal features similar to MPSs should be taken into account (eg, multiple sulfatase deficiency, ML, fucosidosis, α-mannosidosis, and skeletal dysplasia of non-LSD origin).

Because diagnosis is tricky and might be difficult and confusing because of the rareness of the diseases and their differential diagnosis, the authors recommend referring any suspicious patient to a specialized center (**Box 3**).

TREATMENT

Because MPSs are progressive diseases characterized by complex pathophysiologic mechanisms and multisystemic deterioration, the disease may give rise to different symptoms and clinical manifestations, some of which are not easily reversible. For this reason, response to available therapies depends on the severity of the disease, phenotype, and degree of disease progression at treatment initiation.[53] Timely diagnosis and early treatment can improve the outcome. Besides supportive therapy and pain management for MPSs I, II, and VI (in clinical trials, MPS IV A and VII), effective but unfortunately not curative treatments, such as ERT, and, particularly for MPS I, HSCT, are available.[53–56]

Enzyme Replacement Therapy

The efficacy and safety of ERT with recombinant human enzyme is well accepted and confirmed by many clinical trials. Enzyme infusion, however, which is a life-long therapy, is administered intravenously once a week over approximately 4 hours and can be associated with immune reactions and thus could have a negative impact on disease management.[57] Nevertheless, the benefits include reduction of liver spleen size, improved endurance and shoulder mobility, improved respiration, and enhanced quality of life.

So far, ERT efficacy mainly consists of reducing the burden of peripheral diseases; enzymes capable of effectively targeting the bones, especially the CNS, are still to be developed.[58] There are ongoing clinical trials with intrathecal enzyme application in MPS I and MPS III A. ERT is available for MPSs I, II, and VI and in clinical trials in MPS IV A and MPS VII.

Hematopoietic Stem Cell Transplantation

When performed in patients under the age of 2 years and with a developmental quotient greater than or equal to 70%, HSCT is the gold standard treatment of MPS I patients. It was proved that HSCT may preserve cognitive function and extend life expectancy in severely affected MPS I pediatric patients[59] and is under investigation

---

Box 3
Diagnostics in mucopolysaccharidoses

1. Step: screening test	Urinary GAG excretion (pitfall: urinary GAG excretion can be in normal range in attenuated patients and in adults)
2. Step: gold standard	Enzyme measurement in leukocytes, plasma, heparin blood, or fibroblasts
3. Step: genetic testing as an additional diagnostic test and to facilitate prenatal testing and is mandator in x-linked diseases to detect carriers	Dried blood spot testing for MPSs I, II, and VI available
	Newborn screening under development
	Families at risk: prenatal testing (chorionic villi and amniocentesis) is available

for several other MPS disorders.[53] Considering the importance of quickly selecting the optimal treatment choice (ERT or HSCT) that is often related to the phenotypical severity of the disorder, a consensus scale for phenotypically classifying MPS I patients was developed to facilitate treatment decisions and patient communication.[60] Unfortunately, data from the international observational database, the MPS I Registry, underlines that diagnosis is still delayed and that it is necessary to increase awareness about MPS I signs and symptoms to shorten the time frame between first manifestations of the disease and treatment initiation.[61] It is important to emphasize that available treatments for MPSs, although offering benefit and delaying disease progression when initiated early, are not curative and have little impact on associated skeletal malformations and spinal cord compression at the craniocervical junction.[62]

Supportive Therapy and Observation of Disease Progression

The multisystemic course of MPSs requires a multidisciplinary team, at its best coordinated by an experienced metabolic physician. Patient disease progression should be observed by regular follow-up examinations at least annually. In addition to pain management, typical comorbidities often need surgical intervention, such as hernia repair, adenoidectomy or tympanostomy tube implantation, orthopedic surgeries (correction of skeletal changes), neurosurgical procedures (carpal tunnel release or craniocervical or thoracolumbar decompression), heart valve replacement, and corneal clouding. Because of the GAG accumulation in all tissues, anesthesia complications are much higher than in unaffected population; thus, every surgical intervention should be considered carefully.[63,64]

In particular, spinal cord compression at the craniocervical junction caused by thickening of the surrounding soft tissues and/or atlantoaxial instability should be recognized as a life-threatening complication.

Other specialists (eg, cardiologists; pulmologists; ophthalmologists; ear, nose, and throat physicians; physiotherapists; and psychologists) are essential for giving consideration to patients' needs and improving quality of life, including patients with types of MPSs for which no causal therapy is available.

OTHER LYSOSOMAL STORAGE DISEASES

Apart from MPSs, there are other LSDs that manifest with musculoskeletal symptoms. Because symptoms can mimic rheumatologic disorders, rheumatologists play a key role in diagnosis.

Fabry Disease

Fabry disease is an X-linked inherited disorder due to a deficiency of the enzyme α-galactosidase, resulting in accumulation of globotriaosylceramide and other sphingolipids within lysosomes of almost all cells and tissues, leading to a variability of progressive clinical signs and symptoms.[65] Although the disease is X-linked inherited, women are also affected with, in general, higher variability, a later onset of the disease, and a slower disease progression, but the disease course can also present as severe as in men. The frequency of concerned women can be as high as 60% to 70% of all women heterozygous for Fabry disease.[66]

In all probability, Fabry disease is underdiagnosed. Neonatal screening programs have shown a much higher birth prevalence than the estimated 0.21/100,000 to 0.85/100,000 derived from diagnostic laboratory data.[67]

Diagnosis is made by demonstrating enzyme deficiency in plasma or leukocytes (male patients) or by genotyping (female patients, where a false high enzyme activity might be registered).

Symptoms arise in a time-dependent manner: in children, pain, altered temperature sensitivity, and gastrointestinal symptoms (including abdominal pain) are the most prevalent manifestations.[68] The pain consists of burning and prickling in hands and feet (acroparesthesia), worsened by changes of temperature and emotional stress (**Fig. 7**).[69]

Pain crises caused by fever, fatigue, changes in temperature, and stress with excruciating pain intensity also are described. These features may lead to seeking a rheumatologist[69] and can be wrongly diagnosed as a rheumatic disease, such as juvenile rheumatoid arthritis or rheumatic fever.[12] Other prominent manifestations of neurologic involvement are hypohidrosis/hyperhidrosis, heat intolerance, and signs of autonomic involvement. Further common symptoms include angiokeratoma, corneal changes, and tinnitus or hearing loss.

Later in life, patients develop renal failure, stroke at young age, pulmonary symptoms, and cardiac involvement, all of which are life limiting. Osteopenia has also been reported as a frequent phenomenon[70,71] and, in single cases, avascular femur head necrosis. Prominent dysmorphic features are not part of the disease. Considering that presumably many patients suffer from Fabry disease without proper diagnosis, the life-threatening complications, in particular, the availability of a causal therapy, underline the importance of timely diagnosis and early initiation of treatment.

As discussed previously, treatment consists of ERT. The neuropathic pain is treated with antiepileptic drugs (carbamazepine or pregabalin) or antidepressants and with

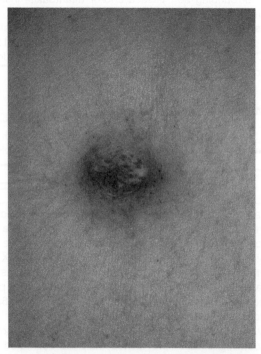

Fig. 7. Very discrete angioceratoma in a 27-year-old patient with Fabry disease.

avoidance of triggers. Guidelines for the management of neuropathic pain in Fabry disease have been published recently.[72]

A complete survey of all features of this disease is beyond the scope of this article; interested readers can find comprehensive information in 2 reviews by Zarate and Hopkin[65] and Germain.[67]

Gaucher Disease

Gaucher disease is one of the most common LSDs, caused by a defect in the GBA gene, leading to accumulation of glucocerebroside in macrophages of the tissue of multiple organs due to a defect of the lysosomal enzyme, β-glucocerebrosidase.[34] The most prevalent phenotype is Gaucher disease type 1 (approximately 94%),[73] which lacks serious involvement of the CNS. Despite type 1 sometimes referred to as adult type, most patients are diagnosed in the first 2 decades of life.[73] Gaucher type 2 and type 3 have a neuronopathic disease course (rapidly progressive in type 2 and more prolonged in type 3). This article focuses on Gaucher disease type 1.

Gaucher disease type 1 is characterized by multisystemic manifestations: progressive cytopenia, hepatosplenomegaly, and destructive bone disease, but, because there is a high phenotypic heterogeneity, especially among the non-neuronopathic form (type 1), affected children often are mainly asymptomatic or manifest general symptoms that do not immediately raise suspicion of a serious condition.[74] In a study of 887 children, 95% showed mild to severe splenomegaly, 87% hepatomegaly, 50% thrombocytopenia, and 40% anemia. Another finding was growth retardation (34%). Symptomatic involvement of the skeleton was found in 27% (bone pain) and 9% (bone crisis), but radiologic evidence of bone destruction was found in approximately 81%.[75]

The involvement of the skeletal system in children and adults consists of decreased bone mineral density,[76,77] bone marrow infiltration by macrophages, Erlenmeyer flask deformity of the tubular bones (mostly the femur), osteonecrosis, osteosclerosis, and pathologic fractures (**Fig. 8**).[78]

Bone pain is a common complaint of patients, with Gaucher disease not necessarily associated with pathologic radiologic findings; bone crisis is an important

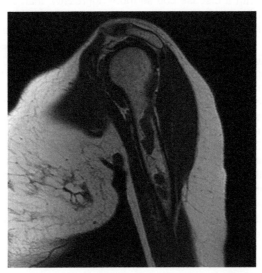

Fig. 8. Bone marrow infiltration of the humerus in a 42-year-old patient with Gaucher disease.

aspect of Gaucher disease, sometimes mimicking but not to be confused with acute osteomyelitis or sickle cell crisis.[78,79] Alarming arthritis-like symptoms, such as joint effusions, localized warmth and swelling, and pain that can be manifested with sub-chondral infiltration of Gaucher cells and further inflammatory tissue changes, also should be considered. Associate manifestations, such as leukocytosis, increased level of ESR, and fever, can sometime misleadingly lead a physician to consider juvenile idiopathic arthritis, rheumatoid arthritis, or rheumatic fever instead of an LSD.[80]

Another main radiologic feature that should induce physicians to suspect Gaucher disease is the presence of the characteristic Erlenmeyer flask deformities (present in approximately 46% of cases), mainly affecting the distal femur and proximal tibia.[12]

Osteopenia is a frequent phenomenon in Gaucher disease, affecting half of all pa-tients, with a peak prevalence in adolescence.[81]

Bone involvement is a hallmark feature in 70% to 100% of cases.[82] Recurrent infec-tions and delayed puberty are also often noted.[83–85]

There are other rheumatologic aspects of Gaucher disease. In a study of 109 patients with Gaucher disease, the diagnosis of fibromyalgia was made in 6 patients; the investigators state that they were not able to distinguish whether this was due to Gaucher disease and the patients' comorbidities or an independent finding but stress the importance of careful examination of trigger points and treatment of symptoms of fibromyalgia.[86] Patients with myopathy have also been reported[87] as anecdotal re-ports of single cases of uveitis.[88,89]

The importance of early diagnosis lies in the availability of ERT and substrate reduc-tion therapy.

Mucolipidosis II and III

Mucolipidosis (ML) II and ML III, in particular ML II, resemble MPS, which has led to the term, *pseudo-Hurler polydystrophy*, for ML III.

The diseases are allelic and caused by an autosomal recessive inherited defect in *N*-acetylglucosaminylphosphotransferase.[90] The clinical picture is a wide continuum, including patients with a disease course more aggressive than any MPS to almost healthy individuals,[91] with no more severe signs than bilateral hip dysplasia (mainly ML III) reported.[92] ML II indicates the more severe disease, manifesting in the neonatal period or infancy, whereas the first symptoms of ML III prevail in toddlers or even later[93]; thus, ML III may be mistaken for juvenile rheumatoid arthritis. There seems to be no clear distinction between ML II and ML III, so many patients show an interme-diate type of disease. In patients with ML II, suspicion of an underlying disease is at hand, due to classic dysmorphic features and delayed development, but patients with typical ML III may show normal speech and intellectual development and minimal dysmorphology and present mainly with pain and joint stiffness.[93]

The course of LSDs is determined by 2 parameters as many LSDs: type of the dis-ease and time. Patients with ML II show signs of neonatal hyperparathyroidism and patients with ML III an osteochondrodystrophy, which has many features in common with hyperparathyroidism but lacks elevated levels of parathormone.[92] In the later course of the disease, stiffness of joints (hips, shoulders, and phalangeal joints of the hands) and pain are predominating; CTS in childhood is also a common feature and should be taken as a red flag.

To make a long and maybe oversophisticated presented story short, ML II, ML III, and MPS have much in common (not only musculoskeletal symptoms but also, for example, corneal clouding) and cannot always be differentiated by clinical features.

Patients with ML IV do not exhibit signs or symptoms of rheumatologic disease.[94]

Although there is no basic treatment available for ML, supportive therapy leads to improved patient quality of life. In particular, life-threatening complications, such as spinal cord compression at the craniocervical junction, should be detected and have to be treated surgically.

Joint pain, possibly due to the osteochondrodystrophy, has been ameliorated by bisphosphonates[92,95] in case reports.

Farber Disease

Farber disease is a rare, autosomal recessive inherited disease. Seven subtypes with a wide variability are described. The main features consist of painful nodules, which are located near the joints, mostly at the interphalangeal joints, wrist, and elbow, and a characteristic hoarseness. Other manifestations are progressive neurologic deterioration, pneumonia, and hepatosplenomegaly, although subtypes 2 and 3 have no CNS involvement. The symptoms (ie, the painful nodules) start usually during the first year of life. These lipogranulomatous nodules lead to progressive destruction of the joints and stiffness[90,96] and might be misdiagnosed as juvenile rheumatoid arthritis. In cases of no CNS involvement, allogeneic HSCT has shown promising results in some patients: in 4 patients, the progression of the disease could be stopped and even function regained.[97]

Oligosaccharidoses

The oligosccharidoses are rare diseases. Although in most cases, the diagnosis of LSD is made before rheumatologic symptoms evolve, many patients suffering from mental retardation seeking medical advice for a problem seemingly not related to their underlying condition may receive no accurate diagnosis. Furthermore, their prevalence is higher in certain populations, for instance, in the population of southern Italy (fucosidosis)[98] and, as recently shown, in Cuba (fucosidosis and α-mannosidosis).[99] Diagnosis is made by measuring the enzyme activity in blood and concentration of oligosaccharides in urine.

The autosomal recessive inherited diseases, fucosidosis (decreased activity of α-fucosidase) and α-mannosidosis (decreased activity of acid α-mannosidase), share some aspects of MPS, especially mild dysostosis multiplex, recurrent infections, and organomegaly, but progressive neurologic impairment predominates.[100] In the largest overview of patients with fucosidosis, 48% of all patients suffered from joint contractures and 66% from kyphoscoliosis; mental retardation was found in 95%.[98] Patients with α-mannosidosis commonly exhibit, besides scoliosis and sternum deformity, genua valga, sometimes needing orthopedic correction[100]; in older patients, deforming and destructive arthropathy of large joints has been described.[101,102] Bone marrow transplantation in the first decade of life seems to promise some benefit in α-mannosidosis[100] and has been performed in fucosidosis.[103,104] Other oligsaccharidoses do not exhibit rheumatologic features.

SUMMARY

Accurate and timely diagnosis of LSDs may be difficult and demands high clinical suspicion, physical examination, and appropriate investigations. This is particularly true for patients with more attenuated phenotypes. In these cases, diagnosis is often missed or delayed. Because commonly, patients affected by LSDs seek rheumatologists' attention because their presenting symptoms mainly consist of pain, stiffness, and contractures of the joints; tendon alterations without inflammation; CTS; and hip dysplasia, rheumatologists play a key role and should be aware of the clinical

> **Box 4**
> **Rheumatologists' take-home message**
>
> - Think of MPS in any patient with
>   - Dysostosis multiplex
>   - CTS
>   - Bilateral hip dysplasia
>   - Joint stiffness or contractures, tendon alterations without inflammation

characteristics of LSDs that may vary largely between patients. In particular, they should know how to make a differential diagnosis for differentiating LSDs from the more common rheumatologic diseases, for example, inflammatory arthritis.

Special consideration should be given to musculoskeletal manifestations and related presence of extraskeletal abnormalities. Radiologic and molecular investigations facilitate the timely diagnosis and appropriate management of these patients. An interdisciplinary approach, which includes a collaborative consultation with metabolic specialists, clinical geneticists, and/or laboratory physicians, is fundamental for a definitive diagnosis (**Box 4**).

REFERENCES

1. National Institutes of Health, Office of Rare Disease Research, Rare Diseases and Related Terms. Available at: http://rarediseases.info.nih.gov/RareDiseaseList.aspx?PageID=1, ~http://rarediseases.info.nih.gov/RareDiseaseList.aspx?PageID=1/.
2. Vitner EB, Platt FM, Futerman AH. Common and uncommon pathogenic cascades in lysosomal storage diseases. J Biol Chem 2010;285:20423–7.
3. Wilcox WR. Lysosomal storage disorders: the need for better pediatric recognition and comprehensive care. J Pediatr 2004;144:S3–14.
4. Walkley SU. Pathogenic cascades in lysosomal disease: why so complex? J Inherit Metab Dis 2009;32:181–9.
5. Parkinson-Lawrence EJ, Shandala T, Prodoehl M, et al. Lysosomal storage disease: revealing lysosomal function and physiology. Physiology (Bethesda) 2010;25(2):102–15.
6. Ballabio A, Gieselmann V. Lysosomal disorders: from storage to cellular damage. Biochim Biophys Acta 2009;1793:684–96.
7. Wraith JE. Lysosomal disorders. Semin Neonatol 2002;7:75–83.
8. Futerman AH, van Meer G. The cell biology of lysosomal storage disorders. Nat Rev Mol Cell Biol 2004;5:554–65.
9. Vellodi A. Lysosomal storagedisorders. Br J Haematol 2005;128:413–31.
10. Filocamo M, Morrone A. Lysosomal storagedisorders: molecularbasis and laboratorytesting. Hum Genomics 2011;5(3):156–69.
11. Wenger DA, Coppola S, Liu SL. Insightsinto the diagnosis and treatment of lysosomal storagediseases. Arch Neurol 2003;60:322–8.
12. Aldenhoven M, Sakkers RJ, Boelens J, et al. Musculoskeletalmanifestations of lysosomal storagedisorders. Ann Rheum Dis 2009;68(11):1659–65.
13. Baehner F, Schmiedeskamp C, Krummenauer F, et al. Cumulative incidence rates of themucopolysaccharidoses in Germany. J Inherit Metab Dis 2005;28(6):1011–7.

14. Clarke LA. The mucopolysaccharidoses: a success of molecular medicine. Expert Rev Mol Med 2008;10:e1.
15. Clarke LA. Pathogenesis of skeletal and connective tissue involvement in the mucopolysaccharidoses: glycosaminoglycan storage is merely the instigator. Rheumatology (Oxford) 2011;50(Suppl 5):v13–8.
16. Coutinho MF, Lacerda L, Alves S. Glycosaminoglycan storage disorders: a review. Biochem Res Int 2012;2012:471325. http://dx.doi.org/10.1155/2012/471325.
17. Kloska A, Tylki-Szymańska A, Wegrzyn G. Mucopolysaccharidoses–biochemical mechanisms of diseases and therapeutic possibilities. Postepy Biochem 2011;57(2):133–47 [in Polish].
18. Guarany NR, Schwartz IV, Guarany FC, et al. Functional capacity evaluation of patients with mucopolysaccharidosis. J Pediatr Rehabil Med 2012;5(1):37–46.
19. Cimaz R, Coppa GV, Koné-Paut I, et al. Joint contractures in the absence of inflammation may indicate mucopolysaccharidosis. Pediatr Rheumatol Online J 2009;7:18.
20. Simonaro CM, D'Angelo M, He X, et al. Mechanism of glycosaminoglycan-mediated bone and joint disease: implications for the mucopolysaccharidoses and other connective tissue diseases. Am J Pathol 2008;172(1):112–22.
21. Simonaro CM, Ge Y, Eliyahu E, et al. Involvement of the Toll-like receptor 4 pathway and use of TNF-alpha antagonists for treatment of the mucopolysaccharidoses. Proc Natl Acad Sci U S A 2010;107(1):222–7.
22. Pastores G. Musculoskeletal complications encountered in the lysosomal storage disorders. Best Pract Res Clin Rheumatol 2008;22:937–47.
23. Wilson S, Hashamiyan S, Clarke L, et al. Glycosaminoglycan-mediated loss of cathepsin K collagenolytic activity in MPS I contributes to osteoclast and growth plate abnormalities. Am J Pathol 2009;175:2053–62.
24. Coppa GV. Why should rheumatologists be aware of the mucopolysaccharidoses? Rheumatology (Oxford) 2011;50(Suppl 5):v1–3.
25. White KK, Sousa T. Mucopolysaccharide disorders in orthopaedic surgery. J Am Acad Orthop Surg 2013;21(1):12–22.
26. Vijay S, Wraith JE. Clinical presentation and follow-up of patients with the attenuated phenotype of Mucopolysaccharidosis type I. Acta Paediatr 2005;94:872–7.
27. Lampe C. Attenuated mucopolysaccharidosis: are you missing this debilitating condition? Rheumatology (Oxford) 2012;51(3):401–2.
28. Lachman R, Martin KW, Castro S, et al. Radiologic and neuroradiologic findings in the mucopolysaccharidoses. J Pediatr Rehabil Med 2010;3(2):109–18.
29. Beck M, Muenzer J, Scarpa M. Evaluation of disease severity in mucopolysaccharidoses. J Pediatr Rehabil Med 2010;3(1):39–46.
30. Morishita K, Petty RE. Musculoskeletal manifestations of mucopolysaccharidoses. Rheumatology (Oxford) 2011;50(Suppl 5):v19–25.
31. Wraith JE. The clinical presentation of lysosomal storage disorders. Acta Neurol Taiwan 2004;13(3):101–6.
32. Polgreen LE, Miller BS. Growth patterns and the use of growth hormone in the mucopolysaccharidoses. J Pediatr Rehabil Med 2010;3(1):25–38.
33. Cimaz R, Vijay S, Haase C, et al. Attenuated type I mucopolysaccharidosis in the differential diagnosis of juvenile idiopathic arthritis: a series of 13 patients with Scheie syndrome. Clin Exp Rheumatol 2006;24:196–202.
34. Neufeld EU, Muenzer J. The mucopolysaccharidoses. In: Scriver CR, editor. The metabolic and molecular bases of inherited disease. New York: McGraw-Hill; 2001. p. 3421–52.

35. Jimeno-Ruiz S, Martín-Molina R, García-Pérez A, et al. Carpal tunnel syndrome in childhood. Neurologia 2009;24(10):849–55 [in Spanish].

36. Van Meir N, De Smet L. Carpal tunnel syndrome in children. Acta Orthop Belg 2003;69:387–95.

37. Al-Qatan MM, Thomson HG, Clarke HM. Carpal tunnel syndrome in children and adolescents with no history of trauma. J Hand Surg Br 1996;21:108–11.

38. White K, Kim T, Neufeld JA. Clinical assessment and treatment of carpal tunnel syndrome in the mucopolysaccharidoses. J Pediatr Rehabil Med 2010;3(1):57–62.

39. Yuen A, Dowling G, Johnstone B, et al. Carpal tunnel syndrome in children with mucopolysaccaridoses. J Child Neurol 2007;22:260–3.

40. Meyer-Marcotty MV, Kollewe K, Dengler R, et al. Carpal tunnel syndrome in children with mucopolysaccharidosis type 1H: diagnosis and therapy in an interdisciplinary centre. Handchir Mikrochir Plast Chir 2012;44(1):23–8 [in German].

41. Haddad FS, Jones DH, Vellodi A, et al. Carpal tunnel syndrome in the mucopolysaccharidoses and mucolipidoses. J Bone Joint Surg Br 1997;79:576–82.

42. Haddad FS, Hill RA, Jones DH. Triggering in the mucopolysaccharidoses. J Pediatr Orthop B 1998;7:138–40.

43. Mankin HJ, Jupiter J, Trahan CA. Hand and foot abnormalities associated with genetic diseases. Hand (N Y) 2011;6(1):18–26.

44. Chen SJ, Li YW, Wang TR, et al. Bony changes in common mucopolysaccharidoses. Zhonghua Min Guo Xiao Er Ke Yi Xue Hui Za Zhi 1996;37:178–84.

45. Montaño AM, Tomatsu S, Gottesman GS, et al. International Morquio A Registry: clinical manifestations and natural course of Morquio A disease. J Inherit Metab Dis 2007;30:165–74.

46. Mikles M, Stanton RP. A review of Morquio syndrome. Am J Orthop 1997;26: 533–40.

47. Lehman TJ, Miller N, Norquist B, et al. Diagnosis of the mucopolysaccharidoses. Rheumatology (Oxford) 2011;50(Suppl 5):v41–8.

48. Civallero G, Bender F, Gomes A, et al. Reliable detection of mucopolysacchariduria in dried-urine filter paper samples. Clin Chim Acta 2013;415:334–6.

49. Brusius-Facchin AC, Kubaski F, Giugliani R, et al. Important aspects in the molecular diagnosis of mucopolysaccharidoses. J Inherit Metab Dis 2012. [Epub ahead of print].

50. Wang RY, Bodamer OA, Watson MS, et al, ACMG Work Group on Diagnostic Confirmation of Lysosomal Storage Diseases. Lysosomal storage diseases: diagnostic confirmation and management of presymptomatic individuals. Genet Med 2011;13(5):457–84.

51. de Ruijter J, de Ru MH, Wagemans T, et al. Heparan sulfate and dermatan sulfate derived disaccharides are sensitive markers for newborn screening for mucopolysaccharidoses types I, II and III. Mol Genet Metab 2012;107(4):705–10.

52. Zhang H, Young SP, Millington DS. Quantification of glycosaminoglycans in urine by isotope-dilution liquid chromatography-electrospray ionization tandem mass spectrometry. Curr Protoc Hum Genet 2013;17. Unit17.12.

53. Valayannopoulos V, Wijburg FA. Therapy for the mucopolysaccharidoses. Rheumatology (Oxford) 2011;50(Suppl 5):v49–59.

54. Peters C. Hematopoietic cell transplantation for storage diseases. In: Blume KG, Forman SJ, Appelbaum FR, editors. Hematopoietic stem cell transplantation. Malden (MA): Blackwell Science; 2004. p. 1455–70.

55. McGill JJ, Inwood AC, Coman DJ, et al. Enzyme replacement therapy for mucopolysaccharidosis VI from 8 weeks of age—a sibling control study. Clin Genet 2010;77:492–8.

56. Schulze-Frenking G, Jones SA, Roberts J, et al. Effects of enzyme replacement therapy on growth in patients with mucopolysaccharidosis type II. J Inherit Metab Dis 2011;34:203–8.

57. Ohashi T. Enzyme replacement therapy for lysosomal storage diseases. Pediatr Endocrinol Rev 2012;10(Suppl 1):26–34.

58. Wraith JE. Enzyme replacement therapy for the management of the mucopolysaccharidoses. Int J Clin Pharmacol Ther 2009;47(Suppl 1):S63–5.

59. de Ru MH, Boelens JJ, Das AM, et al. Enzyme replacement therapy and/or hematopoietic stem cell transplantation at diagnosis in patients with mucopolysaccharidosis type I: results of a European consensus procedure. Orphanet J Rare Dis 2011;6:55.

60. de Ru MH, Teunissen QG, van der Lee JH, et al. Capturing phenotypic heterogeneity in MPS I: results of an international consensus procedure. Orphanet J Rare Dis 2012;7:22.

61. D'Aco K, Underhill L, Rangachari L, et al. Diagnosis and treatment trends in mucopolysaccharidosis I: findings from the MPS I Registry. Eur J Pediatr 2012; 171(6):911–9.

62. White KK. Orthopaedic aspects of mucopolysaccharidoses. Rheumatology (Oxford) 2011;50(Suppl 5):v26–33.

63. Muenzer J, Beck M, Eng CM, et al. Multidisciplinary management of Hunter syndrome. Pediatrics 2009;124(6):e1228–39.

64. Muenzer J, Wraith JE, Clarke LA. International Consensus Panel on Management and Treatment of Mucopolysaccharidosis I. Mucopolysaccharidosis I: management and treatment guidelines. Pediatrics 2009;123(1):19–29.

65. Zarate YA, Hopkin RJ. Fabry's disease. Lancet 2008;372:1427–35.

66. Pinto LL, Vieira TA, Giugliani R, et al. Expression of the disease on female carriers of X-linked lysosomal disorders: a brief review. Orphanet J Rare Dis 2010;5:14.

67. Germain DP. Fabry disease. Orphanet J Rare Dis 2010;5:30.

68. Ramaswami U, Parini R, Pintos-Morell G. Natural history and effects of enzyme replacement therapy in children and adolescents with Fabry disease. In: Mehta A, Beck M, Sunder-Plassmann G, editors. Fabry disease: perspectives from 5 Years of FOS. Oxford: Oxford Pharma Genesis; 2006. Chapter 31.

69. Ries M, Gupta S, Moore DF, et al. Pediatric Fabry disease. Pediatrics 2005; 115(3):e344–55.

70. Germain DP, Benistan K, Boutouyrie P, et al. Osteopenia and osteoporosis: previously unrecognized manifestations of Fabry disease. Clin Genet 2005;68(1): 93–5.

71. Mersebach H, Johansson JO, Rasmussen AK, et al. Osteopenia: a common aspect of Fabry disease. Predictors of bone mineral density. Genet Med 2007;9(12):812–8.

72. Burlina AP, Sims KB, Politei JM, et al. Early diagnosis of peripheral nervous system involvement in Fabry disease and treatment of neuropathic pain: the report of an expert panel. BMC Neurol 2011;11:61.

73. Charrow J, Andersson HC, Kaplan P, et al. The Gaucher registry: demographics and disease characteristics of 1698 patients with Gaucher disease. Arch Intern Med 2000;160(18):2835–43.

74. Elstein D, Abrahamov A, Dweck A, et al. Gaucher disease: pediatric concerns. Paediatr Drugs 2002;4(7):417–26.

75. Kaplan P, Andersson HC, Kacena KA, et al. The clinical and demographic characteristics of nonneuronopathic Gaucher disease in 887 children at diagnosis. Arch Pediatr Adolesc Med 2006;160(6):603–8.

76. Bembi B, Ciana G, Mengel E, et al. Bone complications in children with Gaucher disease. Br J Radiol 2002;75(Suppl 1):A37–44.
77. Andersson H, Kaplan P, Kacena K, et al. Eight-year clinical outcomes of long-term enzyme replacement therapy for 884 children with Gaucher disease type 1. Pediatrics 2008;122(6):1182–90.
78. Wenstrup RJ, Roca-Espiau M, Weinreb NJ, et al. Skeletal aspects of Gaucher disease: a review. Br J Radiol 2002;75(Suppl 1):A2–12.
79. Roca Espiau M. Bone disease in Gaucher's disease. Med Clin (Barc) 2011; 137(Suppl 1):23–31 [in Spanish].
80. Brisca G, Di Rocco M, Picco P, et al. Coxarthritis as the presenting symptom of Gaucher disease type 1. Arthritis 2011;2011:361279.
81. Mistry PK, Weinreb NJ, Kaplan P, et al. Osteopenia in Gaucher disease develops early in life: response to imiglucerase enzyme therapy in children, adolescents and adults. Blood Cells Mol Dis 2011;46(1):66–72.
82. Guggenbuhl P, Grosbois B, Chalès G. Gaucher disease. Joint Bone Spine 2008; 75(2):116–24.
83. Wijburg FA. Early recognition and diagnosis of treatable lysosomal storage disorders. Eur Obstet Gynaecol 2006;1–7.
84. Tomatsu S, Montaño AM, Ohashi A, et al. Enzyme replacement therapy in a murine model of Morquio A syndrome. Hum Mol Genet 2008;17(6):815–24.
85. Tomatsu S, Vogler C, Montaño AM, et al. Murine model (Galns(tm(C76S)slu)) of MPS IVA with missense mutation at the active site cysteine conserved among sulfatase proteins. Mol Genet Metab 2007;91(3):251–8.
86. Brautbar A, Elstein D, Pines B, et al. Fibromyalgia and Gaucher's disease. QJM 2006;99(2):103–7.
87. Tsai LK, Chien YH, Yang CC, et al. Myopathy in Gaucher disease. J Inherit Metab Dis 2008. [Epub ahead of print].
88. Dweck A, Rozenman J, Ronen S, et al. Uveitis in Gaucher disease. Am J Ophthalmol 2005;140(1):146–7.
89. vom Dahl S, Niederau C, Häussinger D. Loss of vision in Gaucher's disease and its reversal by enzyme-replacement therapy. N Engl J Med 1998;338(20): 1471–2.
90. Moser HW, Linke I, Fensom AH, et al. In: Scriver CR, editor. The metabolic and molecular bases of inherited disease. 8th edition. New York: McGraw-Hill; 2001. p. 3573–85.
91. Tylki-Szymańska A, Czartoryska B, Groener JE, et al. Clinical variability in mucolipidosis III (pseudo-Hurler polydystrophy). Am J Med Genet 2002;108(3): 214–8.
92. David-Vizcarra G, Briody J, Ault J, et al. The natural history and osteodystrophy of mucolipidosis types II and III. J Paediatr Child Health 2010;46(6):316–22.
93. Cathey SS, Leroy JG, Wood T, et al. Phenotype and genotype in mucolipidoses II and III alpha/beta: a study of 61 probands. J Med Genet 2010;47(1):38–48.
94. Bach G. Mucolipidosis type IV. Mol Genet Metab 2001;73(3):197–203.
95. Robinson C, Baker N, Noble J, et al. The osteodystrophy of mucolipidosis type III and the effects of intravenous pamidronate treatment. J Inherit Metab Dis 2002; 25(8):681–93.
96. Jameson RA, Holt PJ, Keen JH. Farber's disease (lysosomal acid ceramidase deficiency). Ann Rheum Dis 1987;46(7):559–61.
97. Ehlert K, Frosch M, Fehse N, et al. Farber disease: clinical presentation, pathogenesis and a new approach to treatment. Pediatr Rheumatol Online J 2007;5:15.

98. Willems PJ, Gatti R, Darby JK, et al. Fucosidosis revisited: a review of 77 patients. Am J Med Genet 1991;38(1):111–31.
99. Menéndez-Sainz C, González-Quevedo A, González-García S, et al. High proportion of mannosidosis and fucosidosis among lysosomal storage diseases in Cuba. Genet Mol Res 2012;11(3):2352–9.
100. Malm D, Nilssen Ø. Alpha-mannosidosis. Orphanet J Rare Dis 2008;3:21.
101. Gerards AH, Winia WP, Westerga J, et al. Destructive joint disease in alpha-mannosidosis. A case report and review of the literature. Clin Rheumatol 2004;23(1):40–2.
102. DeFriend DE, Brown AE, Hutton CW, et al. Mannosidosis: an unusual cause of a deforming arthropathy. Skeletal Radiol 2000;29(6):358–61.
103. Vellodi A, Cragg H, Winchester B, et al. Allogeneic bone marrow transplantation for fucosidosis. Bone Marrow Transplant 1995;15(1):153–8.
104. Miano M, Lanino E, Gatti R, et al. Four year follow-up of a case of fucosidosis treated with unrelated donor bone marrow transplantation. Bone Marrow Transplant 2001;27(7):747–51.

Noninflammatory Myopathies

Alan N. Baer, MD[a],*, Robert L. Wortmann, MD[b]

KEYWORDS

- Myopathy • Metabolic myopathy • Differential diagnosis • Polymyositis
- Mitochondrial myopathy • Muscle glycogenoses

KEY POINTS

- Noninflammatory myopathies have diverse causes, including inherited or acquired metabolic abnormalities, toxins and drugs, and infections, as well as heritable defects in structural proteins (muscular dystrophies).
- This group of diseases should be considered in the differential diagnosis of autoimmune-mediated idiopathic inflammatory myopathies, because they can present with proximal muscle weakness, increased serum levels of muscle enzymes, and in some cases, endomysial inflammation.
- The primary metabolic myopathies are inherited disorders of muscle glycogen, lipid, or mitochondrial metabolism characterized by episodic exercise intolerance, occasionally with myoglobinuria, or progressive proximal muscle weakness.
- Drugs commonly used in rheumatology practice, including statins, antimalarials, and colchicine, can induce myopathies via diverse mechanisms.

The noninflammatory myopathies are a diverse group of diseases distinct from the autoimmune-mediated idiopathic inflammatory myopathies. They include the metabolic, toxic, and infectious myopathies, as well as the muscular dystrophies. Certain forms of these diseases can present with muscle weakness or pain and thus must be considered in the differential diagnosis of a patient being evaluated for polymyositis or other autoimmune-mediated muscle disease (**Table 1**).[1] The term noninflammatory is a misnomer, because some forms of muscular dystrophy and a variety of infectious myopathies may have inflammatory muscle infiltrates, and some forms of statin-induced myopathies may involve autoimmune mechanisms. In addition, inclusion body myositis is traditionally categorized as an idiopathic inflammatory myopathy but may not be autoimmune in origin. For the purposes of this review, the focus is on those noninflammatory myopathies that may mimic adult or pediatric forms of idiopathic inflammatory myopathy.

The authors report no relationships with commercial companies that have a direct financial interest in the subject matter discussed in this article.
[a] Division of Rheumatology, Johns Hopkins University School of Medicine, Suite 4000, Mason Lord Center Tower, 5200 Eastern Avenue, Baltimore, MD 21224, USA; [b] Rheumatology Section, Geisel School of Medicine at Dartmouth, One Medical Center Drive, Lebanon, NH 03756, USA
* Corresponding author.
E-mail address: alanbaer@jhmi.edu

Rheum Dis Clin N Am 39 (2013) 457–479
http://dx.doi.org/10.1016/j.rdc.2013.02.006
0889-857X/13/$ – see front matter
rheumatic.theclinics.com

Table 1
Differential diagnosis of idiopathic inflammatory myopathies and commonly encountered mimics

	Idiopathic Inflammatory Myopathy	Myophosphorylase Deficiency	CPT2 Deficiency (adult form)	Mitochondrial Myopathy	Dysferlinopathy	Fascioscapulohumeral Muscular Dystrophy	Proximal Myotonic Dystrophy Type 2
Typical age of onset	Childhood Midadult life	Childhood and adolescence	Young adulthood	Most often childhood, young adulthood	Adolescence and young adulthood	Before age 20 y	Young adulthood
Muscle symptoms	Proximal weakness	Pain early during exercise, especially if intense Late proximal weakness	Pain ± myoglobinuria, triggered by prolonged exercise or fasting	Premature fatigue with submaximal exercise Ocular muscle weakness	Proximal weakness	Facial and shoulder weakness; Eventual pelvic girdle weakness	Minimal or absent myotonia on examination Proximal weakness
Rash	Photosensitive Gottron Heliotrope Mechanic's hands	None	None	Lipomas	None	None	Hyperhidrosis
Other extramuscular involvement	Fever Arthritis Interstitial lung disease Raynaud Cardiomyopathy	None	None	Axonal neuropathy Ataxia Seizures Pigmentary retinopathy Sensorineural hearing loss	None	Retinal vasculopathy Sensorineural hearing loss	Cardiomyopathies and conduction defects Cataracts Diabetes Testicular failure
Family history	Autoimmunity	Same syndrome	Same syndrome	Possible symptoms in mother (mtDNA disorders)	Same syndrome	Same syndrome	Same syndrome in forebearers but more severe in proband (anticipation)
CK levels	Usually 2–30 × normal	Always increased	Normal between attacks	Less than 1500 IU/mL	10–70 × normal	2–7 × normal	Normal or slightly increased

DIAGNOSTIC EVALUATION

The evaluation of a suspected muscle disease begins with a careful patient history, focusing on the temporal pattern of onset and characteristics of the muscle symptoms, presence and distribution of muscle weakness, other organ system involvement, and family history. The physical examination should include an assessment of proximal and distal muscle strength and a search for neurogenic signs, such as spasticity, altered deep tendon reflexes, impaired sensation, muscle fasciculation, and atrophy. Subsequent testing usually involves measurement of serum levels of muscle enzymes, electromyography (EMG), magnetic resonance imaging (MRI), and muscle biopsy. The evaluation of metabolic myopathies often requires additional tests, including measurement of serum lactate and other metabolic intermediates, exercise testing, quantitative analysis of enzyme activity in muscle or blood lymphocytes, and molecular genetic analyses. An increasing number of metabolic myopathies and muscular dystrophies may now be diagnosed with molecular genetic testing, thereby obviating a muscle biopsy.

Increased serum levels of creatine kinase (CK), aldolase, aspartate aminotransferase, alanine aminotransferase, and lactate dehydrogenase (LDH) characterize many forms of myopathy, both inflammatory and noninflammatory. An increased CK level is the most sensitive of these tests. Some noninflammatory myopathies, including certain metabolic myopathies and electrolyte disorders, may develop without an increase in muscle enzymes. Myositis-specific autoantibodies support the presence of an idiopathic inflammatory myopathy. A diagnostic test for statin-associated autoimmune necrotizing myopathy will also be available soon.

EMG can facilitate the differentiation of myopathic or neuropathic processes, determine the distribution of a myopathy, and pinpoint an affected muscle group for biopsy. The signs of a myopathy include spontaneous electrical activity at rest from single muscle fibers (fibrillation potentials and positive sharp waves); short, small-amplitude polyphasic motor unit action potentials during muscle contraction; and the inability to identify individual motor unit potentials (interference pattern) with lower than normal forces of contraction (early recruitment). The presence of abnormal spontaneous electrical activity in the resting muscles indicates an irritable myopathy and is postulated to reflect the presence of an active necrotizing myopathic process or unstable muscle membrane potential. However, this finding has poor sensitivity and specificity for predicting the presence of an inflammatory myopathy on biopsy.[2]

MRI of patients with inflammatory myopathies shows increased muscle signal on fast spin echo T2 fat-saturated or short-tau inversion recovery sequences, which indicates edema. In the noninflammatory myopathies, MRI is normal or may show atrophy, sometimes of characteristic musculature. MRI and spectroscopy of the brain often show findings that help establish a diagnosis of mitochondrial disease.[3]

A muscle biopsy remains a critical test, unless the diagnosis can be secured with genetic testing. The best specimen is obtained from muscle that is moderately weak but not affected by end-stage atrophy, fibrosis, or replacement by fat, as judged by clinical examination, EMG, or MRI. The tissue should be analyzed in a reference muscle histopathology laboratory, where a comprehensive panel of immunohistochemical and histochemical stains can be performed. The histologic analyses depend in part on the clinical history, so it is important that this information be forwarded to the laboratory. The protocol for handling the tissue should be made available to the surgeon and the local pathologist in advance. If a metabolic myopathy is suspected, a portion of the specimen should be snap frozen in liquid nitrogen and stored at −70°C for future quantitative enzyme analyses at a reference laboratory.

Mitochondrial myopathies are often associated with defects in multiple metabolic pathways, and assays of these provide diagnostic information. An increased fasting plasma lactate level may be a useful indicator of a mitochondrial myopathy, but it is not uniformly present. Assays of plasma and cerebrospinal fluid (CSF) amino acids and urinary organic acids can also provide useful information in the diagnosis of mitochondrial disorders, primarily in pediatric patients with profound metabolic disturbances.[4] A decrease in plasma levels of free carnitine and a relative increase in acylcarnitine species are often observed in fatty acid oxidation disorders and mitochondrial myopathies related to mutations in mitochondrial DNA (mtDNA).

The forearm ischemic exercise test screens for defects in the glycogenolysis, glycolysis, and myoadenylate deaminase pathways (**Box 1**, **Fig. 1**). When normal skeletal muscle becomes ischemic, anaerobic glycolysis and the purine nucleotide cycle become essential sources of energy. Both lactate and ammonia levels increase 3-fold to 5-fold.[5] Individuals with myophosphorylase (McArdle disease) and phosphofructokinase deficiency can increase ammonia but not lactate production. Patients with debrancher, phosphoglycerate mutase, phosphoglycerate kinase, and LDH deficiencies have a blunted increase in lactate, whereas patients with deficiencies of acid maltase, branching enzyme, and phosphorylase b kinase have normal responses.[6] Patients with myoadenylate deaminase deficiency increase their serum lactate but not ammonia. Because exercise under ischemic conditions can cause painful muscle contractures and occasional rhabdomyolysis in patients with myophosphorylase deficiency, a forearm exercise test without tourniquet occlusion of blood flow is now advocated by some investigators.[7,8] The Forearm Ischemic Exercise Test (FIET) may yield false-positive results in individuals who cannot or do not exercise vigorously enough to increase lactate production. Accordingly, any positive test must be followed by biochemical analysis of muscle or molecular studies of blood cells to identify the putative enzyme defect.

Aerobic exercise testing can be used in the diagnostic evaluation of patients with suspected fatty acid oxidation defects or mitochondrial myopathies. A high respiratory

---

Box 1
FIET

Method

- Venous blood is collected for measurements of lactate and ammonia, preferably from the nondominant arm without using a tourniquet.

- A blood pressure cuff is inflated around the dominant upper arm and maintained at a pressure of 20 to 30 mm Hg higher than systolic pressure while the patient vigorously exercises the dominant forearm by squeezing a tennis ball or a rolled-up, partially inflated blood pressure cuff. The cuff is kept inflated around the arm for 2 minutes or until exercise causes complete exhaustion of the extremity (whichever is longer), at which point it is released.

- Two minutes later, blood is sampled for repeat lactate and ammonia levels from the dominant arm using a tourniquet.

Results

- Normal: at least a 3-fold increase over baseline in venous lactate and ammonia.

- Glycogenoses (except for deficiency of acid maltase, phosphorylase b kinase, or branching enzyme): ammonia levels increase but lactate levels remain at baseline.

- Myoadenylate deaminase deficiency: lactate levels increase but ammonia levels remain at baseline.

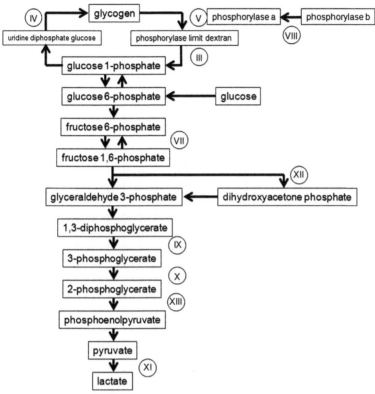

Fig. 1. Pathways of cytosolic glycogen metabolism. Deficiencies of numbered enzymes are recognized to cause a specific type of glycogen storage disease: VIII, phosphorylase b kinase; IV, branching enzyme; V, myophosphorylase; III, debrancher enzyme; VII, phosphofructoki-nase; XII, aldolase A; IX, phosphoglycerate kinase; X, phosphoglycerate mutase; XIII, β-enolase; XI, LDH. Note: acid maltase is not included because it is a lysozomal enzyme. (*Adapted from* Wortmann RL, DiMauro S. Differentiating idiopathic inflammatory myopa-thies from metabolic myopathies. Rheum Dis Clin North Am 2002;28:760.)

exchange ratio, low maximal level of oxygen consumption, and a high postexercise level of serum lactate[7] are findings that provide strong support for a mitochondrial myopathy.

Molecular genetic testing is now available for many of the more common metabolic myopathies and muscular dystrophies (**Table 2**). These tests are costly and are thus best used to confirm rather than screen for a diagnosis of a specific myopathy. The laboratories that offer these genetic tests are listed on the Web site http://www.genetests.org.

METABOLIC MYOPATHIES

The metabolic myopathies are a heterogeneous group of diseases defined by the inability of skeletal muscle to produce or maintain adequate levels of adenosine triphosphate (ATP) for contraction and relaxation (**Box 2**). Primary metabolic myopa-thies are associated with known or postulated biochemical defects in glycogen, lipid, or mitochondrial metabolism that render the muscle unable to maintain adequate concentrations of ATP. They are classified according to their underlying metabolic

Table 2
Molecular genetic analysis of selected adult myopathies[a]

Disease	Gene	Analysis of Entire Coding Region[b]	Targeted Mutation Analysis	Deletion/Duplication Analysis
Myophosphorylase	PYGM	X	X	X
Phosphoglycerate kinase	PGK	X		X
Phosphofructokinase	PFKM	X	X	
Debrancher	AGL	X		
Phosphorylase b kinase	PHKA1, PHKA2, PHKB, PHKG2	X		X
Phosphoglycerate mutase	PGAM	X		X
Acid maltase	GAA	X		X
Myoadenylate deaminase	AMPD1	X	X	
Carnitine palmitoyltransferase II	CPT2	X	X	X
Mitochondrial myopathies mtDNA deletion syndromes (KSS, PEO, Pearson syndrome)				X
MELAS, MERRF, LHON		X	X	
Leigh syndrome, NARP		X	X	X

Category	Gene (Protein)		
LGMDs			
LGMD1B	Lamin A/C (LMNA)	X	
LGMD2A	Calpain-3 (CAPN3)	X	
LGMD2B	Dysferlin (DYSF)	X	
LGMD1C	Caveolin-3 (CAV3)	X	
LGMD2C, LGMD2D, LGMD2E, LGMD2F	α-sarcoglycan, β-sarcoglycan, δ-sarcoglycan, γ-sarcoglycan (SGCA-D)	X	X
LGMD2I	Fukutin-related protein (FKRP)	X	
Dystrophinopathies	DMD	X	X
Facioscapulohumeral dystrophy	Likely DUX4		X
Proximal myotonic dystrophy 2	CNBP		X

Abbreviations: KSS, Kearns-Sayre syndrome; LGMD, limb-girdle muscular dystrophy; LHON, Leber hereditary optic neuropathy; MELAS, mitochondrial-encephalopathy–lactic acidosis–stroke; MERRF, myoclonic epilepsy associated with ragged red fibers; NARP, neurogenic muscle weakness, ataxia, and retinitis pigmentosa; PEO, progressive external ophthalmoplegia.

a The availability of these tests is listed at http://www.genetests.org.
b With sequence analysis or mutation scanning.

Box 2
Metabolic myopathies

Disordered glycogen metabolism
- Myophosphorylase deficiency (McArdle disease)
- Phosphorylase b kinase deficiency
- Phosphofructokinase deficiency
- Debrancher enzyme deficiency
- Branching enzyme deficiency
- Phosphoglycerate kinase deficiency
- Phosphoglycerate mutase deficiency
- LDH deficiency
- Acid maltase deficiency
- Aldolase deficiency
- β-Enolase deficiency

Disordered lipid metabolism
- Carnitine deficiencies
- Carnitine palmitoyltransferase (CPT) deficiency
- Myopathy with secondary coenzyme Q10 (CoQ10) deficiency
- Neutral lipid storage diseases (NLSDs)
- Fatty acid acyl–coenzyme A (CoA) dehydrogenase deficiencies
- Mitochondrial trifunction protein deficiency

Mitochondrial myopathies
- MtDNA mutations
- Nuclear DNA mutations
- Acquired defects

Endocrine
- Acromegaly
- Hypothyroidism
- Hyperthyroidism
- Hyperparathyroidism
- Cushing disease
- Addison disease
- Hyperaldosteronism

Metabolic-nutritional
- Uremia
- Hepatic failure
- Malabsorption
- Periodic paralysis
- Vitamin D deficiency
- Vitamin E deficiency

Electrolyte disorders

- Hypernatremia and hyponatremia
- Hyperkalemia and hypokalemia
- Hypercalcemia and hypocalcemia
- Hypophosphatemia
- Hypomagnesemia

defect. Secondary metabolic myopathies arise from various endocrine or electrolyte abnormalities. Many of these diseases present clinically with muscle weakness, pain, or increased muscle enzyme levels, thereby engendering concern for an idiopathic inflammatory myopathy.

Pain, cramping, stiffness, and weakness of exercising muscles are characteristic symptoms of many metabolic myopathies. This so-called exercise intolerance varies as a function of which biochemical pathway is impaired. Glycogen, free fatty acids, and amino acids are all muscle fuel sources, and their relative use depends on the intensity and duration of exercise.

At rest, free fatty acids are almost the exclusive source of fuel for muscles. At low to moderate exercise levels, glucose derived from glycogen supplements free fatty acids as a fuel source, with the relative proportion of each varying with exercise duration. With longer activity, less glucose and more fatty acid is used. With increasing intensity of exercise, more energy is derived from glycogen through aerobic glycolysis. However, intense exercise involving sustained isometric contraction (such as lifting a heavy object or pushing a stalled car) limits blood flow and oxygen delivery to the exercising muscles, prompting anaerobic metabolism. The glucose moieties, derived from muscle glycogen stores, are metabolized by the glycolytic pathway in the sarcoplasm to produce ATP and pyruvate. Under these conditions, pyruvate is reduced to lactate and diffuses out of the muscle into the systemic circulation. When oxygen is available to muscle under conditions of less intense exercise, the pyruvate is transported into mitochondria, where it is decarboxylated to acetyl-CoA (see **Fig. 1**). The β-oxidation of fatty acids that have been transported into mitochondria is also a source of acetyl-CoA. Energy is generated from acetyl-CoA by oxidation through the Krebs (tricarboxylic acid) cycle and respiratory chain.

Primary Metabolic Myopathies

Disorders of glycogen metabolism

The muscle glycogenoses constitute 11 different diseases characterized by an underlying defect in muscle glycogenolysis, glycolysis, or glycogen synthesis (**Fig. 2**).[9,10] These enzyme deficiency states result in an abnormal accumulation of glycogen in skeletal muscle and are thus considered glycogen storage diseases. Acid maltase is a lysosomal enzyme and is often classified separately from the other glycogenoses, where cytosolic enzymes are deficient. The key features of these muscle glycogenoses are summarized in **Table 3**. Seven types of muscle glycogenoses present predominantly with exercise intolerance, whereas 4 present with fixed muscle weakness.

The most common of the muscle glycogenoses is myophosphorylase deficiency (McArdle disease), with an estimated prevalence of 1 case in 100,000 people.[11] Symptoms of exercise intolerance may begin at any age, but usually before the age of 15 years. These symptoms may be described by the patient as muscle pain, fatigue,

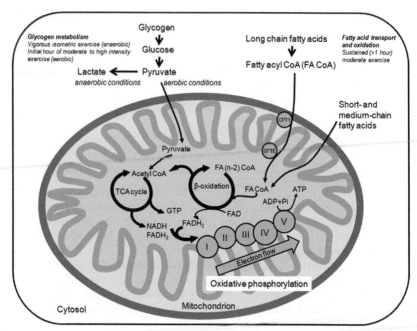

Fig. 2. Oxidative metabolism in muscle. The oxidative metabolism of both cellular glucose and free fatty acids occurs in the mitochondria. Acetyl-CoA is the key metabolic intermediate, derived both from pyruvate and as an end product of the mitochondrial β-oxidation of fatty acids. Pyruvate, generated from the glycolytic pathway in the sarcoplasma, diffuses across the mitochondrial membrane and is then converted to acetyl-CoA by pyruvate dehydrogenase. The fatty acids are activated by ATP to fatty acyl-CoA derivatives, within the mitochondrion for those with short and medium chains and in the sarcoplasma for those with long chains. Short-chain and medium-chain fatty acids enter the mitochondrion by passive diffusion, but the long-chain fatty acyl-CoA derivatives require facilitated transport via the carnitine shuttle. The long-chain fatty acids are first transferred to carnitine by the enzyme CPT-I, located in the outer mitochondrial membrane. The fatty acid is then transferred into the mitochondrial matrix by a carnitine acylcarnitine translocase (not shown), located in the inner mitochondrial membrane. A second enzyme in this membrane, CPT-II, regenerates the fatty acyl-CoA, releasing free carnitine. Within the mitochondrion, the fatty acyl-CoA are oxidized in a 4-step cycle of reactions (β-oxidation) in which the β-carbon is oxidized to a ketone followed by cleavage between the α- and β-carbons, yielding acetyl-CoA and a fatty acyl-CoA with 2 fewer carbon atoms. The 4 enzymes of this cycle include 1 of 3 acyl-CoA dehydrogenases (specific for short-chain, medium-chain, and long-chain fatty acyl-CoAs), an enoyl-CoA hydratase, a nicotinamide adenine dinucleotide (NAD$^+$) dependent dehydrogenase and a thiolase. Each cycle of β-oxidation yields 1 mol each of acetyl-CoA, flavin adenine dinucleotide (FADH$_2$) and NAD reduced (NADH) (not shown); for a 16-carbon fatty acid such as palmitate the cycle is repeated 7 times, yielding 8 mol of acetyl-CoA and 7 mol of FADH$_2$ and NADH. Acetyl-CoA is oxidized in the tricarboxylic acid cycle (or Krebs cycle) (TCA), a series of 8 enzymatic reactions. Each mole of acetyl-CoA yields 3 mol of NADH and 1 mol of FADH$_2$. These reduced nucleotide coenzymes subsequently transfer electrons to molecular oxygen via the electron transport chain, in the process generating ATP from adenosine diphosphate (ADP) and inorganic phosphate (Pi). The electron transport chain consists of 5 large protein complexes (I–V) located in the inner mitochondrial membrane and 2 small independent components, cytochrome c and ubiquinone (not shown). Electrons move sequentially from 1 protein complex to the next (in the order of I–V) down an energy gradient. In the process, protons are pumped by complexes I, III, and IV across the inner mitochondrial membrane into the intermembrane space, creating a membrane potential. The controlled influx of protons through complex V (ATP synthase) powers the synthesis of ATP. (*Adapted from* Baer AN. Metabolic, drug-induced and other non-inflammatory myopathies. In: Hochberg M, Silman A, Smolen J, et al, editors. Rheumatology. 5th edition. London: Elsevier; 2010. p. 1485; and Baer AN. Metabolic myopathies. In: Klippel JH, Stone JH, Crofford LJ, et al, editors. Primer on the rheumatic diseases. 13th edition. New York: Springer-Verlag; 2007. p. 384.)

stiffness, weakness, or intense cramping. They are relieved by rest and are commonly associated with myoglobinuria. Most afflicted persons are asymptomatic at rest and during low levels of physical activity, such as walking on level ground. Symptoms develop after brief and intense exercise (such as pushing or lifting heavy objects) or less intense, sustained exercise (such as climbing stairs or walking uphill), times during which most energy for muscular work is derived from carbohydrate.

Many patients report a second wind, whereby they note an increase in exercise capacity if they rest briefly after the initial onset of muscle symptoms. This phenomenon is attributed to the exercise-induced mobilization and delivery of glucose and free fatty acids of nonmuscle origin. Some patients develop fixed weakness in late stages of the disease. Patients with this presentation may not seek medical attention until middle age and may be initially misdiagnosed as having polymyositis.

Phosphofructokinase deficiency closely resembles that of myophosphorylase in its clinical presentation. However, affected patients typically lack the second wind phenomenon and may have evidence of a concomitant hemolytic anemia.

Four of the glycogenoses present with fixed muscle weakness, including acid maltase, branching and debrancher enzyme, and aldolase deficiencies. In contrast to the muscle glycogenoses that cause exercise intolerance and myoglobinuria, these glycogenoses are caused by enzyme defects that are not restricted to muscle. Acid maltase deficiency is the most prevalent of these disorders and can present in infantile, childhood, or adult forms. The adult form typically presents after age 20 years with proximal muscle weakness or respiratory failure. Diaphragmatic weakness may be disproportionately severe. Respiratory involvement eventually occurs in all adults and is the usual cause of death.

Serum CK levels are increased at all times in myophosphorylase deficiency and variably increased in the other muscle glycogenoses. The EMG may be normal or show nonspecific myopathic changes. Adult acid maltase deficiency causes characteristic EMG changes of intense electrical irritability and myotoniclike discharges in the absence of clinical myotonia. The FIET is a useful screening method for most glycogenoses (see earlier discussion). Subsarcolemmal deposits of glycogen are the characteristic histologic abnormality of the muscle glycogenoses, but vary in extent and sometimes are evident only with electron microscopy. In acid maltase deficiency, electron microscopy shows the glycogen deposits to be membrane-bound within lysosomes. Myophosphorylase and phosphofructokinase deficiencies can be assessed in muscle biopsy specimens with histochemical analysis of enzyme activities. All of the glycogenoses are amenable to biochemical analysis of the relevant enzyme activities using muscle biopsy specimens. Testing for the more common genetic mutations that account for up to 90% of myophosphorylase deficiency can be performed using whole blood. Similarly, the diagnosis of acid maltase deficiency can be confirmed with showing deficient α-glucosidase activity in dried blood spots on filter paper or genetic analysis of peripheral blood samples.

Patients with myophosphorylase deficiency should avoid bursts of high-intensity exercise. Regular, submaximal aerobic exercise should be encouraged, because it increases oxidative capacity. Ingestion of sucrose before exercise can markedly improve exercise tolerance in myophosphorylase deficiency but worsen it in patients with glycolytic defects (phosphofructokinase, phosphoglycerate kinase, and phosphoglycerate mutase deficiencies).[11] A carbohydrate-rich diet, vitamin B_6, and low-dose creatine supplementation (60 mg/kg/d) have each been shown to be beneficial in myophosphorylase deficiency.[12] Enzyme replacement therapy with α-glucosidase is available for patients with acid maltase deficiency. Its efficacy is well established for infants and children with the classic phenotype.[12]

Table 3
Muscle glycogenoses

Enzyme or Biochemical Defect	Genetics	Infantile or Early Childhood Presentation	Adolescent or Adult Presentation	Special Testing
Acid maltase (type II)	Autosomal recessive	Infantile: weakness, hypotonia, enlargement of heart, liver, and tongue Childhood: myopathy, respiratory failure	Proximal myopathy Respiratory insufficiency	Increased resting serum CK Myotonic discharges on EMG Normal FIET Deficient α-glucosidase in leucocytes and muscle
Debrancher (type III)	Autosomal recessive	Hepatomegaly, growth retardation, hypoglycemia, seizures Myopathy Subclinical cardiomyopathy	Myopathy: distal or generalized Subclinical cardiomyopathy Hepatomegaly	Increased resting serum CK Diabetic glucose tolerance test Myopathic and neuropathic EMG findings Abnormal FIET
Branching (type IV)	Autosomal recessive	Hepatic failure Nonprogressive liver disease Myopathy Cardiomyopathy	Myopathy Polyglucosan body disease (dementia, upper and lower motor neuron disease)	Variable increase in resting CK Irritative myopathic EMG findings Normal FIET
Aldolase (type XII)	Autosomal recessive	Exercise intolerance Hemolytic anemia	None	Increased resting serum CK
Phosphofructokinase (type VII)	Autosomal recessive	Arthrogryposis and weakness Seizures, cortical blindness, cardiomyopathy	Exercise intolerance; myoglobinuria Out-of-wind phenomenon Hemolytic anemia Gout	Increased resting serum CK Abnormal FIET

Disease	Inheritance	Associated features	Clinical features	Laboratory findings
Myophosphorylase (type V)	Autosomal recessive	Rare	Exercise intolerance; myoglobinuria; Second wind phenomenon	Increased resting serum CK; Normal EMG; Abnormal FIET
Phosphorylase b kinase (type VIII)	Autosomal or X-linked recessive	Hepatomegaly, hypoglycemia; Hepatomegaly and myopathy; Cardiomyopathy	Exercise intolerance; myoglobinuria	Variable increase in resting serum CK; Normal FIET
Phosphoglycerate kinase (type IX)	X-linked	Hemolytic anemia; Mental retardation, seizures, strokes	Exercise intolerance; myoglobinuria	Variable increase in resting serum CK; Abnormal FIET
Phosphoglycerate mutase (type X)	Autosomal recessive	None	Exercise intolerance; myoglobinuria; Most often in African Americans	Increased resting serum CK; Abnormal FIET
LDH (type XI)	Autosomal recessive	None	Exercise intolerance; myoglobinuria; Dystocia; Rash	Serum LDH does not increase proportionally to CK during attack of myoglobinuria; Abnormal FIET
β-enolase (type XIII)	Autosomal recessive	None	Exercise intolerance	Increased resting serum CK; Abnormal FIET

Disorders of lipid metabolism

The disorders of lipid metabolism result from defects in the catabolism of endogenous triglyceride stores, fatty acid transport into mitochondria, and intramitochondrial fatty acid β-oxidation. Two clinical forms of muscle disease may result: progressive muscle weakness or recurrent episodes of myoglobinuria.[13] In the first form, markedly increased numbers of lipid droplets are present in the muscle fibers. These lipid storage myopathies include primary carnitine deficiency, multiple acyl-CoA dehydrogenase deficiency (MADD), myopathy with secondary CoQ10 deficiency, and various forms of neutral lipid storage disease (NLSD). In the second form, histopathologic evidence of increased lipid storage is minimal or absent. These disorders include defects of mitochondrial fatty acid transport and β-oxidation, such as deficiencies of CPT, very long-chain acyl-CoA dehydrogenase (VLCAD), and mitochondrial trifunctional protein.

The lipid storage myopathies are multisystemic and usually diagnosed in infancy or childhood. A deficiency in carnitine, the amino acid required for the transport of long-chain fatty acids into mitochondria, can result from inherited or acquired causes. Primary carnitine deficiency is a rare autosomal recessive disorder caused by the lack of a functional plasma membrane carnitine transporter (OCTN2). It may have a predominantly metabolic or cardiomuscular presentation. The metabolic type develops before age 2 years, with severe fasting hypoglycemia leading to coma. The cardiomuscular type presents most often between the ages of 2 and 4 years, with a progressive hypertrophic or dilated cardiomyopathy and a myopathy. Both types respond well to high doses of oral L-carnitine. Carnitine deficiency may be secondary to other metabolic disorders (fatty acid oxidation disorders, organic acidemias), pregnancy, long-term hemodialysis, renal Fanconi syndrome, and chronic treatment with valproate or pivampicillin. In carnitine deficiency, serum CK levels are increased in more than 50% of patients and the EMG often reveals myopathic changes. Biochemical analysis of carnitine levels in muscle is required to establish the diagnosis of the myopathic type of carnitine deficiency. Free and acylated plasma carnitine levels are extremely reduced. Plasma carnitine levels are less than 10% of normal in the systemic form of primary carnitine deficiency.

MADD, also known as glutaric academia type II, is an autosomal-recessive disorder resulting from defects in intramitochondrial acyl-CoA dehydrogenation stemming from impaired electron transport. Most patients present in the first few days of life with hypoglycemia and metabolic acidosis, but rare patients can present in their childhood or adult years with a lipid storage myopathy. Urinary organic acid and blood acylcarnitine profiles show characteristic abnormalities. Primary CoQ10 deficiency may present as an isolated lipid storage myopathy in children or adults, associated with proximal muscle weakness, exercise intolerance, and increased serum CK and lactate levels.[14] In the muscle tissue, CoQ10 levels are low and the activity of respiratory chain complexes I and III is impaired. NLSD arises from defects in 2 enzymes, adipose triglyceride lipase (ATGL) and α/β-hydrolase domain-containing protein 5 (ABHD5), leading to impaired triglyceride metabolism and massive triglyceride storage in muscle and other tissues. Mutations in ABHD5 are associated with several phenotypes, the most prominent being Chanarin-Dorfman syndrome, a disease marked by an ichthyosiform nonbullous erythroderma, a mild proximal myopathy, and hepatomegaly (NLSD with ichthyosis). Hearing loss, mild mental retardation, short stature, and various ophthalmologic symptoms occur inconstantly. Mutations in ATGL are associated with a clinical syndrome characterized by a proximal and distal myopathy and cardiomyopathy (NLSD with myopathy).[15,16] CK levels in both forms of NLSD are mild to moderately increased. There are no characteristic biochemical abnormalities in blood and urine tests, but intracytoplasmic lipid storage can be detected in leucocytes (Jordan anomaly).

Recurrent myoglobinuria is a characteristic of certain defects in mitochondrial fatty acid transport and β-oxidation. The most common of these is CPT deficiency. Two distinct acyltransferases transport long-chain fatty acid–carnitine complexes into mitochondria. The first, CPT1, is located on the inner side of the outer mitochondrial membrane, and the second, CPT2, is located on the inner side of the inner mitochondrial membrane. Deficiencies of both CPT1 and CPT2 occur but muscle disease is confined to the latter. CPT2 deficiency is an autosomal-recessive disorder with clinical presentations in juvenile or adult life (muscle form), in infancy (hepatocardiomuscular form) and at birth (hepatic form). The muscle form of CPT2 deficiency is the most common cause of hereditary recurrent myoglobinuria. It occurs most often in adolescent or young adult men. The primary clinical feature of CPT2 deficiency is paroxysmal myoglobinuria, usually precipitated by prolonged exercise and less often by fasting, infection, or exposure to cold. Patients typically notice dark urine several hours after completion of the exercise. Soreness of their muscles develops during the exercise and then persists for several days. True cramps do not occur. Serum CK concentrations, EMG, and muscle histology are normal, except during episodes of symptomatic rhabdomyolysis. The diagnosis is made by assaying muscle tissue for enzyme activity. Genetic analysis of whole blood can be used to screen for approximately 80% of known mutant alleles. Patients with CPT2 deficiency should avoid fasting and maintain regular carbohydrate intake during periods of infection. Bezafibrate may be beneficial in patients with mild forms of the disease.[12] Intravenous glucose should be infused during general anesthesia.

VLCAD deficiency has early-onset and late-onset phenotypes; the latter closely resembles CPT2 deficiency in adults. The diagnosis is aided by showing an abnormal plasma increase of long-chain acylcarnitines. Mitochondrial trifunctional protein deficiency may have a late-onset form characterized by recurrent exercise-induced myoglobinuria, pigmentary retinopathy, cardiomyopathy, and a progressive sensorimotor axonal peripheral neuropathy. Respiratory failure may accompany the episodes of myoglobinuria.

Mitochondrial myopathies

The mitochondrial myopathies are a clinically heterogeneous group of disorders that arise from a primary defect in electron transport chain function and oxidative phosphorylation.[17] The mitochondrial myopathies are usually part of a multisystem disease with involvement of tissues that are highly dependent on oxidative metabolism, such as skeletal muscle, heart, brain, retina, endocrine glands, and renal tubules. Mitochondrial diseases have an estimated prevalence of 9 to 15 cases per 100,000 persons.[18,19] They may present at any age. Mitochondrial myopathies may be caused by mutations in mtDNA or in the nuclear DNA that encodes proteins involved in oxidative phosphorylation. The mtDNA disorders are inherited through maternal transmission, impair the respiratory chain exclusively, and account for approximately half of mitochondrial diseases in adults. The nuclear DNA disorders have Mendelian inheritance patterns (usually autosomal recessive), may impair a variety of mitochondrial functions, and account for approximately 80% of the mitochondrial diseases in children. Pathogenic mutations of mtDNA usually affect only some of the numerous copies of mtDNA in each cell (heteroplasmy). Because this proportion varies widely, there is a spectrum of clinical severity among individuals with a pathogenic mtDNA mutation. In addition, the heteroplasmy of a mitochondrial mutation may vary within and between tissues, resulting in marked variation of the phenotypic manifestations.

The clinical spectrum of mitochondrial diseases is diverse. They are typically multi-systemic, but may present with manifestations restricted to 1 organ system and involve other organs only slowly over time. They may present as distinct clinical syndromes, such as Kearns-Sayre syndrome; chronic progressive external ophthal-moplegia; myoclonic epilepsy associated with ragged red fibers; mitochondrial myop-athy, encephalopathy, lactic acidosis and strokelike episodes (MELAS); Leber hereditary optic neuropathy; infantile subacute necrotizing encephalopathy (Leigh syndrome); and sideroblastic anemia of childhood with exocrine pancreatic failure (Pearson syndrome). However, many patients, particularly children, present with symptoms and signs that overlap 1 or more syndromes.

Muscle involvement with exercise intolerance is present in most mitochondrial diseases. Many adult patients report exercise intolerance, marked by premature fatigue, headaches, nausea, and vomiting after submaximal exercise, such as walking up a flight of stairs. Patients can generally resume their activity after brief rest, but the symptoms then recur. In contrast to patients with glycogenoses, exercise-induced cramps or myoglobinuria are rare. The muscle symptoms are often aggravated by fasting or the presence of an infection. Mild weakness of the proximal limb muscula-ture may be present. The hip girdle musculature is primarily affected, leading to a waddling gait and difficulty climbing stairs.

Chronic progressive external ophthalmoplegia and eyelid ptosis often accompany the skeletal muscle disease in adults.[20] Diverse types of organ involvement may be present and should be clues to the diagnosis. These types include endocrine (eg, diabetes mellitus, hypopituitarism with growth retardation, diabetes insipidus, hypo-parathyroidism, amenorrhea), heart (conduction disorder, hypertrophic or dilated cardiomyopathy, and left ventricular hypertrabeculation or noncompaction), central nervous system (seizures, strokelike episodes, ataxia, myoclonus, dementia, migraine, encephalopathy, and spasticity), peripheral nervous system (peripheral neuropathy), eye (pigmentary retinopathy, optic atrophy), ears (sensorineural hearing loss), kidney (Fanconi syndrome, polycystic kidneys) and gastrointestinal tract (dysphagia, hepatic steatosis, recurrent diarrhea from small bowel villous atrophy).

The diagnosis of a mitochondrial disease may be based on the recognition of a char-acteristic phenotype, such as MELAS, with molecular genetic confirmation. In the absence of a fully developed syndrome, the occurrence of myopathy in association with other organ involvement, such as neuropathy, diabetes, cardiomyopathy, or deafness should prompt screening for a mitochondrial disorder. An increased fasting serum lactate level is present in approximately 70% of patients,[17] but is nonspecific and may be spurious in origin.[4] Other screening tests may include CSF lactic acid levels, plasma acylcarnitines, and urinary organic acids. Algorithms for diagnostic testing depend heavily on the clinical findings and setting, and may be different with juvenile versus adult presentations. Useful discussions of these issues have been published.[4,17,21,22]

The serum CK level is usually normal or increased by no more than 5 x upper limit of normal (ULN). The EMG is often normal, but may show myopathic or mixed myopathic and neuropathic changes. Muscle biopsy or genetic testing is required for confirmation of the diagnosis. The characteristic histopathologic findings include ragged red fibers (subsarcolemmal accumulation of mitochondria on modified Gomori trichrome stain), muscle fibers with reduced or absent cytochrome c oxidase activity, and accumulation of neutral lipids. Electron microscopy may also show mitochondria in increased numbers or with abnormal morphology. Deficiencies in respiratory chain enzyme func-tion can be sought with biochemical assays using muscle tissue that was snap frozen at the time of biopsy. Confirmation of a diagnosis of a mitochondrial disorder is best achieved with molecular genetic testing for mutations believed most likely to be present based on clinical and laboratory features.

Myoadenylate deaminase deficiency

Myoadenylate deaminase deficiency is found in 2% of the general population and is not believed to cause myopathy. The deficiency is often detected in the context of ischemic forearm exercise testing, in which there is a characteristic increase in lactate, but not ammonia. Affected patients have normal muscle strength, serum CK concentrations, EMG, and muscle histology. If an individual with this deficiency has muscle weakness, myalgia, or fatigue, then another diagnosis should be sought to explain these symptoms.

Secondary Metabolic Myopathies

Proximal muscle weakness may accompany endocrine and metabolic disorders, including Cushing syndrome, hypothyroidism, hyperthyroidism, and hyperparathyroidism. Thyroid and parathyroid diseases may be associated with high serum CK levels and myopathic EMG findings. Disorders that disturb sodium, potassium, calcium, magnesium, or phosphorus balance can also cause muscle weakness, fatigue, pain, or cramps.

DRUG-INDUCED MYOPATHIES

Many drugs may injure muscle via different mechanisms (**Table 4**). The offending drugs discussed herein are used commonly in rheumatology practice.

Statin-Induced Myopathy

The prescription of statins (3-hydroxy-3-methylglutaryl-CoA reductase inhibitors) for dyslipidemia may be associated with varying forms of muscle symptoms and toxicity, including myalgia, myositis (defined by muscle symptoms with increased CK levels), and rhabdomyolysis (CK increases greater than 10 × ULN with evidence of acute pigment-induced renal injury).[23] It is now known that statin use may rarely be associated with the development of an immune-mediated necrotizing myopathy that persists long after the cessation of statin use.[24,25] This form of myopathy is marked by the

Table 4
Drug-induced myopathies

Type of Myopathy	Drugs
Autoimmune necrotizing myopathy	3-Hydroxy-3-methylglutaryl CoA reductase inhibitors (statins)
Necrotizing myopathy	3-Hydroxy-3-methylglutaryl CoA reductase inhibitors (statins), fibrates, alcohol
Inflammatory myopathy	Penicillamine, interferon α, procainamide
Mitochondrial myopathy	Zidovudine, clevudine
Hypokalemic myopathy	Diuretics, laxatives, licorice, amphotericin B, alcohol
Microtubular myopathy	Colchicine, vincristine
Lysosomal storage myopathy	Chloroquine, hydroxychloroquine, quinacrine, amiodarone, perhexilene
Steroid myopathy	Corticosteroids, especially fluorinated
Myofibrillar myopathy	Ipecac syrup, emetine

presence of serum antibodies to 3-hydroxy-3-methylglutaryl-CoA reductase[26] and requires immunosuppressive therapy.

Myalgia is reported by 1% to 5% of participants in statin clinical trials, with a frequency equal in statin and placebo-treated groups. However, muscle symptoms were reported by 10.5% of patients in a prospective observational study of 7924 patients receiving high-dose statin treatment in general practice, and prompted discontinuation of the statin in 20%.[27] Serious muscle toxicity in the form of rhabdomyolysis occurs in 0.1% to 0.5% of patients on statin monotherapy.[28]

Symptoms of statin-induced myopathy include any combination of aching, cramping, tenderness, or weakness,[27] often arising in the pectoral, quadriceps, biceps, abdominal, low back, and gluteal muscles.[29] With exercise, the muscle symptoms are typically more widespread and intense. In some patients, muscle symptoms may persist long after the cessation of statin therapy, and this should prompt an evaluation for a previously unrecognized neuromuscular disorder or an immune-mediated necrotizing myopathy.

The muscle tissue from patients with statin myopathy does not usually show histopathologic abnormalities[30] but may show changes that indicate mitochondrial dysfunction.[31] Rarely, the muscle biopsies may show a necrotizing myopathy, even in patients who have discontinued statin use for prolonged periods of time.[32]

Statin myotoxicity is determined primarily by pharmacokinetic factors, which lead to higher drug levels in the blood or tissues. These factors include drug dose, dependence on hepatic cytochrome P450 (CYP450) metabolism, propensity for drug-drug interactions, and genetic factors. The frequency of myotoxicity increases with higher doses of most statins, implying the presence of a dose effect.[33] With the exception of pravastatin and rosuvostatin, the statins are metabolized primarily by the hepatic CYP450 system. Coadministration of a statin and another drug that is metabolized by the same CYP450 isozyme can lead to increased levels of the statin and a heightened risk for myotoxicity. Such drug interactions can occur with cyclosporine, macrolide antibiotics, azole antifungals, amiodarone, nondihydropyridine calcium channel blockers, protease inhibitors, nefazodone, and grapefruit juice. Myotoxicity may be more common when statins are taken together with a fibrate in an effort to optimize lipid profiles.

The risk of statin myopathy may have a genetic contribution. In a recent genome-wide association scan, statin myopathy had a single strong association with the rs4363657 single-nucleotide polymorphism located within the SLCOB1 gene on chromosome 12.[34] This gene encodes the organic anion-transporting polypeptide OATP1B1, which mediates the hepatic uptake of most statins and other drugs. Other genetic factors that have been implicated include polymorphisms of the CYP450 isozymes and serotonin receptors, heritable defects of muscle energy metabolism, and traits that alter fatty acid oxidative metabolism.

Various pathogenetic mechanisms have been postulated for statin myotoxicity.[35] The most prominent is the depletion of isoprenoid intermediary metabolites, which are essential for prenylation, a fundamental element of posttranscriptional lipid modification of proteins and other compounds. Others include depletion of membrane cholesterol, disturbed calcium homeostasis, inhibition of CoQ10 production, and induction of muscle autoimmunity.[36]

Glucocorticoid Myopathy

Most patients treated with corticosteroids eventually develop some degree of muscle weakness, usually after a period of at least 4 weeks. Painless weakness of the proximal muscles, preferentially those of the lower extremities, and neck flexors is characteristic.

Respiratory muscle weakness may occur in severe cases. The weakness is more severe and may develop more rapidly in those treated with high-dose corticosteroids and with fluorinated preparations, such as dexamethasone, triamcinolone, and betamethasone.[37] Women are more likely than men to develop the myopathy. Glucocorticoid myopathy is usually accompanied by other features of iatrogenic Cushing syndrome, including a moon facies, fragile skin, and suprascapular fat pad. Muscle enzymes are normal. EMG shows low-amplitude motor unit potentials and the absence of any spontaneous electrical activity. Selective atrophy of type 2 muscle fibers and the absence of inflammation or muscle necrosis are characteristic histologic features. The myopathy typically improves with tapering of the corticosteroid dose or switching to a nonfluorinated preparation. Avoidance of starvation or protein deprivation is also important.

Colchicine Myopathy

A neuromyopathy may develop in patients taking standard doses of colchicine for prolonged periods, particularly if they have impaired or recently changed renal function. The concomitant use of cyclosporine or a statin may be a predisposing factor. Affected patients develop proximal muscle weakness, distal sensory loss, and areflexia. Serum CK levels are almost always increased, usually in the range of 2 to 20 times higher than normal.[38] The myopathy improves quickly after discontinuation of the colchicine, but the axonal neuropathy is slower to resolve. Muscle biopsy shows a vacuolar myopathy without prominent necrosis or inflammation.

Chloroquine and Hydroxychloroquine Myopathy

A myopathy may develop in patients treated chronically with chloroquine, and to a lesser extent with hydroxychloroquine. Patients develop slowly progressive muscle weakness, first in the lower extremities and later in the upper limbs and rarely the face. The myopathy is often accompanied by a polyneuropathy. Muscle enzyme levels are mildly increased, most often that of LDH.[39] Chloroquine myopathy most often develops with sustained use of higher doses, such as 500 mg per day for a year or more. The myopathy and neuropathy both resolve within several months after discontinuation of the antimalarial agent. The muscle biopsy show a vacuolar myopathy, often evident only with electron microscopy.[39] The vacuoles contain concentric lamellar structures (myeloid bodies) and curvilinear bodies.

MUSCULAR DYSTROPHIES

The muscular dystrophies are a group of inherited disorders characterized clinically by progressive muscle weakness and wasting and pathologically by muscle fiber size variation, necrosis and regeneration, and fatty and fibrous tissue replacement. They arise primarily from mutations in genes encoding structural proteins of muscle. Certain forms may mimic an idiopathic inflammatory myopathy. Thus Becker, limb-girdle, facioscapulohumeral, and myotonic dystrophies may present in late adolescence or adult life with muscle weakness and increased muscle enzymes. In addition, the dysferlinopathies (limb-girdle muscular dystrophy [LGMD] type 2B [LGMD2B]), facioscapulohumeral dystrophies, and dystrophinopathies may have endomysial inflammation. The muscular dystrophies have clinical features that help differentiate them from the idiopathic inflammatory myopathies (see **Table 1**).

The dystrophinopathies arise from mutations in the dystrophin gene on the X-chromosome and include Duchenne muscular dystrophy (DMD) and Becker muscular dystrophy (BMD). DMD is diagnosed in the first few years of a boy's life and invariably results in the loss of his ability to ambulate before age 13 years. BMD usually presents in childhood with shoulder and pelvic girdle muscle weakness, but affected boys remain ambulatory beyond the age of 16 years. Some patients with BMD do not develop symptoms until after the age of 30 years and can continue to walk until the seventh decade of life. Female carriers of DMD and BMD may present with early cardiomyopathy and mild muscle weakness in later life; their CK levels are typically increased 2-fold to 10-fold. Other forms of dystrophinopathy include young men with painful muscles and exercise-induced cramps (occasionally with myoglobinuria), isolated quadriceps myopathy, and isolated hyperCKemia. Molecular genetic analysis of the dystrophin gene is the first step in confirming a diagnosis. If no mutation is found, a muscle biopsy should be performed with immunohistochemical staining for dystrophin or Western blot analysis of the tissue.

LGMDs are a heterogeneous group of disorders distinct from the more common X-linked dystrophinopathies and characterized by progressive proximal muscle weakness. The inheritance is autosomal, most frequently recessive. Affected patients usually present in the second or third decade of life, initially with weakness of the proximal leg muscles and later with upper limb involvement. The onset may be delayed to the third or fourth decade of life. The progression of muscle weakness is slower than in DMD. The LGMDs are mostly related to mutations in structural muscle protein genes, including those for the various sarcoglycans, dysferlin, caveolin, telethonin, and lamin. One form of LGMD arises from a mutation in the gene for calpain 3, a calcium-dependent protease.

LGMD2B and Myoshi distal myopathy result from mutations in the dysferlin gene and are known as dysferlinopathies. LGMD2B is characterized by weakness and atrophy of the pelvic and shoulder girdle muscles, developing in adolescence or young adulthood and progressing slowly thereafter. Weakness begins in the lower extremities and may not progress to the upper extremities until 10 or more years later.[40] Upper extremity involvement usually begins with weakness of the biceps muscles. Some patients may have both proximal and distal muscle weakness at onset. Scapular winging does not occur. LGMD2B may mimic polymyositis because of its onset in adult life, marked increase of serum CK level, and the presence of inflammatory infiltrates in the muscle biopsy.[41,42] Confirmation of the diagnosis begins with a muscle biopsy, showing dystrophic changes as well as reduced levels or absence of dysferlin in the muscle sarcolemma with immunohistochemical staining. Molecular genetic studies are needed to confirm and define the character of the mutation.

The sarcoglycanopathies are forms of LGMD (types 2C, D, E, and F) caused respectively by mutations in the γ-sarcoglycan, α-sarcoglycan, β-sarcoglycan, and δ-sarcoglycan genes and primarily affect Whites. Onset is most often in early childhood and loss of ambulation generally occurs before the age of 16 years. However, milder phenotypes do occur, with proximal muscle weakness first developing in young adulthood. Muscle weakness is initially detectable in the pelvic girdle, and later involves the shoulders, with scapular winging. Respiratory muscle involvement occurs late in the disease and frequently leads to respiratory failure and death. Serum CK levels are increased 10 to 100 × ULN, typically higher than in other forms of LGMD. Immunostaining of muscle biopsy specimens can establish the diagnosis.

Facioscapulohumeral muscular dystrophy is an autosomal-dominant disorder that predominantly affects the facial, scapulohumeral, pelvic girdle, and anterior tibial muscles. Patients first develop symptoms in the first to fifth decades of life. Facial weakness usually begins first; patients are unable to close their eyes tightly or whistle. Medical attention is usually sought after weakness of scapular fixation precludes abduction of the arm beyond 90°. Scapular winging is a prominent feature. Sensorineural hearing loss and a retinal vasculopathy are frequently present. The serum CK level may be normal or mildly increased. The disease arises from mutations in the 4q35 gene and can be confirmed by molecular genetic testing.

Proximal myotonic dystrophy, type 2 (DM2) is an autosomal-dominant disorder characterized by proximal muscle weakness, muscle pain, cataracts, myotonia, tremors, cardiac disturbances, and hypogonadism.[43] The neck flexors, hip flexors, and triceps muscles are most commonly affected. This disease is distinct from myotonic dystrophy, having no temporal atrophy, wasting of the sternocleidomastoid muscles, or ptosis and either minimal or no distal weakness. The myotonia is also atypical in DM2, being commonly asymmetric, variable in severity, and intermittent in occurrence. The onset of DM2 is typically in the third decade, but may be delayed until after the age of 50 years.[44] Serum CK levels are increased 2 to 4 × ULN. The muscle biopsy shows myopathic features but no inflammation.

INFECTIOUS MYOPATHIES

Some infections can cause a chronic myopathy that may resemble polymyositis.[45] Patients with human immunodeficiency virus infection may develop a slowly progressive myopathy with symmetric weakness of the proximal legs and arms and increase of the serum CK levels. In addition to myopathic changes, there may be electrodiagnostic evidence of an axonal sensory neuropathy. Muscle biopsies show endomysial, perimysial, or perivascular mononuclear cell infiltrates with muscle fiber necrosis and phagocytosis. In some patients, the muscle biopsies show nemaline rod bodies (expansion of Z bands and loss of thick filaments) with variable amounts of inflammation, moth-eaten fibers, type 2 fiber atrophy, and neuropathic changes. Toxoplasmosis can cause an inflammatory myopathy in immunocompromised hosts, often accompanied by fever, encephalitis, and other organ involvement. Rarely, trichinosis can produce a clinical syndrome resembling polymyositis. Eosinophilia is an important diagnostic clue; serologic testing confirms the diagnosis. Myositis can also be seen in Lyme disease.

SUMMARY

The noninflammatory myopathies are a diverse group of diseases, some of which may mimic the autoimmune-mediated idiopathic inflammatory myopathies in their clinical presentation. They include certain metabolic, toxic, and infectious myopathies as well as muscular dystrophies. In addition to muscle weakness, these forms of myopathy may present with exercise intolerance and muscle pain. Most of the metabolic myopathies and muscular dystrophies cause medical conditions that manifest in infancy or childhood. However, certain forms of these diseases may first become clinically apparent during the teenage years and adulthood and are thus pertinent to the evaluation of adults presenting with a myopathy. The diagnosis of a noninflammatory myopathy should be considered in patients who seem to have polymyositis but lack the characteristic changes of inflammation found on EMG, MRI, or muscle histology, present in early adulthood, have normal or unusually high CK levels, report a family history of muscle disease, or have proved refractory to immunosuppressive therapy. A directed evaluation using the clinical, laboratory, and genetic approaches summarized in this article should allow for the differentiation of most noninflammatory myopathies from polymyositis and other forms of idiopathic inflammatory myopathy.

REFERENCES

1. Baer AN. Differential diagnosis of idiopathic inflammatory myopathies. Curr Rheumatol Rep 2006;8:178–87.

2. Lyu RK, Cornblath DR, Chaudhry V. Incidence of irritable electromyography in inflammatory myopathy. J Clin Neuromuscul Dis 1999;1:64–7.

3. Friedman SD, Shaw DW, Ishak G, et al. The use of neuroimaging in the diagnosis of mitochondrial disease. Dev Disabil Res Rev 2010;16:129–35.

4. Mitochondrial Medicine Society's Committee on Diagnosis, Haas RH, Parikh S, et al. The in-depth evaluation of suspected mitochondrial disease. Mol Genet Metab 2008;94:16–37.

5. Livingstone C, Chinnery PF, Turnbull DM. The ischaemic lactate-ammonia test. Ann Clin Biochem 2001;38:304–10.

6. Haller RG, Vissing J. Functional evaluation of metabolic myopathies. In: Engel AG, Franzini-Armstrong C, editors. Myology. 3rd edition. New York: McGraw Hill; 2004. p. 665–79.

7. Tarnopolsky M. Exercise testing in metabolic myopathies. Phys Med Rehabil Clin N Am 2012;23:173–86, xii.

8. Kazemi-Esfarjani P, Skomorowska E, Jensen TD, et al. A nonischemic forearm exercise test for McArdle disease. Ann Neurol 2002;52:153–9.

9. DiMauro S, Lamperti C. Muscle glycogenoses. Muscle Nerve 2001;24:984–99.

10. Di Mauro S. Muscle glycogenoses: an overview. Acta Myol 2007;26:35–41.

11. Vissing J, Haller RG. The effect of oral sucrose on exercise tolerance in patients with McArdle's disease. N Engl J Med 2003;349:2503–9.

12. Angelini C, Semplicini C. Metabolic myopathies: the challenge of new treatments. Curr Opin Pharmacol 2010;10:338–45.

13. Bruno C, Dimauro S. Lipid storage myopathies. Curr Opin Neurol 2008;21:601–6.

14. Horvath R, Schneiderat P, Schoser BG, et al. Coenzyme Q10 deficiency and isolated myopathy. Neurology 2006;66:253–5.

15. Ohkuma A, Nonaka I, Malicdan MC, et al. Distal lipid storage myopathy due to PNPLA2 mutation. Neuromuscul Disord 2008;18:671–4.

16. Fischer J, Lefevre C, Morava E, et al. The gene encoding adipose triglyceride lipase (PNPLA2) is mutated in neutral lipid storage disease with myopathy. Nat Genet 2007;39:28–30.

17. van Adel BA, Tarnopolsky MA. Metabolic myopathies: update 2009. J Clin Neuromuscul Dis 2009;10:97–121.

18. DiMauro S, Schon EA. Mitochondrial respiratory-chain diseases. N Engl J Med 2003;348:2656–68.

19. Schaefer AM, McFarland R, Blakely EL, et al. Prevalence of mitochondrial DNA disease in adults. Ann Neurol 2008;63:35–9.

20. Nardin RA, Johns DR. Mitochondrial dysfunction and neuromuscular disease. Muscle Nerve 2001;24:170–91.

21. Rahman S, Hanna MG. Diagnosis and therapy in neuromuscular disorders: diagnosis and new treatments in mitochondrial diseases. J Neurol Neurosurg Psychiatry 2009;80:943–53.

22. Haas RH, Parikh S, Falk MJ, et al. Mitochondrial disease: a practical approach for primary care physicians. Pediatrics 2007;120:1326–33.

23. Pasternak RC, Smith SC Jr, Bairey-Merz CN, et al. ACC/AHA/NHLBI clinical advisory on the use and safety of statins. Stroke 2002;33:2337–41.

24. Christopher-Stine L, Casciola-Rosen LA, Hong G, et al. A novel autoantibody recognizing 200-kd and 100-kd proteins is associated with an immune-mediated necrotizing myopathy. Arthritis Rheum 2010;62:2757–66.

25. Mammen AL, Pak K, Williams EK, et al. Rarity of anti-3-hydroxy-3-methylglutaryl-coenzyme A reductase antibodies in statin users, including those with self-limited musculoskeletal side effects. Arthritis Care Res (Hoboken) 2012;64:269–72.

26. Mammen AL, Chung T, Christopher-Stine L, et al. Autoantibodies against 3-hydroxy-3-methylglutaryl-coenzyme A reductase in patients with statin-associated autoimmune myopathy. Arthritis Rheum 2011;63:713–21.
27. Bruckert E, Hayem G, Dejager S, et al. Mild to moderate muscular symptoms with high-dosage statin therapy in hyperlipidemic patients–the PRIMO study. Cardiovasc Drugs Ther 2005;19:403–14.
28. Graham DJ, Staffa JA, Shatin D, et al. Incidence of hospitalized rhabdomyolysis in patients treated with lipid-lowering drugs. JAMA 2004;292:2585–90.
29. Grupp C. A pain in the tuches. JAMA 2012;308:2467–8.
30. Lamperti C, Naini AB, Lucchini V, et al. Muscle coenzyme Q10 level in statin-related myopathy. Arch Neurol 2005;62:1709–12.
31. Gambelli S, Dotti MT, Malandrini A, et al. Mitochondrial alterations in muscle biopsies of patients on statin therapy. J Submicrosc Cytol Pathol 2004;36:85–9.
32. Grable-Esposito P, Katzberg HD, Greenberg SA, et al. Immune-mediated necrotizing myopathy associated with statins. Muscle Nerve 2010;41:185–90.
33. Davidson MH, Clark JA, Glass LM, et al. Statin safety: an appraisal from the adverse event reporting system. Am J Cardiol 2006;97:32C–43C.
34. The SEARCH Collaborative Group. SLCO1B1 variants and statin-induced myopathy–a genomewide study. N Engl J Med 2008;359:789–99.
35. Baker SK. Molecular clues into the pathogenesis of statin-mediated muscle toxicity. Muscle Nerve 2005;31:572–80.
36. Abd TT, Jacobson TA. Statin-induced myopathy: a review and update. Expert Opin Drug Saf 2011;10:373–87.
37. Hanaoka BY, Peterson CA, Horbinski C, et al. Implications of glucocorticoid therapy in idiopathic inflammatory myopathies. Nat Rev Rheumatol 2012;8:448–57.
38. Wilbur K, Makowsky M. Colchicine myotoxicity: case reports and literature review. Pharmacotherapy 2004;24:1784–92.
39. Casado E, Gratacos J, Tolosa C, et al. Antimalarial myopathy: an underdiagnosed complication? prospective longitudinal study of 119 patients. Ann Rheum Dis 2006;65:385–90.
40. Argov Z, Sadeh M, Mazor K, et al. Muscular dystrophy due to dysferlin deficiency in Libyan Jews. Clinical and genetic features. Brain 2000;123(Pt 6):1229–37.
41. Kissel JT. Misunderstandings, misperceptions, and mistakes in the management of the inflammatory myopathies. Semin Neurol 2002;22:41–51.
42. Confalonieri P, Oliva L, Andreetta F, et al. Muscle inflammation and MHC class I up-regulation in muscular dystrophy with lack of dysferlin: an immunopathological study. J Neuroimmunol 2003;142:130–6.
43. Ricker K. Myotonic dystrophy and proximal myotonic myopathy. J Neurol 1999; 246:334–8.
44. Turner C, Hilton-Jones D. The myotonic dystrophies: diagnosis and management. J Neurol Neurosurg Psychiatry 2010;81:358–67.
45. Crum-Cianflone NF. Bacterial, fungal, parasitic, and viral myositis. Clin Microbiol Rev 2008;21:473–94.

Lipid-Associated Rheumatologic Syndromes

Eyal Kedar, MD, Gregory C. Gardner, MD*

KEYWORDS

- Hyperlipidemia • Tendon xanthoma • Lipid liquid crystals • Arthritis

KEY POINTS

- Tendon xanthomas are associated with Type II and III hyperlipidemia and their presence is a marker for an increase the risk of cardiovascular disease.
- Arthritis associated with hyperlipidemia may affect one or multiple joints and is likely a peri-arthritis in most cases.
- Lipid liquid crystal arthritis is self-limited inflammatory arthritis characterized by the presence of positively birefringent spherules in the synovial fluid.
- There is an association between hyperlipidemia and gout that is likely both environmental and genetic.
- Statins have been implicated in the development of autoimmune disease including a recently described necrotizing myopathy.

INTRODUCTION

Lipid-associated musculoskeletal syndromes are uncommon problems seen in the rheumatologist's office. The rheumatologist, however, may be the first clinician to recognize the manifestations of a lipid-associated syndrome and initiate proper investigation and therapy. Khachadurian[1] was one of the first to report that patients with hyperlipidemia experienced musculoskeletal symptoms. The single-author article from the American University in Beirut reported that 10 of 18 patients homozygous for familial type II hyperlipidemia had attacks of acute migratory polyarthritis lasting up to a month that resembled acute rheumatic fever, as well as tendon xanthomata. No other explanation for the arthritis was uncovered, and the implication was that the hyperlipidemia was the cause of the attacks.[1] Since then a variety of reports covering this topic and expanding on the musculoskeletal manifestations of hyperlipidemia has been published. This article reviews the current literature regarding

Disclosures: Dr Kedar is supported by an NIH training grant. Dr Gardner has no disclosures related to this article.
Division of Rheumatology, University of Washington, Box 356428, Seattle, WA 98195, USA
* Corresponding author.
E-mail address: rheumdoc@uw.edu

lipid-associated syndromes involving joints and tendons, and also reviews the data regarding the relationship of hyperlipidemia with hyperuricemia and gout. Finally, drug-induced rheumatologic illness related to lipid-lowering therapy is briefly discussed.

LIPOPROTEINS AND THE CURRENT CLASSIFICATION OF DYSLIPIDEMIA

The 5 major types of hyperlipidemia are classified by their relevant forms of lipoprotein dysmetabolism under the Fredrickson classification system (**Table 1**).[2] A proper understanding of this system requires a brief review of the 5 major lipoproteins and their basic functions.[3]

Lipoproteins are assemblies of lipids (triglycerides and/or cholesterol, in the case of the lipoproteins discussed in this article) and protein (referred to as apolipoproteins or apoproteins), which serve to transport lipids in the body. Lipid metabolism can be broadly characterized as being under the control of both endogenous and exogenous pathways. The lipoprotein associated with exogenous (dietary) lipid metabolism is the chylomicron, which is mainly a carrier of triglycerides but which also carries, to a significantly lesser extent, cholesterol esters. Chylomicrons are formed in enterocytes and are transported through the lymphatic system to the circulation, where they are broken down by lipoprotein lipase into free fatty acids (from triglycerides) and apoproteins. Ultimately, the remaining chylomicron remnants are taken up by hepatocytes and their contents reprocessed (eg, remaining triglycerides can be packaged for reexport into the circulation as part of very low-density lipoproteins [VLDLs]).

Endogenous pathways of lipid metabolism refer to the processing of hepatically derived lipids, and begin with export of VLDLs from the liver. As with chylomicrons, VLDLs carry triglycerides and, to a lesser extent, cholesterol, and are broken down in the periphery by lipoprotein lipase to yield, among other elements, a combination of free fatty acids and apoproteins. The result is the formation of smaller, denser VLDL "remnants" (also referred to as intermediate-density lipoproteins [IDLs]), which in turn can be broken down further by hepatic lipase to yield IDL remnants known as low-density lipoproteins (LDLs). As the VLDL is broken down, it becomes denser and more enriched in cholesterol, as evidenced by LDL's main role as a carrier of cholesterol rather than triglycerides.

High-density lipoprotein (HDL), like LDL, is chiefly a carrier of cholesterol. Its main role is to absorb excess cholesterol from intracellular pools and to transport this

Table 1
Fredrickson/World Health Organization classification of dyslipidemias

Type	Elevated Lipoprotein(s)	Lipids Elevated
I	Chylomicrons	Triglycerides
IIa	LDL	Cholesterol
IIb	LDL, VLDL	Cholesterol > triglycerides
III	IDL (VLDL remnants), chylomicrons	Cholesterol and triglycerides
IV	VLDL	Triglycerides
V	VLDL, chylomicrons	Triglycerides > cholesterol

Abbreviations: IDL, intermediate-density lipoprotein; LDL, low-density lipoprotein; VLDL, very low-density lipoprotein.

Data from Fredrickson DS. An international classification of hyperlipidemias and hyperlipoproteinemias. Ann Intern Med 1971;75(3):471–2; and Durrington P. Dyslipidaemia. Lancet 2003; 362(9385):717–31.

cholesterol, via a combination of direct and indirect pathways, back to the liver or to steroidogenic tissues such as the adrenals, ovaries, and testes. This transport can be done directly via interaction with scavenger cholesterol receptors on target tissues, or indirectly via initial transfer of cholesterol esters to LDL, which in turn delivers these esters to the tissues.

The roles of the 5 major lipoproteins (in order of decreasing size and increasing density) can be summarized as follows:

- Chylomicrons: large lipoproteins that carry dietary, or exogenous, lipids (triglycerides > cholesterol)
- VLDLs: carriers of hepatically derived, or endogenous, lipids (triglycerides > cholesterol)
- IDLs (also referred to as VLDL remnants): carriers of endogenous cholesterol and triglycerides
- LDLs: carriers of endogenous cholesterol
- HDLs: absorb excess cholesterol from intracellular pools and return this cholesterol to the liver and steroidogenic tissues (adrenals, ovaries, and testes)

HYPERLIPIDEMIA AND TENDINOPATHY

Of the major classes of hyperlipidemia, types II and III have been shown to be associated with xanthomatous disease, and type II has been associated with tendinopathy.[4] Type II hyperlipidemia is characterized by elevation of LDL levels (see **Table 1**) and has 2 known subtypes (types IIa and IIb). It can be inherited as a familial disease or present as a polygenic or sporadic disorder. Patients homozygous for familial type II hyperlipidemia have mutations in both LDL receptor (LDLR) alleles, and develop tendon xanthomata that can be either symptomatic or asymptomatic.[4,5] These xanthomata are collections of lipid-laden macrophages that typically develop over the Achilles tendons (although other tendon areas, including the triceps tendons, may also be involved) and that, in homozygotes, typically develop in childhood.[6] In addition, type II homozygotes may develop fever and a migratory polyarthritis that mimics rheumatic fever, which was first reported by Khachadurian[1] and is discussed in more depth in the next section. Of note, there was no clear relationship between the observed joint pains and the locations of xanthomata.[1,5]

Tendon xanthomata are also found in patients who have type II heterozygous hyperlipidemia (**Fig. 1**). Xanthomata present later in life than in homozygotes (who typically die of cardiovascular disease before the age of 30 years), are present at

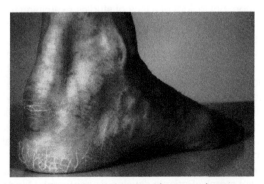

Fig. 1. Achilles tendon xanthoma in a patient with type II heterozygous hyperlipidemia. (*From* Durrington P. Dyslipidaemia. Lancet 2003;362(9385):719; with permission.)

a comparatively lower frequency, and are not present in all patients.[7] As with their homozygous counterparts, these xanthomata can be asymptomatic. The Achilles tendon is the most common location of xanthomata in patients with type II hyperlipidemia, and Mathon and colleagues[7] reported that 18% of 73 patients with familial heterozygous type II hyperlipidemia had Achilles pain and 11% had evidence of Achilles tendinitis.[8] In a controlled cross-sectional study, Beeharry and colleagues[9] reported that 46.6% of 133 patients with familial heterozygous type II hyperlipidemia had had 1 or more episodes of Achilles pain, compared with 6.9% of 87 unaffected controls. The patients were also significantly much more likely to report the pain as severe or very severe, with pain lasting an average of 4 days, and more likely than the controls to seek medical attention for the Achilles symptoms. One of the early studies of symptomatic Achilles tendon involvement reported that tendinitis could be unilateral or bilateral, that patients could have up to 12 attacks per year, and that one patient had 4 to 5 attacks per year for 40 years.[10] The presence of tendon xanthomata is an independent risk factor for cardiovascular disease and indicates the need for more aggressive lipid-lowering therapy.[11] In a meta-analysis of xanthoma formation, heterozygous type II hyperlipidemia, and cardiovascular risk, Oosterveer and colleagues[12] found that the presence of xanthomata conferred a 3.2-fold higher risk for cardiovascular disease. Increasing age, male gender, and levels of LDL cholesterol and triglycerides increased the risk of developing xanthomata. The xanthoma has a composition similar to that of atheroma, and treatment-associated regression of xanthomata with either statins or fibrates may be a marker of atheroma regression.[8] Achilles tendon xanthomata are easily detected by ultrasonography or magnetic resonance imaging (MRI) before they may be detectable clinically. Ultrasonography, in turn, is the easiest and most cost-effective way of detecting xanthomata, and can also be used to quantitatively measure treatment-associated xanthoma regression.[8]

Type III hyperlipidemia (familial dysbetalipoproteinemia) is an autosomal recessive disorder involving 2 apoprotein E2 alleles that results in elevated levels of IDL (VLDL remnants) and chylomicrons and, in turn, elevated cholesterol and triglyceride levels. Tuberoeruptive xanthomata (which typically involve the extensor surfaces) and plantar crease xanthomata (xanthomata palmare striatum) are typical of this disorder.[3,4] These xanthomata are asymptomatic and do not involve joint or tendon areas.[3,13] Of note, reports have shown that close to half of these patients have asymptomatic hyperuricemia, with actual gout attacks being rare.[4,14]

Beyond familial forms of hyperlipidemia, secondary forms (such as hyperlipidemia secondary to diabetes or thyroid disease) can also present with xanthomata.[15] Rheumatic symptoms (such as joint pains) associated with several of the secondary hyperlipidemias are common, but in light of a lack of studies examining the causes of these symptoms as well as the clinical heterogeneity and genetic complexity of the underlying diseases, clear associations have not been found.[5]

Two final entities that deserve note are cerebrotendinous xanthomatosis and sitosterolemia, both of which are rare autosomal recessive disorders of lipid metabolism associated with tendon xanthomata but not actual tendinitis or arthritis.[6] Cerebrotendinous xanthomatosis involves a mutation in the sterol 27-hydroxylase gene, which leads to accumulation of dihydrocholesterol (cholestanol). It is associated with asymptomatic xanthomata of the Achilles tendons that appear in the second to fourth decades of life, as well as a variety of other symptoms including cataracts, diarrhea, vascular disease, cerebellar ataxia, and dementia.[6,16]

Sitosterolemia involves excessive intestinal absorption, and subsequent increased plasma levels, of plant sterols. Patients develop asymptomatic tendon xanthomata as well as accelerated atherosclerosis.[6]

HYPERLIPIDEMIA-ASSOCIATED ARTHRITIS

The 1968 report of Khachadurian has been the basis for the association of hyper-lipidemia with arthritis.[1] Of 18 young homozygous patients with familial type II hyper-lipidemia, 10 were reported to develop self-limited attacks of migratory polyarthritis that could be severe enough to cause the sufferer to be bedridden. In the 10 affected patients, Khachadurian ruled out acute rheumatic fever and hyperuricemia in all cases as a cause of the arthritis. Sedimentation rates and C-reactive protein could be elevated and the patient could be febrile as well. The sedimentation rate often remained elevated between attacks of arthritis. The joints were described as being swollen, but the one attempted arthrocentesis from a swollen knee was unsuccessful in that no fluid was obtained. A photo of a patient's hands included in the report shows marked fullness around the metacarpophalangeal joints, and proximal interphalangeal (PIP) joints in particular are described as being xanthomatous. All of the patients included in this report had xanthomata. The lack of obtainable synovial fluid and the appearance of the hands raise the question of a periarthritis rather than a true arthritis.

A much more detailed report of the arthritis of hyperlipidemia was published in 1978 by Rooney and colleagues.[17] These investigators followed 41 patients with familial hyperbetalipoproteinemia for up to 4 years, noting the symptoms and joints involved, and reporting on fluid obtained during arthrocentesis and even doing xenon clearance from joints assumed to be inflamed. Again a transient migratory polyarthritis was noted, which affected both large and small joints in up to 10 of these patients, lasting 3 to 12 days. The pain was moderate to severe and in no case was the arthritis attribut-able to acute rheumatic fever of gout. Synovial fluid was obtained from 6 swollen joints; in all cases the fluid had 200 or fewer white blood cells (WBCs) per cm^3 and was reported to have normal viscosity. Bacteriologic and crystal analyses were nega-tive in all patients. Xenon clearance for affected joints was also normal, suggesting to the investigators that the arthritis was in all cases actually a periarthritis. In a case report of a male patient with swelling of PIP joints and familial hypercholesterolemia, MRI revealed periarticular fat deposition, which by appearance may have been capsular in location but certainly not intra-articular.[18] Fine-needle aspiration of the periarticular lipid accumulation at the PIP joints in a young girl with familial hypercho-lesterolemia demonstrated the presence of abundant foam cells (ie, macrophages laden with lipids and found in atherosclerotic plaques as well as xanthomata of skin and tendons).[6,19] Foam cells are metabolically active and may produce cytokines and other proinflammatory molecules, or possibly metabolize the internalized lipid to cause it to become phlogistic.[20] These activities may contribute to periarticular inflammation seen in affected patients. A patient with a similar periarticular deposition of lipid is shown in **Fig. 2**.

Although the weight of evidence favors a periarthritis, at least one report has docu-mented an inflammatory synovial fluid in a patient with type II hyperlipidemia arthritis.[10] The patient was a 23-year-old with episodes of oligoarthritis affecting the knees and ankles beginning at age 20 years. Synovial fluid analysis from a swollen knee demonstrated 5400 WBCs with the majority being neutrophils, and with no other apparent cause of the arthritis.

Patients who develop arthritis/periarthritis typically have familial type II hyperlipid-emia. As previously mentioned, these patients are also those who have a tendency to develop tendon xanthomata. Many of the early reports were in patients with the rare homozygous form of disease. Mathon and colleagues,[7] in a cross-sectional study of patients with heterozygous familial hypercholesterolemia, found that 7% of 73 affected patients reported at least 1 episode of a monoarthritis or an oligoarthritis,

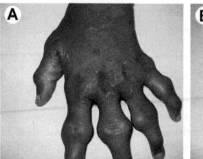 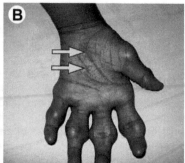

Fig. 2. (*A*) Dorsal view of the hand showing marked periarticular fullness around he PIP joints in a patient with Type II hyperlipidemia. (*B*) Palmar view of the same hand showing palmar xanthomata (*arrows*) in addition to the periarticular fullness. (*From* Sharma A, Dogra S, Mahajan R, et al. An unusual cause of joint swelling. Lancet 2010;375:1109; with permission.)

whereas 4% reported a more classic migratory polyarticular syndrome. The onset is not generally before age 20 years in these patients, in comparison with childhood onset in patients with homozygous disease. In addition, at the time the patients were examined there was no evidence of joint abnormality, despite numerous attacks in some patients, confirming the nondestructive nature of the arthritis/periarthritis.

Although the majority of the case report/case series literature has focused on type II patients, type IV patients have also been reported to develop episodic arthritis. Twenty-four patients with type IV hyperlipidemia described by Goldman and colleagues[21] and Buckingham and colleagues[22] were reported to have an acute to subacute pauciarthritis of large and small joints that could not be explained by another cause (in particular, gout). In some cases of the Goldman series pain could be severe, but in others it was mild and persistent. Goldman and colleagues also reported that the evidence of inflammation was often less than the reported level of pain. The synovial fluid was noninflammatory in 2 knee effusions aspirated by Goldman and colleagues, whereas synovial fluid obtained from 2 patients in the Buckingham series was described as mildly inflammatory.

The results of epidemiologic studies give a mixed picture of arthritis and hyperlipidemia. In 1978 Welin and colleagues[23] reported on a relatively large cohort of men from Sweden born in either 1913 or 1923, and included data on their lipid profiles and clinical information. In a comparison with men with normal lipid levels they could not find a relationship between any of the subtypes of hyperlipidemia and increased musculoskeletal manifestations, although the overall numbers in each subtype of hyperlipidemia were small. Wysenbeek and colleagues[24] reported an increase in foot and ankle pain in 69 patients with type IIa hyperlipidemia compared with 33 controls, but no increase in inflammatory-type manifestations. Klemp and colleagues[25] conducted a comparison between 88 patients with adult and juvenile familial forms of hyperlipidemia (type II) or a mixed form (elevated cholesterol and triglycerides) and 88 controls. Adults with familial forms of hyperlipidemia were found to have an excess of xanthomata and Achilles tendinitis, whereas the mixed form of hyperlipidemia demonstrated an excess of xanthomata, Achilles tendinitis, and oligoarthritis compared with controls. The juvenile form of hyperlipidemia was not found to have excess musculoskeletal manifestations in comparison with controls, and migratory polyarthritis, though reported by 5 patients in the adult group and none of the controls, was reported to be not significant. It is possible that the small number in each group

(48 adult type II, 16 juvenile type II, and 24 mixed) was too inadequate to reveal this rare complication. Large well-controlled studies aimed at answering prevalence questions regarding hyperlipidemia and arthritis are currently lacking.

Anecdotal experience regarding treatment further implicates hyperlipidemia as a cause of joint symptoms. In general, arthritis and musculoskeletal symptoms have been reported to respond to lipid-lowering therapy in both type II and type IV patients.[5,6,19]

LIPID LIQUID CRYSTAL ARTHRITIS

Lipid liquid crystal arthritis is an uncommonly reported cause of acute arthritis. The attacks have a gout-like quality in that they usually affect single, typically large joints, and resolve within days without therapy or in response to nonsteroidal anti-inflammatories (NSAIDs), colchicine, or corticosteroid injections. Acute-phase reactants are often elevated during the attack as well.[26,27] Lipid liquid crystals are identified in synovial fluid under compensated polarized light as strongly positively birefringent spherules resembling beach balls (**Fig. 3**).[28] Such crystals are found both extracellularly and intracellularly in association with, in most cases, a neutrophil-predominant synovial fluid leukocytosis. The crystals stain with Sudan black, dissolve with alcohol/ether 1:1 mixture or xylol, are resistant to urate and ethylenediaminetetraacetic acid, and are alizarin red–negative, implicating lipids as the source of the spherules (rather than the usual causes of gout-like joint swelling).[26,28,29] The positively birefringent spherules do have some resemblance to talc crystals, but at least one report compared talc crystals under polarizing compensated microscopy and pointed out that talc can be easily distinguished from the lipid liquid spherules. The etiology and incidence of this unusual syndrome are still uncertain.

There have been at least 14 cases reported in the English literature, and 7 additional cases from Swiss and Mexican publications (**Table 2**). The first case was described by Weinstein in 1980 in a 48-year-old woman who was hospitalized with an acutely swollen knee, which on arthrocentesis demonstrated 27,800 WBCs, 90% neutrophils, and 8200 red blood cells (RBCs).[30] With polarized light microscopy, up to 10% of the synovial fluid neutrophils contained Maltese-cross inclusions that were Sudanophilic. No other crystals or abnormalities were noted in the synovial fluid or culture, nor were

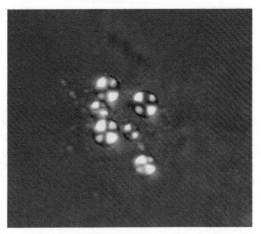

Fig. 3. Lipid liquid crystal in synovial fluid. (*Courtesy of* G. Gardner, MD, Seattle, WA.)

Table 2
Details of 21 cases of lipid liquid arthritis

Case No., Authors,[Ref.] Year	Demographics	Joint or Joints	Course
1. Weinstein,[30] 1980	48-y-old Female	Knee	Resolved in 5 d without therapy
2. Schlesinger et al,[36] 1982	14-y-old Male	Polyarthritis of small and large joints	Acute symptoms improved with NSAIDs; spherules present at 2 mo
3. Reginato et al,[31] 1985	41-y-old Female	Wrist	Resolved in 5 d with colchicine
4. Reginato et al,[31] 1985	21-y-old Female	Knee	Resolved by day 14 with NSAID
5. Reginato et al,[31] 1985	54-y-old Female	Knee	Resolved by day 10 with NSAID
6. Trostle et al,[33] 1986	33-y-old Female	Knee	Resolved in 5 d with colchicine
7. Ugai et al,[34] 1988	36-y-old Male	Knee (PVNS)	Surgery to remove PVNS
8. Ugai et al,[34] 1988	30-y-old Female	Knee (PVNS)	Surgery to remove PVNS
9. Gardner and Terkeltaub,[28] 1989	58-y-old Female	Knee	Resolved in 5 d with NSAID
10. Astorga and Carvajal,[26] 1990	34-y-old Female	Knee	Resolved in 10 d with NSAID
11. Rivest et al,[29] 1992	52-y-old Female	Polyarthritis of MCPs, wrists, elbows (history of RA)	Resolved by day 14 with NSAID; spherules still present at 1 mo
12. Park et al,[37] 1997	Male	Left third MTP then left transverse tarsal joint	Resolved in 14 d with NSAID
13. Hackeng et al,[27] 2000	31-y-old Male	Knee	Resolved in 14 d with NSAID
14. Dylewski,[38] 2005	44-y-old Female	Knee	NSAID followed by steroid injection with resolution in 8 d
15–21	Uncertain	Monoarthritis	Uncertain

Abbreviations: MCP, metacarpophalangeal joint; MTP, metatarsophalangeal joint; NSAID, nonsteroidal anti-inflammatory drug; PVNS, pigmented villonodular synovitis; RA, rheumatoid arthritis.
Cases 15–20 *from* Van Linthoudt D. L'arthrite a cristaux de lipids liquids. Rev Med Suisse 2010;6:2034–7; and Koya P, Marin E, Ricardo R, et al. Monoarthritic asosiada a critales liquidos lipidicos: reporte de seis casos y estudio in vitro de fagocitosis inducida por lipomas artificiales [abstract]. Rev Mex Reumatol 1990;5(Suppl 1):52.

there any serologic data to explain the acute arthritis. Repeat arthrocentesis on day 2 of hospitalization found that the cell count had risen to 38,000, but by day 4 the synovial fluid cell count had dropped to 10,600. Pain and swelling lasted a total of 5 days and resolved without any specific therapy other than the repeated arthrocenteses. The patient reported intermittent swelling in the knee that lasted 2 days per episode (over 2 years of follow-up). Most of the subsequent cases are similar, and the data regarding these are summarized in **Table 2**.

In addition to using laboratory methods to demonstrate the lipid nature of the Maltese crosses, some literature included additional investigation. Reginato and colleagues[31] described 3 cases of acute arthritis associated with intracellular and extracellular Maltese-cross lipid spherules. On electron microscopy of synovial fluid cells, they reported gray lipid droplets and multilayered lamellated inclusions in phagocytic vacuoles that were similar to lipid liquid crystals reported by others. These investigators were the first to refer to the Maltese crosses as lipid liquid crystals. Liquid crystals have properties between those of a liquid and those of solid crystal.[32] A liquid crystal may flow like a liquid, but its molecules may be oriented in a crystalline fashion. Using a polarized light microscope, different liquid crystal phases will appear to have distinct textures, indicating that the molecules of the liquid crystal may be oriented in different, phase-specific directions.

Trostle and colleagues[33] extended the observations of Reginato and colleagues when they performed a synovial biopsy on a patient with acute lipid liquid crystal arthritis. The biopsy showed nonspecific lining cell hyperplasia, with rare lymphocytes and some prominence of the endothelium and perivascular cells. Maltese-cross bodies and irregularly shaped birefringent rod-like material was seen in the neutrophils adherent to the synovium. Some of the irregular birefringent rod-like material was also seen in the synovial lining cells. On electron microscopy, the neutrophils contained lipid droplets as well as multilaminated concentric arrays within phagocytic vacuoles, and some lipid droplets were coated with finely granular protein-like material. Both groups noted that there were lipid droplets as well as lipids in the form of lipid liquid crystals in phagocytic cells.

Two cases reported by Ugai and colleagues[34] may provide further insight into the etiology of lipid liquid crystals. Both patients had pigmented villonodular synovitis with associated abundant RBCs, and the presence of positively birefringent Maltese-cross spherules both in the synovial fluid and inside macrophages. Neither patient had an acute arthritis, but both had chronic joint swelling. The synovial fluids did have a leukocytosis but the cell differentials were different to those seen in patients with the more acute form of the arthritis. The predominant cells were lymphocytes and macrophages, with small numbers of neutrophils noted as well. The investigators speculated that the source of the lipid liquid crystals were the lipid membranes from the degenerating RBCs. Indeed, Choi and colleagues[35] were able to induce an acute synovitis in rabbits by injecting autologous RBCs in knee joints, with subsequent demonstration of lipid liquid crystal formation within the synovial fluid.

Although the majority of patients reported had an acute monoarthritis, 2 patients presented with a polyarthritis. One patient had poorly controlled rheumatoid arthritis and presented a pseudoseptic characterization involving multiple joints, with WBCs as numerous as $120,000/cm^3$.[29] The polyarthritis responded symptomatically to naproxen, but 1 month later synovial fluid continued to show intracellular and extracellular lipid liquid crystals. The other patient with polyarthritis had an undefined chronic illness.[36] The inflammatory cells in the synovial fluid were 100% macrophages, and lipid liquid crystals persisted at 2 months after initial presentation (by which point the severe initial symptoms had subsided). These 2 patients illustrate the point that the lipid liquid crystals, like both pyrophosphate crystals and urate crystals, may be present in synovial fluid without being overtly phlogistic.

The authors suspect that lipid liquid crystal–associated arthritis is more common than the 21 cases suggest. Its self-limited nature in most patients and its response to NSAIDs mean that many cases probably go unrecognized, given the requirement that synovial fluid in affected patients must be examined under polarized light to make the diagnosis. The mechanism of formation of lipid liquid crystals is not entirely clear, but they have been seen in the synovial fluid of patients with rheumatoid arthritis along with cholesterol crystals, suggesting that local lipid saturation may be an important requirement for formation.[39] The source of the lipids my well be the breakdown of cell membranes, as suggested by their presence in the patients with pigmented villonodular synovitis and the data advocating that experimental hemarthrosis leads to the development of lipid liquid crystals.[35] Injecting liposomes into knee joints of rabbits results in acute synovitis and the formation of lipid liquid crystals, suggesting a direct phlogistic potential of the lipids.[40] In addition, Simkin and colleagues[41] have reported on 2 patients with pancreatitis-associated arthritis characterized by elevated intra-articular free fatty acids. Like Choi and colleagues,[40] they were able to induce an acute arthritis in rabbit knees by injecting them with free fatty acids, suggesting that it is this component of the lipid that (at least in part) causes the acute arthritis. Like other crystalline causes of acute arthritis, lipid liquid crystals can be seen in asymptomatic joints as well, therefore factors other than the presence of the spherules/lipids likely contribute to the inflammatory process.

HYPERLIPIDEMIA AND GOUT

There is a known association between hyperlipidemia (and the metabolic syndrome in general) and gout.[42] A recent prospective cohort study of 1606 Chinese patients with gout showed a significant association of hyperlipidemia (as well as both hypertension and obesity) with gout, with hazard ratios of 1.12 and 1.7, respectively, for men and women with hyperlipidemia.[43] In another recent multicenter study of 312 patients with gout in Turkey, 30.1% of the patients had some form of hyperlipidemia.[44]

The association of gout with the metabolic syndrome, and hyperlipidemia in particular, is likely the result of a combination of genetic and environmental factors.[44] Recently, the particular association with coronary artery disease, as well the increased risk of myocardial infarction in young patients with gout, has come to increased attention,[45] as has the long-known association of diet and gout.[46]

Beyond the association of gout with secondary hyperlipidemia, there is also a known relationship with some of the primary hyperlipidemias. As noted earlier, reports have shown that half of patients with type III hyperlipidemia (familial dysbetalipoproteinemia) have asymptomatic hyperuricemia.[4,14] Even better described, however, is the association with type IV hyperlipidemia whereby there are elevated levels of VLDL and, in turn, hypertriglyceridemia. When this disorder occurs in a family it is termed familial hypertriglyceridemia.[3,4] These patients can experience recurrent gout attacks,[4,47] although it is unclear whether the hyperlipidemia is a cause of or merely an association with gout, and vice versa.[5]

RHEUMATOLOGIC DISEASE INDUCED BY LIPID-LOWERING THERAPY

Beyond the well-known association of statins with myalgias and myopathy, these medications have also been implicated as a cause of drug-induced autoimmune disease. In a 1993 review of musculoskeletal manifestations of hyperlipidemia, Careless and Cohen[5] noted that there had been several cases of drug-induced lupus associated with statins and 1 case ascribed to clofibrate. These cases were associated with antihistone antibodies, and resolved with immunosuppressive therapy and withdrawal of the medication. Autoantibodies resolved over time as well, suggesting a drug-associated syndrome.

In a 2005 review of the literature for reports of autoimmune disease associated with statins, 28 cases of statin-induced autoimmune diseases were identified.[48] This cohort included 10 cases of systemic lupus erythematosus, 3 cases of subacute cutaneous lupus erythematosus, 14 cases of dermatomyositis and polymyositis, and 1 case of lichen planus pemphigoides. Autoimmune hepatitis was also noted in

2 patients with coexisting systemic lupus erythematosus. Patients were treated for a mean of 12.8 months before symptoms appeared within a range of 1 month to 6 years. Most required immunosuppressive therapy, and 2 patients died of pulmonary complications as a result of their drug-induced syndrome (1 lupus, 1 myositis). More recently, de Jong and colleagues[49] preformed a case/noncase study based on individual case safety reports listed in the World Health Organization global individual case safety reports database (VigiBase). This study identified 3362 cases of lupus-like syndrome in the database, and found that statins were associated with 3.2% of these. As statin use increases, such rare manifestations may be seen in larger numbers and will become important for rheumatologists to recognize.

Finally, a recently described immune-mediated necrotizing myopathy associated with antibodies directed against 3-hydroxy-3-methyl-glutaryl coenzyme-A (HMG CoA) reductase has been described and associated with statin use.[50,51] The myopathy is characterized as a subacute, severe, symmetric, proximal myopathy with elevated creatine kinase levels, which shows little inflammation on biopsy and requires immunosuppressive therapy for control. This form of myopathy is reported to respond to steroids and methotrexate, but in some cases has required rituximab or intravenous immunoglobulin. Manifestations persist after withdrawal of the drugs. Up to 6% of patients treated with statins may demonstrate antibodies, although most do not have evidence of myopathy. Statins upregulate the expression of HMG CoA reductase in muscle cells, and regenerating muscle cells express high levels of these molecules, perpetuating the syndrome even when the statin is no longer present. Patients with other rheumatologic diseases can also express these antibodies, and an HMG CoA reductase antibody-associated myopathy may also spontaneously occur without exposure to statins. More information on this form of myopathy is certain to be forthcoming.

SUMMARY

Although patients with lipid-associated rheumatologic disorders present relatively infrequently, it is likely that most clinical rheumatologists will encounter these conditions during their career. The proper diagnosis and treatment of these patients will relieve their suffering, and in some cases, prevent future complications of hyperlipidemia. However, a complete understanding of the pathophysiologic mechanisms by which these conditions develop remains to be elucidated.

REFERENCES

1. Khachadurian AK. Migratory polyarthritis in familial hypercholesterolemia (type II hyperlipoproteinemia). Arthritis Rheum 1968;11(3):385–93.
2. Fredrickson DS. An international classification of hyperlipidemias and hyperlipoproteinemias. Ann Intern Med 1971;75(3):471–2.
3. Durrington P. Dyslipidaemia. Lancet 2003;362(9385):717–31.
4. Fishel B, Rosenbach TO, Yaron M, et al. Hyperlipidemias and rheumatic manifestations. Clin Rheumatol 1986;5(1):75–9.
5. Careless DJ, Cohen MG. Rheumatic manifestations of hyperlipidemia and antihyperlipidemia drug therapy. Semin Arthritis Rheum 1993;23(2):90–8.
6. Handel ML, Simons L. Rheumatic manifestations of hyperlipidaemia. Best Pract Res Clin Rheumatol 2000;14(3):595–8.
7. Mathon G, Gagné C, Brun D, et al. Articular manifestations of familial hypercholesterolaemia. Ann Rheum Dis 1985;44(9):599–602.
8. Tsouli SG, Kiortsis DN, Argyropoulou MI, et al. Pathogenesis, detection and treatment of Achilles tendon xanthomas. Eur J Clin Invest 2005;35(4):236–44.

9. Beeharry D. Familial hypercholesterolaemia commonly presents with Achilles tenosynovitis. Ann Rheum Dis 2006;65(3):312–5.
10. Glueck CJ, Levy RI, Frederickson DS. Acute tendinitis and arthritis. A presenting symptom of familial type II hyperlipoproteinemia. JAMA 1968;206(13):2895–7.
11. Civeira F. Tendon xanthomas in familial hypercholesterolemia are associated with cardiovascular risk independently of the low-density lipoprotein receptor gene mutation. Arterioscler Thromb Vasc Biol 2005;25(9):1960–5.
12. Oosterveer DM, Versmissen J, Yazdanpanah M, et al. Differences in characteristics and risk of cardiovascular disease in familial hypercholesterolemia patients with and without tendon xanthomas: a systematic review and meta-analysis. Atherosclerosis 2009;207(2):311–7.
13. Sharma D, Thirkannad S. Palmar xanthoma—an indicator of a more sinister problem. Hand (N Y) 2009;5(2):210–2.
14. Morganroth J, Levy RI, Fredrickson DS. The biochemical, clinical, and genetic features of type III hyperlipoproteinemia. Ann Intern Med 1975;82(2):158–74.
15. Parker F. Xanthomas and hyperlipidemias. J Am Acad Dermatol 1985;13(1):1–30.
16. Moghadasian MH, Salen G, Frohlich JJ, et al. Cerebrotendinous xanthomatosis: a rare disease with diverse manifestations. Arch Neurol 2002;59(4):527–9.
17. Rooney PJ, Third J, Madkour MM, et al. Transient polyarthritis associated with familial hyperbetalipoproteinaemia. Q J Med 1978;47(187):249–59.
18. Alfadhli E. Cholesterol deposition around small joints of the hands in familial hypercholesterolemia mimicking "Bouchard's and Heberden's nodes" of osteoarthritis. Intern Med 2010;49(15):1675–6.
19. Chakraborty PP, Mukhopadhyay S, Achar A, et al. Migratory polyarthritis in familial hypercholesterolemia (type IIa hyperlipoproteinemia). Indian J Pediatr 2010;77(3):329–31.
20. McLaren JE, Michael DR, Ashlin TG, et al. Cytokines, macrophage lipid metabolism and foam cells: implications for cardiovascular disease therapy. Prog Lipid Res 2011;50(4):331–47.
21. Goldman JA, Glueck CJ, Abrams NR, et al. Musculoskeletal disorders associated with type-IV hyperlipoproteinaemia. Lancet 1972;2(7775):449–52.
22. Buckingham RB, Bole GG, Bassett DR. Polyarthritis associated with type IV hyperlipoproteinemia. Arch Intern Med 1975;135(2):286–90.
23. Welin L, Larsson B, Svärdsudd K, et al. Serum lipids, lipoproteins and musculoskeletal disorders among 50- and 60-year-old men. An epidemiologic study. Scand J Rheumatol 1978;7(1):7–12.
24. Wysenbeek AJ, Shani E, Beigel Y. Musculoskeletal manifestations in patients with hypercholesterolemia. J Rheumatol 1989;16(5):643–5.
25. Klemp P, Halland AM, Majoos FL, et al. Musculoskeletal manifestations in hyperlipidaemia: a controlled study. Ann Rheum Dis 1993;52(1):44–8.
26. Astorga GP, Carvajal PR. Lipid spherule associated arthritis. J Rheumatol 1990; 17(12):1720.
27. Hackeng CM, de Bruijn LA, Douw CM, et al. Presence of birefringent, maltese-cross-appearing spherules in synovial fluid in a case of acute monoarthritis. Clin Chem 2000;46(11):1861–3.
28. Gardner GC, Terkeltaub RA. Acute monoarthritis associated with intracellular positively birefringent Maltese cross appearing spherules. J Rheumatol 1989; 16(3):394–6.
29. Rivest C, Hazeltine M, Gariepy G, et al. Acute polyarthritis associated with birefringent lipid microspherules occurring in a patient with longstanding rheumatoid arthritis. J Rheumatol 1992;19(4):617–20.

30. Weinstein J. Synovial fluid leukocytosis associated with intracellular lipid inclusions. Arch Intern Med 1980;140(4):560–1.
31. Reginato AJ, Schumacher HR, Allan DA, et al. Acute monoarthritis associated with lipid liquid crystals. Ann Rheum Dis 1985;44(8):537–43.
32. Chandrasekhar S. Cholesteric lipid crystals. Liquid crystals. England: Cambridge University Press; 1992.
33. Trostle DC, Schumacher HR, Medsger TA, et al. Lipid microspherule-associated acute monoarticular arthritis. Arthritis Rheum 1986;29(9):1166–9.
34. Ugai K, Kurosaka M, Hirohata K. Lipid microspherules in synovial fluid of patients with pigmented villonodular synovitis. Arthritis Rheum 1988;31(11):1442–6.
35. Choi SJ, Schumacher HR, Clayburne G. Experimental haemarthrosis produces mild inflammation associated with intracellular Maltese crosses. Ann Rheum Dis 1986;45(12):1025–8.
36. Schlesinger PA, Stillman MT, Peterson L. Polyarthritis with birefringent lipid within synovial fluid macrophages: case report and ultrastructural study. Arthritis Rheum 1982;25(11):1365–8.
37. Park YB, Lee SK, Song CH, et al. Acute monoarthritis associated with positively birefringent maltese cross appearing lipid spherules in a hyperlipidemic diabetic patient. Yonsei Med J 1997;38:236–9.
38. Dylewski J. Acute monoarticular arthritis caused by Maltese cross-like crystals. Canadian Medical Association Journal 2005;172:741–2.
39. Ettlinger RE, Hunder GG. Synovial effusions containing cholesterol crystals report of 12 patients and review. Mayo Clin Proc 1979;54(6):366–74.
40. Choi SJ, Schumacher HR, Clayburne G, et al. Liposome-induced synovitis in rabbits. Light and electron microscopic studies. Arthritis Rheum 1986;29(7):889–96.
41. Simkin PA, Brunzell JD, Wisner D, et al. Free fatty acids in the pancreatic arthritis syndrome. Arthritis Rheum 1983;26(2):127–32.
42. Stamp LK, Chapman PT. Gout and its comorbidities: implications for therapy. Rheumatology 2012;52(1):34–44.
43. Chen JH, Yeh WT, Chuang SY, et al. Gender-specific risk factors for incident gout: a prospective cohort study. Clin Rheumatol 2011;31(2):239–45.
44. Oztürk MA, Kaya A, Senel S, et al. Demographic and clinical features of gout patients in Turkey: a multicenter study. Rheumatol Int 2012. [Epub ahead of print].
45. Kuo CF, Yu KH, See LC, et al. Risk of myocardial infarction among patients with gout: a nationwide population-based study. Rheumatology 2012;52(1):111–7.
46. Kedar E, Simkin PA. A perspective on diet and gout. Adv Chronic Kidney Dis 2012;19(6):392–7.
47. Struthers GR, Scott DL, Bacon PA, et al. Musculoskeletal disorders in patients with hyperlipidaemia. Ann Rheum Dis 1983;42(5):519–23.
48. Noël B. Lupus erythematosus and other autoimmune diseases related to statin therapy: a systematic review. J Eur Acad Dermatol Venereol 2007;21(1):17–24.
49. de Jong HJ, Cohen Tervaert JW, Saldi SR, et al. Association between statin use and lupus-like syndrome using spontaneous reports. Semin Arthritis Rheum 2011;41(3):373–81.
50. Liang C, Needham M. Necrotizing autoimmune myopathy. Curr Opin Rheumatol 2011;23(6):612–9.
51. Mammen AL, Chung T, Christopher-Stine L, et al. Autoantibodies against 3-hydroxy-3-methylglutaryl-coenzyme A reductase in patients with statin-associated autoimmune myopathy. Arthritis Rheum 2011;63(3):713–21.

Index

Note: Page numbers of article titles are in **boldface** type.

A

ACCESS (A Case Control Etiologic Study of Sarcoidosis), 279
N-Acetylglucosaminylphosphotransferase deficiency, in mucolipidoses, 448–449
Achilles tendonopathy, in hyperlipidemia, 483–484
Acid maltase deficiency, 462, 467–468
Acne
    in Behçet's syndrome, 248
    in SAPHO syndrome, **401–418**
Acne conglobata, 407
Acropachy, 384
Adalimumab
    for Behçet's syndrome, 254
    for relapsing polychondritis, 272
    for SAPHO syndrome, 411–412
    for sarcoidosis, 289
Adipose triglyceride lipase deficiency, 470
Adrenal gland
    enlargement of, in Erdheim-Chester disease, 304
    fibrosis of, 367
Aerobic exercise testing, for myopathies, 460–461
Aldolase deficiency, 468
Alendronate, for SAPHO syndrome, 412
5-Aminosalicylic acid, for Behçet's syndrome, 255
Amyloidosis, **323–345**
    AA (inflammation), 326–327
        detection of, 327
        epidemiology of, 327
        identification of, 329–330
        imaging for, 334
        treatment of, 335–336
    Aβ_2M (dialysis), 326–327
        clinical manifestations of, 332
        imaging for, 332
        treatment of, 335–336
    AL (light chain), 326–327
        clinical manifestations of, 331–332
        detection of, 327
        epidemiology of, 327–328
        imaging for, 333–334
        treatment of, 335–337, 339
    amyloid in
        detection of, 328–329

Rheum Dis Clin N Am 39 (2013) 495–513
http://dx.doi.org/10.1016/S0889-857X(13)00036-7
0889-857X/13/$ – see front matter © 2013 Elsevier Inc. All rights reserved.

Moving?

Make sure your subscription moves with you!

To notify us of your new address, find your **Clinics Account Number** (located on your mailing label above your name), and contact customer service at:

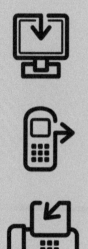

Email: journalscustomerservice-usa@elsevier.com

800-654-2452 (subscribers in the U.S. & Canada)
314-447-8871 (subscribers outside of the U.S. & Canada)

Fax number: 314-447-8029

Elsevier Health Sciences Division
Subscription Customer Service
3251 Riverport Lane
Maryland Heights, MO 63043

*To ensure uninterrupted delivery of your subscription, please notify us at least 4 weeks in advance of move.

Printed and bound by CPI Group (UK) Ltd, Croydon, CR0 4YY

13/10/2024

01773499-0003